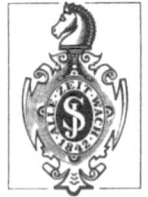

H. D. Becker · W. F. Caspary

Postgastrectomy and Postvagotomy Syndromes

With 84 Figures (Mainly in Two Colors)

Springer-Verlag
Berlin Heidelberg New York 1980

Professor Dr. med. H. D. Becker
Klinik und Poliklinik für Allgemeinchirurgie, Robert-Koch-Str. 40,
D-3400 Gottingen, Federal Republic of Germany

Professor Dr. med. W. F. Caspary
II. Medizinische Klinik, Stadtkrankenhaus, Leimenstraße 20,
D-6450 Hanau, Federal Republic of Germany

ISBN-13: 978-3-642-67352-8   e-ISBN-13: 978-3-642-67350-4
DOI: 10.1007/978-3-642-67350-4

Library of Congress Cataloging in Publication Data. Becker, Horst-Dieter, 1941,
Postgastrectomy and postvagotomy syndromes. Includes bibliographies and index.
1 Postgastrectomy syndromes. 2. Postvagotomy syndromes. I Caspary, Wolfgang
F , 1940, joint author. II. Title. [DNLM: 1. Postgastrectomy syndromes. 2. Vagotomy – Adverse effects 3 Stomach – Surgery WI380 B395p] RD540 5 B45
617:55301 80-11186

© by Springer-Verlag Berlin · Heidelberg 1980
Softcover reprint of the hardcover 1st edition 1980

Illustrations: Adrian Cornford.

To our wifes and children

Hedda, Christian, Tina,
Brigitte, Ulrike, Martin

Foreword

Besides the mortality rate the value of an operative procedure is measured against the incidence and the degree of undesirable postoperative sequelae. In the surgical treatment of gastroduodenal ulcerations vagotomy is now competing with the successfully established resection therapy. Since this latter method has been further developed during the last years and late results are rare, a comparison between both types of operation is difficult. Meritoriously, the authors have tried to perform a comprehensive analysis.

Due to the complexity of postoperative syndromes the diagnostic procedure and treatment can be successful only after integrated cooperation by gastroenterologists and surgeons. This is documented by the current monograph which originates from a cooperation of several years and an active exchange of scientific and practical experience. The monograph will facilitate the indication for the primary surgical procedure by critical confrontation of the postoperative syndromes and provide advice in treating postoperative complaints.

We hope that the monograph will have the expected impact, which means the spreading of the actual knowledge of postgastrectomy and postvagotomy syndromes.

W. Creutzfeldt   H. J. Peiper

Contents

Part I
Gastric Surgery and its Results

1 Short Historical Survey

When on 29 January 1881 Theodor Billroth [1] performed his first successful gastric resection for stenosing antral cancer and reconstructed the continuity by creating a gastroduodenostomy, modern gastro-intestinal surgery had begun. After several insufficiencies at the gastroduodenostomy had occurred, Billroth in further operations closed the resection line at the stomach and duodenum and anastomosed the first jejunal loop to the gastric stump; this is now known as the Billroth II anastomosis. This operative procedure was initiated by Wölfler, who in September 1881 performed a gastrojejunostomy in a patient with a stenosing unresectable antral tumour [2].

The first gastric resection for benign peptic ulcer disease was done by Rydygier [3] in 1882, who performed a Billroth I gastroduodenostomy in a patient with stenosing pyloric ulcer. During the following decades, discussion mainly concerned technical aspects of gastric surgery.

Gastric resection for peptic ulcer disease has been widely used in Germany and France, whereas in Britain and North America simple gastro-enterostomy was preferred for several years.

Sequelae of gastric resection were described shortly after the introduction of this technique. The first clinical picture described was the afferent-loop syndrome, which von Hacker [4] tried to avoid by a retrocolic gastrojejunostomy; for the same purpose in 1892 H. Braun [5] developed an entero-enterostomy at the lowest point between the afferent and efferent jejunal loops.

In 1899 Braun observed the occurrence of a peptic jejunal ulcer after the construction of a simple gastro-enterostomy [6]. In the following years it became evident that mainly the so-called palliative operations (Eiselberg and Finsterer's antral exclusion operation [7], simple gastrojejunostomy) were troubled by a high incidence of peptic jejunal ulcerations; therefore, the surgeons switched to more extended gastric resection, which was not followed by this complication.

Denéchean [8] and Jonas [9] in 1907 and 1908 described symptoms after food intake in patients with gastro-enterostomy which are now known as the dumping syndrome. In 1913 Hertz [10] observed similar symptoms in a group of patients with gastro-enterostomy, which he explained as signs of fast gastric emptying. Similar observations were made by Hoffmann [11] and Hesse [12]. The term dumping syndrome is referred to Mix [13], who in 1922 observed dumping of food into the small intestine, during postoperative X-ray examination, in a 40-year-old woman who had a gastro-enterostomy for gastric ulcer. The patient complained of nausea, occasional bile vomiting and increasing weight loss, so it seems possible that she mainly had symptoms of a chronic afferent-loop syndrome; nevertheless, the term introduced by Mix is now used for the most frequent post-gastrectomy syndrome.

Following the original description of vagal influences on gastric secretion by Pawlow in the last decade of the ninetheenth century, the vagus nerve became of major interest for surgical interventions in peptic ulcer disease at the beginning of this century. In 1911 Exner and Schwartzmann [14, 15] introduced truncal vagotomy; the occurrence of gastric atony forced them to perform a gastrostomy or gastro-enterostomy at the same time. In 1922 A. Latarjet [16] treated patients with gastritis or duodenal ulcer with an anterior truncal vagotomy, partly combined with gastro-enterostomy, pyloroplasty or pyloric resection. In 1931 Bircher [17] reported good results of vagotomy in treating uncomplicated gastric ulcer.

A scientific basis for vagotomy, however, was given by Dragstedt et al. [18, 19]; in 1943 Dragstedt and Owens [19] reported two duodenal ulcer patients in whom they had performed bilateral supradiaphragmatic vagotomies. Very soon it became clear that atony of the stomach, with concomitant relative pyloric stenosis, occurred after truncal vagotomy, making an additional gastro-enterostomy necessary [18]. In 1951 Weinberg [20] combined truncal vagotomy with pyloro-plasty of the Heinecke-Mikulicz type.

Jackson [21] and Frankson [22] in 1948 described selective gastric vagotomy, which had to be combined with a gastro-enterostomy; this was used in duodenal ulcer patients by Griffith and Harkins [23, 24]. Harkins et al. [25] combined selective gastric vagotomy with antrectomy and reconstructed the continuity by a gastroduodenostomy ("combined operation").

The last step in the technical development of vagotomy was selective proximal vagotomy (also known as parietal cell vagotomy or highly selective vagotomy), which is based on the work of Holle et al. [27, 28]; in this operation the gastric antrum remains fully innervated. While Holle always adds a pyloroplasty, Johnston et al. [28] and Amdrup et al. [29] have shown that dissection, weakening or by-passing of the pylorus is not necessary after selective denervation of the gastric corpus and fundus.

2 Results of Gastric Surgery

2.1 Gastric Resection in Peptic Ulcer Disease

With the development of standardised operative techniques, it is possible for us to compare the different operative procedures. However, an accurate, statistically relevant comparison can be achieved only by prospective randomised studies. This kind of study is rare in the surgical literature and has been used only during the last few years in clinical investigations.

Table 1. Results of gastric resection in peptic ulcer disease

Authors	Walters and Lynn [30]				Borg [31]		Golgher [50]	Postleth-wait [32]	McKeown [33]		
Ulcer type	DU		GU		DU	GU	DU	DU	DU		GU
Type of resection	B I	B II	B I	B II	B I	B II	B II	B II	B I	B II	B I B II
No. of patients	27	449	113	139	211	162	117	222	78	716	12480
Observations time (years)		6–10			5		5–8	5			
Operative death (%)	—		—	—	0.9	0.6	0	1.8	2.5	0.6	0.9
Recurrences (%)	7.4	3.6	4.4	2.9	12.1	3.6	2.0	3.7	—	1.5	0 0
Diarrhoea (%)	—	—	—	—	—	—	0.9	17.1	—	—	—
Dumping (%)	—	—	—	—	18	22.9	21.5	23.2	0	1.3	0 1.3
Vomiting (%) bile	—	—	—	—	—	—	13.1	4.7	0	1.1	0 1.1
ood							5.6				
Visick grading (%) I	37.0	57.0	33.6	64	76	78	49	60.4		80	
II	40.8	34.4		31.7	14	9	28	29.3			
III	11.1	2.5	2.7	1.4	4	6	17	7.7		14	
IV	11.1	5.1	4.4	2.9	6	18 7	6	2.7		6	

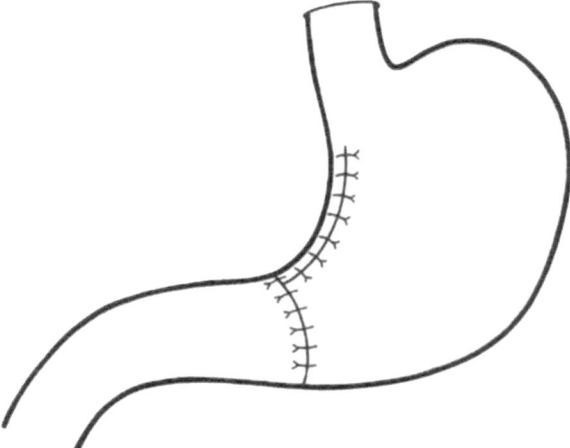

Fig. 1. Billroth I gastroduodenostomy

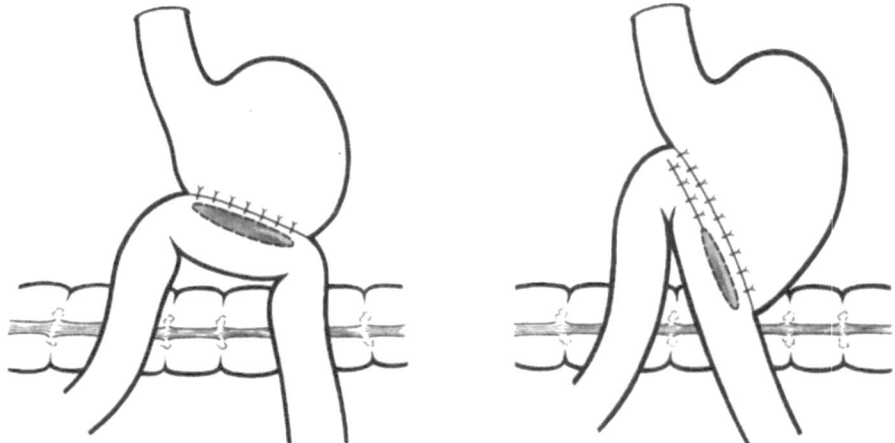

Fig. 2. Billroth II gastrojejunostomy (antecolic)

Table 2. Results of gastric resection in duodenal ulcer

Author	No. of patients	Operative death (%)	Recurrences (%)	Post-gastrectomy-syndromes (%)
Billroth I				
Krause [34]	71	4	19	6.4
Walters + Lynn [30]	27	0	7.4	15
McKeown [33]	78	0.9	2.5	1.6
Billroth II				
Harvey [35]	1,488	2.9	7–10	4.3
Miller [36]	165	—	20.7	24
Salzer [37]	1,704	4.9	—	3.8
Dorn [38]	942	2.05	1 5	8.7

Table 3. Results of gastric resection in gastric ulcer

Author	No. of patients	Operative death (%)	Recurrences (%)	Post-gastrectomy-syndromes (%)
Billroth I				
Salzer [37]	631	4.2	2.0	4.0
Nielsen [39]	97	6.0	5.0	16.0
Sapala [41]	31	3.4	15.0	15.0
Walters [42]	113	0	1.4	4.0
Billroth II				
Nielsen [39]	158	3	5	2
Kraus [43]	112	6	6	3
Welch [44]	424	4.7	1	2.4
Harvey [40]	448	2.9	1.5	1.6

In Table 1 some retro- and prospective studies of the results of resection therapy in gastric and duodenal ulcer disease are listed. The results demonstrate great variation between the different groups. The studies presented seem to indicate that patients with a Billroth I resection (gastroduodenostomy; Fig. 1) will develop postgastrectomy syndromes less frequently than patients with a Billroth II resection (gastrojejunostomy; Fig. 2). If the resection procedures are arranged according to the ulcer type, it becomes evident that duodenal ulcer patients with a Billroth I resection will develop a high rate of recurrent ulcerations (Table 2); however, in gastric ulcer patients Billroth I and Billroth II resections will give similar results in respect of mortality, recurrency and postgastrectomy syndromes (Table 3). The severe complication of gastric resection, gastric stump cancer, will be discussed in Chap. 3.1.10.

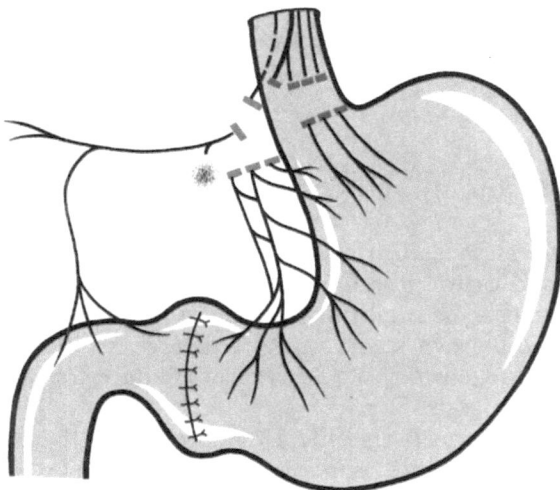

Fig. 3. Truncal subdiaphragmatic vagotomy plus pyloroplasty (Heinecke-Mikulicz type)

Table 4. Results of truncal vagotomy and drainage in the treatment of duodenal ulcer

Authors	Sawyers et al. [45]	Kronborg [46]	Goligher [31]	Kennedy [47]	Postlethwait [32]	Jordan [48]
Type of drainage[a]	PP, antrectomy	PP	PP	PP, GE	PP	PP
No. of patients	90	38	146	50	212	86
Observation time (years)	0.5–2.5	5	5–8	5	5	5–8
Operative death (%)	1.1	0	0.6	0	0.6	1.9
Recurrences (%)	—	13 2	10.9	8.7	6.2	7.8
Diarrhoea (%) mild	21.0	21.6	17.4	0	20.7	19
severe		5.4	4.3			
Dumping (%) mild	20	21.6	11.9	10.9	12.0	14
severe	1	5.4		0		
Visick grading (%) I	64	50	45	63	47.6	60
II	29	27.4	23	23	35 4	34
III	6	10.8	18	4	11.8	
IV	1	11.8	14	10	5 2	6

[a] PP, pyloroplasty; GE, gastro-enterostomy

2.2 Truncal Vagotomy Plus Drainage in Duodenal Ulcer Patients

Based on the studies of Dragstedt, truncal vagotomy (TV) plus drainage has become a standard surgical procedure in uncomplicated duodenal ulcer disease (Fig. 3). In Table 4 several results of prospective studies are summarised. Truncal vagotomy plus drainage has a low mortality, but recurrences are observed in 6%–14%, depending on the observation time. Symptoms induced by operation (postvagotomy syndromes) are mainly diarrhoea and early dumping. While diarrhoea is frequently observed, severe forms of dumping syndrome are rare compared to Billroth II resection. Critical examination of the operative results reveals excellent or good results in 70%–90%; failures are reported in about 6%–10%.

2.3 Comparison of Truncal Vagotomy and Gastric Resection

In recent years, several prospective randomised trials have been performed for comparison of truncal vagotomy and gastric resection in the treatment of un-complicated duodenal ulcer. Table 5 lists the results of Goligher et al. [50] and Postlethwait [33] side by side, since the two studies are comparable. In both studies TV plus drainage was compared with TV plus Billroth I antrectomy (combined operation) or with Billroth II gastrectomy.

In both series the operative mortality was lower after TV plus drainage than after Billroth II gastrectomy. On the other hand, recurrent ulcerations were two to three times more frequent after TV plus drainage than after gastric resection. Furthermore, diarrhoea was observed more often after TV plus drainage, whereas

Table 5. Comparison between truncal vagotomy and gastric resection

Authors	Goligher et al. [50]			Postlethwait [33]			
Type of operation[a]	TV + GE	TV + B I	B II	TV + PP	TV + B I	TV + B II	B II
No. of patients	126	132	117	212	213	248	222
Observation time (years)		5–8			5		
Operative death (%)	0	0	0	0.6	0.9	0 6	1.8
Recurrences (%)	5.9	1.8	2.0	6.2	0.7	0.9	3 7
Diarrhoea (%)	5.1	2.7	0.9	20 7	21.5	21.6	17.1
Dumping (%)	17.9	8.6	21.5	12.0	17.3	19.2	23.2
Vomiting (%) bile	14.5	13.8	13.1	1.8	4.9	3.1	4.7
food	4.3	9.6	5.6	—	—	—	—
Visick grading (%) I	44	50	49	47.6	53.5	60 9	60.4
II	26	28	28	35.7	35.7	32.4	29.3
III	19	14	17	11 8	8.9	4.4	7.7
IV	11	8	6	5.2	1.9	2.4	2.7

[a] GE, gastro-enterostomy; PP, pyloroplasty

dumping syndrome, mainly the severe forms, occurred after Billroth II resection. In the study of the Veterans Administration hospitals [33] signs of an afferent-loop syndrome (bile vomiting) were 2.5-fold more frequent after gastric resection than after TV plus pyloroplasty, whereas in the study of Goligher et al. [50], where TV was combined with gastro-enterostomy, no significant difference was observed. In a further study, Goligher et al. [32] were able to show that using pyloroplasty as the drainage procedure reduced bile vomiting significantly. If the overall results of these various groups are compared, no significant differences in excellent or good clinical results can be demonstrated; however, Billroth II resection is mainly incriminated by its higher operative mortality.

2.4 Comparison of Different Drainage Procedures in Vagotomy

After complete vagal denervation of the stomach (truncal vagotomy, selective gastric vagotomy) a drainage procedure has to be added to achieve adequate gastric emptying. Four main operative procedures have been used for drainage (Fig. 4): gastrojejunostomy; pyloroplasty, Heinicke-Mikulicz type; pyloroplasty, Finney type; and gastroduodenostomy (Jaboulay). In addition, several authors have combined TV with antrectomy (combined operation), which also results in a faster gastric emptying.

From Table 6 the influence of different drainage procedures on the clinical results after TV, selective gastric vagotomy (SGV) or selective proximal vagotomy (SPV) can be seen. The studies of Kennedy et al. [51] and Goligher et al. [32] demonstrate clearly that in patients with TV the recurrence rate is lower after

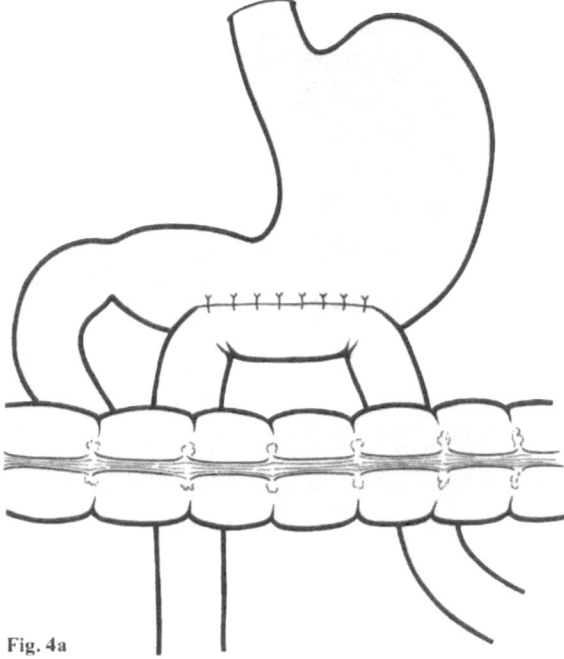

Fig. 4a

Fig. 4a–d. Drainage procedures. **a** retrocolic gastro-enterostomy, **b** Heinecke-Mikulicz type pyloro-plasty; **c** Finney-type pyloroplasty, **d** gastroduodenostomy (Jaboulay)

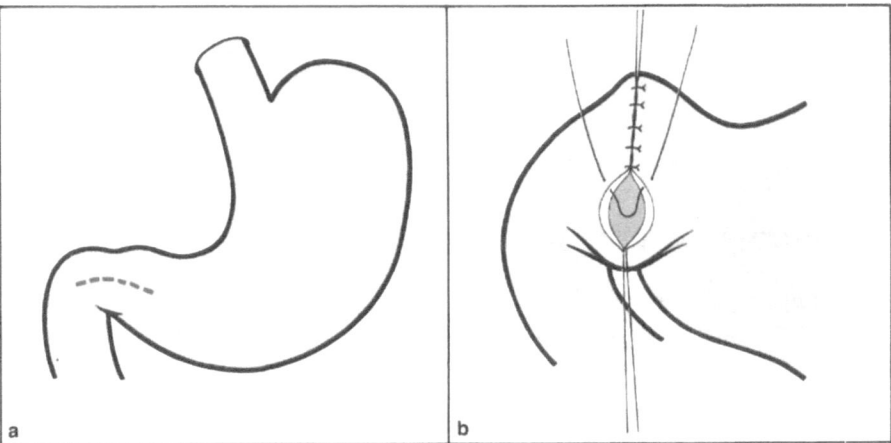

Fig. 4b

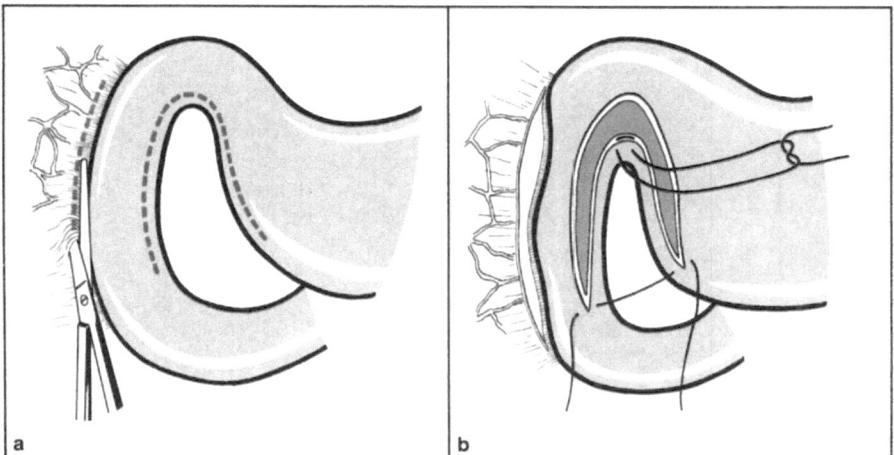

Fig. 4c

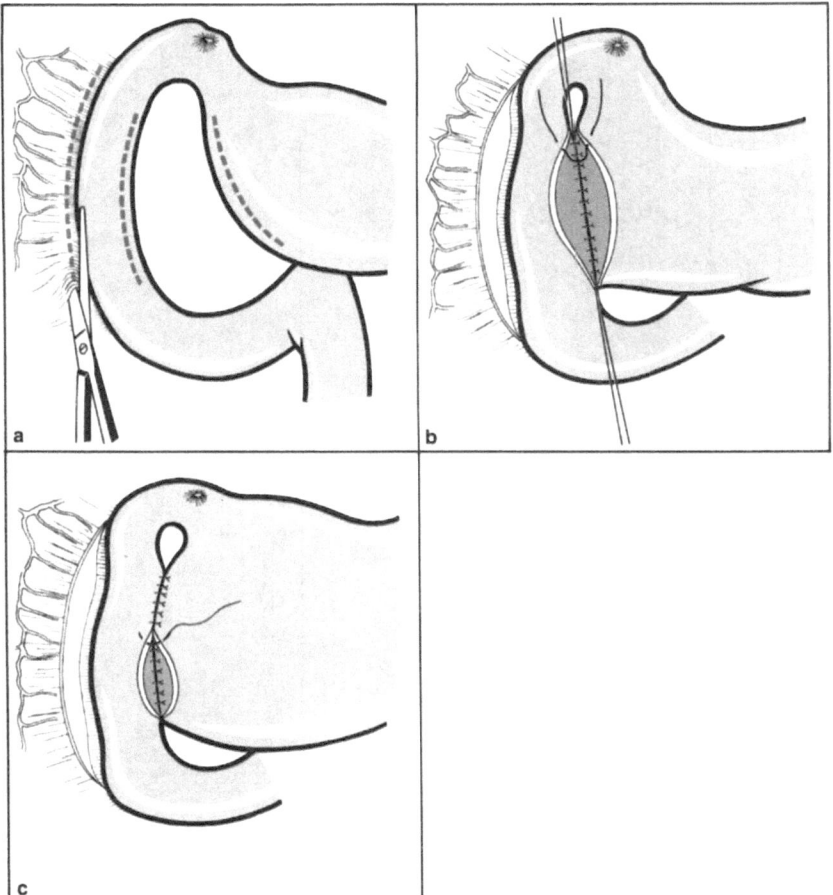

Fig. 4d

Table 6. Comparison of different drainage procedures in vagotomy

| Authors | Golgher et al. [32] | | | Kennedy et al. [51] | | Sawyers and Scott [52] | | Wastell et al. [53] | |
| Type of vagotomy | TV | | | TV | | SGV | | SPV | |
Drainage procedure	GE	PP	Antrectomy	Finney PP	GE	PP	Antrectomy	PP	Without
No. of patients	126	192	132	46	48	40	39	48	52
Operative death	0	0	0	0	0	0	0	0	0
Recurrence (%)	2.5	6.7	0	6.5	4.3	2.6	0	14.6	6.5
Diarrhoea (%)	26.3	21.7	23.2	6.5	10.4	2.6	2.4	10	2
Dumping (%)	17.9	11.9	8.6	39	25	2.4	5.2	5	0
Vomiting (%) bile	14.5	10.1	13.8	8.7	10.4	—	—	22	0
food	4.3	4.4	9.6	4.3	4.2	—	—		
Visick grading (%) I	44	45	50	52	54	55	69	77	78
II	26	23	28	35	37	40	28		
III	19	18	14	6	2	2.5	0	4	14
IV	11	14	8	8	7	2.5	2	9	8

GE, gastro-enterostomy, PP, pyloroplasty

gastro-enterostomy than pyloroplasty; diarrhoea, however, is less frequent after pyloroplasty than after gastro-enterostomy. In the study of Goligher et al. [32] dumping syndrome and bile vomiting are observed less frequently after pyloroplasty than after gastro-enterostomy. The study of Sawyers and Scott [52] compared Heinicke-Mikulicz pyloroplasty with antrectomy in SGV cases. Pyloroplasty resulted in a higher recurrence rate, but dumping symptoms were less frequent. A comparison of the clinical results showed no difference between the two drainage procedures, except for the higher mortality after antrectomy. Wastell et al. [53] compared SPV with and without Heinicke-Mikulicz pyloroplasty. Recurrences were observed more often after pyloroplasty; also, diarrhoea and dumping symptoms were found more often in patients with pyloroplasty. The clinical results tended to be better in patients without pyloroplasty.

2.5 Comparison of Truncal Vagotomy and Selective Gastric Vagotomy

Selective gastric vagotomy, which was introduced by Jackson [21] and Frankson [22], causes a selective denervation of the stomach, whilst all extragastric vagal fibres, to the liver, pancreas, small bowel etc., remain untouched (Fig. 5). It seems reasonable that some of the symptoms, those caused by vagal denervation of these organs, should not occur after SGV. Since 1967, several prospective, partly randomised prospective studies have been performed, comparing SGV with TV. Because of the denervation of the gastric antrum, both operations have to be combined with a drainage procedure; the drainage procedures vary greatly from

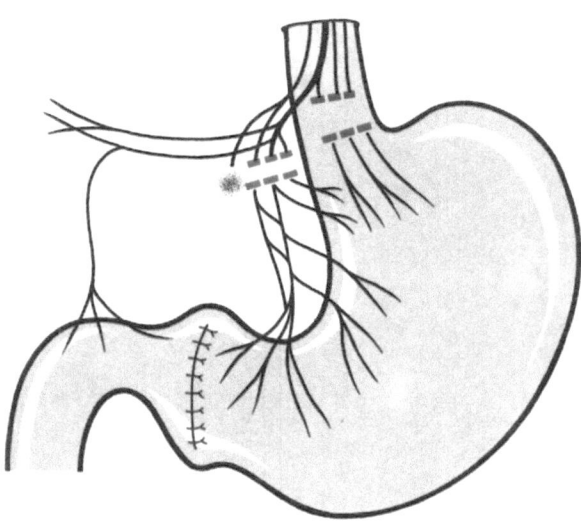

Fig. 5. Selective gastric vagotomy with pyloroplasty (Heinecke-Mikulicz type)

Table 7. Comparison of selective gastric vagotomy and truncal vagotomy

Authors	Kennedy et al. [48]		Sawyers et al. [46]		Kronborg et al. [47]		Kraft et al. [54]	
Type of vagotomy	TV	SGV	TV	SGV	TV	SGV	TV	SGV
Drainage procedure	PP	PP	PP, GE	Antrectomy	PP	PP	PP	
No. of patients	46	49	86	46	38	38	34	42
Observation time (years)	5		1–4		5		3–4	
Operative death (%)	0	0	0	0	0	0	—	—
Recurrence (%)	8.7	2.1	1.4	0	8.0	5.2	12	5
Diarrhoea (%)	28.3	8	21	12	14	0	37	27
Dumping (%)	0	0	1	0	5.7	2.7	29	39
Vomiting (%) bile	4.3	4.2	—	—	—	—	26	20
food	4.3	2.1	—	—	—	—		
Visick grading (%) I	72	57	64	74	55	66	77	88
II	13	40	29	21	31	29	9	5
III	5	—	6	4	—	—		
IV	10	3	1	0	—	—	14	7

PP, pyloroplasty; GE, gastro-enterostomy

study to study: Heinicke-Mikulicz pyloroplasty [47, 48], gastrojejunostomy [46] and Jaboulay gastroduodenostomy [54] have all been used. Several groups have combined SGV with antrectomy [46], termed the "combined operation" by Harkins [25]. This combined operation is characterised by a low recurrence rate but a higher frequency of postgastrectomy symptoms.

The results of the various studies are shown in Table 7. Operative lethality was low in all procedures without gastric resection. All four studies listed agree that the recurrence rate after TV is about three times higher than after SGV. This finding may be explained by technical problems at surgery, since in TV the vagotomy is often incomplete if anterior and posterior vagal trunks are divided above the cardia. Intra-operatively only the larger branches are found and smaller branches remain untouched.

Diarrhoea is less frequent after SGV than after TV. If diarrhoea is further classified according to severity, it can be clearly shown that after SGV the mild forms of diarrhoea are observed, but after TV diarrhoea is usually more severe.

The frequency of dumping symptoms is not different after the two operative procedures. This indicates that for the occurrence of dumping symptoms dissection of extragastric vagal fibres is not important. Also, vomiting of bile or food particles occurs with the same frequency after both types of vagotomy.

Comparison of the clinical results of the two types of vagotomy demonstrates a superiority of SGV over TV; generally excellent or good results are found more often after SGV. Also, failures are observed more often after TV, owing mainly to a higher recurrence rate.

2.6 Selective Proximal Vagotomy

Selective proximal vagotomy (also known as parietal cell vagotomy, highly selective vagotomy etc.) represents the last step in the technical development of vagotomy (Fig. 6). In this procedure, vagal denervation is limited to gastric corpus and fundus, and all vagal fibres to the gastric antrum and pylorus as well as all extragastric fibres remain intact. This type of vagotomy will therefore not disturb the motor activity of the gastric antrum and pylorus. Table 8 lists the results of several prospective studies, based on a follow-up period of 1–12 years.

Operative mortality is low after SPV; in a survey of the literature, operative mortality in 6,500 patients was 0.25% after SPV [55]. The reported recurrence rate varies greatly. The results in Table 8 represent studies done by prominent gastro-intestinal surgeons who have special experience with SPV. In a study on 728 patients performed in several German hospitals, the recurrence rate in duodenal ulcer patients was 3.1% after 1 year and 5.5% after 2 years [59]. For SPV performed in gastric ulcer patients, the recurrence rate after 1 year was 9.3%. On the other hand, the rate of diarrhoea, dumping and bile or food vomiting is lower after SPV than all other operative procedures. Excellent or good clinical results can be expected in about 90% of patients undergoing SPV.

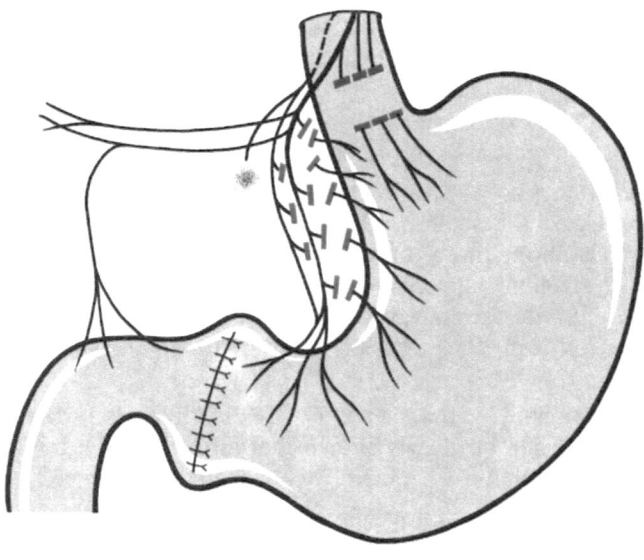

a   with pyloroplasty

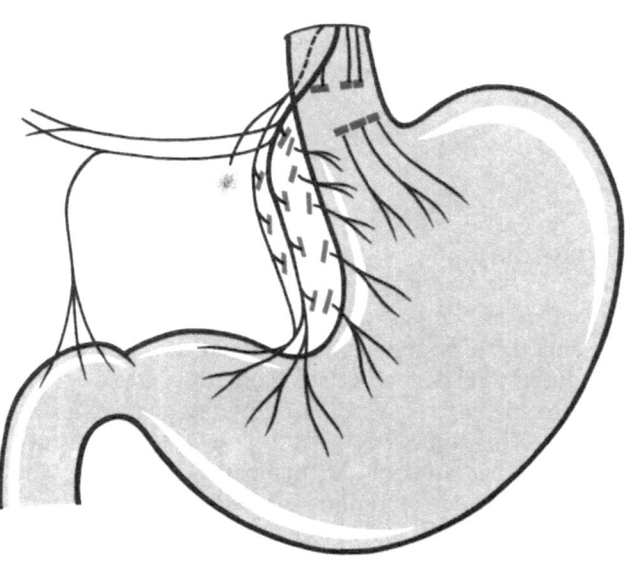

b   without pyloroplasty

Fig. 6a, b. Selective proximal vagotomy: **a** with pyloroplasty (Holle procedure), **b** without drainage procedure (Johnston, Amdrup)

Table 8. Results of selective proximal vagotomy

Authors Type of drainage[a]	Johnston [55] Without	Bauer et al. [56] PP	Grassi et al. [57] Without and with PP	Amdrup [58] Without
No. of patients	107	809	787	109
Observation time (years)	4–7	1–12	1–6	2–4
Operative death (%)	0	0.5	0.3	0
Recurrences (%)	1.0	1.6	1.1	1.8
Diarrhoea (%) mild	4	2	8	6.0
severe	0			0
Dumping (%) mild	6	1	0.4	4.6
severe				1.0
Vomiting (%%) bile	5	1	—	1.8
food	—		—	4.8
Visick grading (%) I	52	90	90	65.8
II	30			22.2
III	10	6	—	7.4
IV	8	4	—	4.6

[a] PP, pyloroplasty

Table 9. Comparison of selective gastric vagotomy and selective proximal vagotomy

Authors Type of vagotomy Drainage procedure[a]	Kronborg et al. [60]		Kennedy et al. [61]		Jordan [62]	
	SPV PP	SGV Without	SPV GE	SPV Without	SGV Antrectomy	SPV Without
No. of patients	50	50	50	50	47	45
Observation time (years)	1–4		1–4		1–2	
Operation death	0	0	0	0	0	0
Recurrence (%)	8	22	2	2	0	2.4
Diarrhoea (%)	12	2	12	4	10	0
Dumping (%)	20	2	37	8	33	16
Vomiting (%) bile	14	4	14	2	6	0
food			10	10		
Visick grading (%) I	68	40	32	60	61	81
II	10	20	42	36	23	11
III	2	24	18	2	16	—
IV	20	8	8	2	—	8

[a] PP, pyloroplasty; GE, gastro-enterostomy

2.7 Comparison of Selective Gastric Vagotomy and Selective Proximal Vagotomy

An exact evaluation of the effectiveness of SPV can be made by comparison with SGV, as shown in Table 9. Three controlled prospective studies have been performed and provide detailed information, but it has to be pointed out that the follow-up period of 1–4 years is relatively short.

Both types of vagotomy have a low operative mortality. The reported recurrence rates after SPV or SGV vary greatly, but the study of Kronborg et al. [60] seems to indicate that after SPV the recurrence rate is higher than after SGV. On the other hand, the frequency of diarrhoea or dumping symptoms is lower after SPV, especially if the SPV was not combined with a drainage procedure. A further analysis of the degree of diarrhoea increases this difference in respect of diarrhoea or dumping. The study of Kennedy [61] demonstrates that bile vomiting is less frequent after SPV than after SGV plus gastro-enterostomy.

The overall clinical results in these controlled studies show a superiority of SPV without drainage over SGV plus drainage; furthermore, the failure rate is significantly lower after SPV.

2.8 Summary

The above results indicate a superiority of vagotomy over gastric resection in the surgical treatment of duodenal ulcer disease. A particular problem in evaluating the different types of vagotomy is the relatively short follow-up period of these studies. There is first evidence that at least after TV the recurrence rate increases to about 30% after a follow-up of 15 years or more [63]. In SGV this tendency could not be shown; the study of Sawyers and Scott [52] demonstrated that 8 years after SGV the recurrence rate was still 2.5%, and there was no tendency to increase.

An interesting aspect of this analysis is the fact that very different surgical procedures lead to very similar clinical results. However, certain facts should be pointed out:
a) After gastric resection the rate of recurrences is low, but the rate of post-gastrectomy symptoms is high.
b) After vagotomy combined with a drainage procedure, the rate of diarrhoea is high, but the rate of dumping is low.
c) Vagotomy combined with antrectomy (combined operation) has the lowest recurrence rate but significantly more postgastrectomy symptoms.
d) Diarrhoea is less frequent after SGV or SPV than after TV, but not compared to gastric resection without vagotomy.
e) All drainage procedures give similiar results.
f) All types of vagotomy result in a lower mortality rate than gastric resection; this finding seems to be the most important advantage of vagotomy over gastric resection.

References

1. Billroth, Th.: Offenes Schreiben an Herrn Dr. Wittelshofer uber die erste mit günstigem Ausgang durchgeführte Pylorektomie. Wien. med. Wschr. *31*, 161 (1881)
2. Wölfler, A.: Gastro-Enterostomie. Zbl. Chir. *8*, 705 (1881)
3. Rydygier, L.: Die erste Magenresektion beim Magengeschwur. Berl. klin. Wschr. *19*, 39 (1882)
4. von Hacker, V.: Zur Kasuistik und Statistik der Magenresektionen und Gastroenterostomien. Arch. klin. Chir. *32*, 616 (1885)

5. Braun, H.: Über Gastro-Enterostomie und gleichzeitig ausgeführte Entero-Anastomose Arch. klin. Chir. *45*, 361 (1893)

6. Braun, H.: Demonstration eines Praparates einer 11 Monate nach Ausführung der Gastroenterostomie entstandenen Perforation des Jejunums. Verh. dtsch. Ges. Chir. *28*, 95 (1899)

7 Eiselsberg, A.: Über Ausschaltung inoperabler Pylorusstrikturen nebst Bemerkungen über die Jejunostomie. Arch. klin. Chir. *50*, 919 (1895)

8. Denèchan, D.: Les suites médicales eloignées de la gastroentérostomie. Diss. Paris (1907)

9. Jonas, S.: Über die nach Gastroenterostomie auftretenden Beschwerden und das rontgenologische Verhalten des anastomosierten Magens. Arch. Verdauungskrh. *14*, 656 (1908)

10. Hertz, A.F.: The cause and treatment of certain unfavorable after effects of gastroenterostomy. Ann. Surg. *58*, 466 (1913)

11 Hoffmann, H.: Unsere Erfahrungen uber die Chirurgie des Magens. Zbl. Chir. 130 (1912)

12. Hesse, X.: Die Gastroenterostomie im Rontgenbild. Zbl. Chir. 1421 (1912)

13. Mix, C.L.: Dumping following gastrojejunostomy. Surg. Clin N. Amer. *2*, 617 (1922)

14. Exner, A.: Ein neues Operationsverfahren bei tabischen Crises gastrique. Dtsch. Z. Chir. *111*, 576 (1911)

15. Exner, A., Schwarzmann, E.: Gastrische Krisen und Vagotomie. Mitt. Grenzgeb. Med Chir. *28*, 15 (1914)

16. Latarjet, A.: Résection des nerfs de l'estomac Technique opératoire. Résultats clinique. Bull. Acad Méd. *87*, 221 (1922)

17. Bircher, E.· Die Behandlung gastrischer Affektionen durch Eingriffe am Nervus vagus und sympathicus. Langenbeck's Arch. Klin. Chir. *167*, 463 (1931)

18. Dragstedt, L.R., Owens, F.M.: Supradiaphragmatic section of vagus nerves in the treatment of duodenal ulcer. Proc. Soc exp. Biol *53*, 152 (1943)

19. Dragstedt, L.R.: Vagotomy for peptic ulcer. Amer. J. Med. *8*, 409 (1950)

20. Weinberg, J.A., Stempien, S.J., Movius, H.J., Dagradi, A.E.: Vagotomy and pyloroplasty in the treatment of duodenal ulcer. Amer. J. Surg. *92*, 202 (1956)

21. Jackson, R.G.: Anatomic study of the vagus nerves with a technic of transabdominal selective gastric vagus resection. Arch. Surg. *57*, 333 (1948)

22. Frankson, C.: Selective abdominal vagotomy. Acta chir. Scand. *96*, 409 (1948)

23. Griffith, C.A., Harkins, H.N.: Partial gastric vagotomy, an experimental study. Gastroenterology *32*, 96 (1957)

24 Griffith, C.A., Stavney, L.S., Kato, T., Harkins, H.N.: Selective gastric vagotomy. Amer. J. Surg. *105*, 13 (1963)

25. Harkins, H.N., Jesseph, J.E., Stevenson, J.K., Nyhus, L.M.: The combined operation for peptic ulcer. Arch. Surg. *80*, 743 (1960)

26. Holle, F., Hart, W.: Form- und funktionsgerechte Operation. Ein Grundsatz moderner Ulcuschirurgie. Arch. klin. Chir. *309*, 205 (1965)

27. Holle, F., Hart, W.: Neue Wege in der Chirurgie des Gastroduodenalulcus. Med. Klin. *62*, 441 (1967)

28. Johnston, D., Wilkinson, A.R.: Selective vagotomy with innervated antrum without drainage procedure for duodenal ulcer. Brit. J. Surg. *56*, 626 (1969)

29. Amdrup, E., Jensen, H.E.: Selective vagotomy of the parietal cell mass preserving innervation of the undrained antrum. Gastroenterology *59*, 522 (1970)

30. Walters, W., Lynn, T.E.: The Billroth I and Billroth II operations. Arch. Surg. *74*, 680 (1957)

31. Borg, I., Borgström, S.: Spatergebnisse der Resektionsbehandlung nach Billroth I und Billroth II in der Ulcuschirurgie. Bruns' Beitr. klin. Chir. *217*, 481 (1970)

32. Goligher, J.C., Pulvertaft, C.N., Irvin, T.T., Johnston, D., Walker, B., Hall, R.A., Willson-Pepper, J., Matheson, T.S.: Five-to eight-year results of truncal vagotomy and pyloroplasty for duodenal ulcer. Brit. med. J. 7 (1972)

33. Postlethwait, R.W.: Five year follow-up results of operations for duodenal ulcer. Surg. Gynec. Obstet. *137*, 387 (1973)

34. McKeown, K.C.: A study of peptic ulcer. Brit. J. Surg. *50*, 220 (1962)

35. Krause, U.: Late prognosis after partial gastrectomy for ulcer. Acta chir. Scand. *114*, 341 (1958)

36. Harvey, H.D.: Twenty-five years of experience with elective gastric resection for duodenal ulcer. Surg. Gynec. Obstet. *112*, 203 (1961)

37. Miller, T.G., Berkowitz, D.: Analysis of results of conservative peptic ulcer therapy. Gastroenterology *29*, 353 (1955)

38. Salzer, G.: Indikationen zur Resektion nach Billroth I und Billroth II einschließlich des hoch-
    sitzenden Ulcus. Klin. Med. 22, 13 (1967)
39. Dorn, P.: Die Ulcuschirurgie in Zürich in den Jahren 1937–1956. Helv Chir. Acta 28, 3 (1961)
40. Nielsen, J., Amdrup, E., Christiansen, P., Fenger, C., Jensen, H E., Lindskov, J., Damgaard-
    Nielsen, A.A.: Gastric ulcer. II. Surgical treatment. Acta chir. Scand. 139, 460 (1973)
41. Harvey, H.D.: Twenty-five years of experience with elective gastric resection for gastric ulcer.
    Surg. Gynec. Obstet. 113, 191 (1961)
42. Sapala, J.A., Ponka, J.L.: Operative treatment of benign gastric ulcers. Amer. J. Surg. 125, 19 (1973)
43. Walters, W.: Six to ten year follow-up of the surgical treatment of duodenal, gastric and gastro-
    jejunal ulcer. Gastroenterology 93, 15 (1960)
44. Kraus, M., Mendeloff, G., Condon, R.E.: Prognosis of gastric ulcer. Ann. Surg. 184, 471 (1976)
45. Welch, C.E., Burke, J.F.: An appraisal of the treatment of gastric ulcer. Surgery 44, 943 (1958)
46. Sawyers, J.L., Scott, H.W., Edwards, W.H., Shull, H.J., Law, D.H.: Comparative studies of the
    clinical effects of truncal and selective gastric vagotomy. Amer. J. Surg. 115, 165 (1968)
47. Kronborg, O., Malmström, J., Christiansen, P.N.: A comparison between the results of truncal
    and selective vagotomy in patients with duodenal ulcer. Scand. J. Gastroent. 5, 519 (1970)
48. Kennedy, T., Connell, A.M., Love, H.G., MacRae, K.D., Sprenger, E.F.A.: Selective or truncal
    vagotomy? Five year results of a double-blind, randomized, controlled trial. Brit. J. Surg. 60,
    944 (1973)
49. Jordan, P.H.: A follow-up report of a prospective evaluation of vagotomy-pyloroplasty and
    vagotomy-antrectomy for treatment of duodenal ulcer. Ann Surg. 180, 259 (1974)
50. Goligher, J.C., de Dombal, F.T., Duthie, H.L., Latchmore, A.J., Smiddy, F.G., Pulverstaft, C.N.,
    Conyers, J.H., Feather, D.B., Shoesmith, J.H., Wilson-Pepper, J.: Five to eight-year results of
    Leeds–York controlled trial of elective surgery for duodenal ulcer. Brit. med. J. 2, 781 (1968)
51. Kennedy, T., Johnston, G.W., Love, A.H.G., Connell, A.M., Spenger, E.F.A.: Pyloroplasty
    versus gastrojejunostomy. Brit. J. Surg. 60, 949 (1973)
52. Sawyers, J.L., Scott, W.H.: Selective gastric vagotomy with antrectomy or pyloroplasty. Ann.
    Surg. 174, 541 (1971)
53. Wastell, C., Colin, J., Wilson, T., Walker, E., Gleeson, J., Zeegen, R.: Prospectively randomised
    trial of proximal gastric vagotomy either with or without pyloroplasty in treatment of un-
    complicated duodenal ulcer. Brit. med. J. 2, 851 (1977)
54. Kraft, R O., Fry, W.J., Wilhelm, G., Ransom, H.K.: Selective gastric vagotomy. Arch. Surg.
    95, 625 (1967)
55. Johnston, D.: Highly selective vagotomy. Progr. Surg. 14, 1 (1975)
56. Bauer, H., Brückner, W., Welsch, K.H., Holle, F.: Die nichtresezierende Chirurgie des
    Gastroduodenalulcus – III. Klinische Resultate. Munch. med. Wschr. 118, 785 (1976)
57. Grassi, G., Orecchia, C, Cantarelli, I., Grassi, G.B.: Development and results of our studies of
    vagotomy, from selective total vagotomy to ultraselective vagotomy. Chir. Gastroent. 9, 23 (1975)
58. Amdrup, E., Jensen, H.E., Johnston, D., Walker, B.E., Goligher, J.C.: Clinical results of parietal
    cell vagotomy (highly selective vagotomy) two to four years after operation. Ann. Surg. 180,
    279 (1974)
59. Zumtobel, V., Engelke, B., Marie, C., Muhe, E.: Proximal-selektive Vagotomie. Resultate einer
    prospektiven Studie. Langenbeck's Arch Chir. 345, 223 (1977)
60. Kronborg, O., Madsen, P.: A controlled, randomized trial of highly selective vagotomy versus
    selective vagotomy and pyloroplasty in the treatment of duodenal ulcer. GUT 16, 268 (1975)
61. Kennedy, T., Johnston, G.W., MacRae, K.D., Sprenger, E.F.A.: Proximal gastric vagotomy.
    Interim results of a randomized controlled trial. Brit. med. J. 2, 301 (1975)
62. Jordan, P.: A prospective study of parietal cell vagotomy and selective vagotomy-antrectomy
    for treatment of duodenal ulcer. Ann. Surg. 183, 619 (1976)
63. Stabile, B.E., Passaro, E.: Recurrent peptic ulcer. Gastroenterology 70, 124 (1976)

Part II
Diagnostic Procedures

3 X-Ray Findings

Radiology of the operated stomach requires special attention by the radiologist since he has to look not only for the usual pathological findings, such as inflammation, ulceration and cancer with their consequences, but also for postoperative changes and their consequences. Knowledge of typical postoperative changes is necessary in order to prevent misinterpretation.

Radiological study is, after endoscopy, the most important procedure in the diagnosis of the postoperative stomach. In order to extract all the available information from this examination the radiologist has to understand an assortment of gastric operations. The large number of eponyms used in the surgical literature and the lack of uniformity of description are both complex and discouraging. Terminologies such as "partial gastrectomy" or "gastroduodenostomy" are readily understood, but whereas the procedures Billroth I and Billroth II are known in many countries, in other countries they may mean little.

The dilemma of a lack of exact description of the surgical procedure performed may be demonstrated by an exaggerated attempt to distribute surgical credits. Ogilvie [1] described the most satisfactory gastrectomy as "the high posterior Finsterer-Lake-Lahey modification of the Mikulicz-Krönlein-Hofmeister-Reichel-Polya improvement of the Billroth II gastrectomy with a large valve and a small stoma".

The information provided by eponyms is neither useful nor precise. A purely descriptive terminology is much more useful. According to the suggestion of Burhenne [2] several basic components of gastric surgery have to be considered when all variants of gastric surgery are analyzed:

1. Extent of gastric resection
2. Kind of anastomosis
2.1. End-to-end anastomosis, side-to-side anastomosis
2.2. Anterior or posterior anastomosis
2.3. Superior or inferior anastomosis
3. Diameter of the stoma
4. Gastric emptying (slow or fast)
5. Ante- or retrocolic gastrojejunostomy
6. Aniso- or isoperistaltic anastomosis
7. Length of jejunal loop (long or short)
8. Situs of anastomosis (horizontal or oblique)
9. Direction of gastric emptying.

Radiology of the operated stomach has to give an information on the *extent* of the stomach *resected*. An estimate based on the roentgenograms of the amount remaining after resection may be misleading because the remnant of the stomach will enlarge with the late emptying and its size will be smaller with mechanical dumping. Depending on the *placement of* the *stoma* (superior or inferior anastomosis) the preference of gastric emptying into either the proximal or distal limb will be influenced. The entire cut end of the stomach may be utilized for a complete stoma (so-called Polya gastrectomy). For a restricted stoma (Hofmeister gastrectomy) the cut end of the stomach is partially closed.

Traditional ulcer surgery removes with the pyloric portion that part of the stomach which is believed to serve an important function in gastric emptying. In addition the gastric reservoir is lost in all patients after gastric resection and rapid emptying into the jejunum is present. Gastric emptying is particularly accelerated with a more extensive gastric resection and creation of a large stoma.

Whether the jejunum is placed in front of the colon (antecolic gastrojejunostomy) or behind it through a surgical opening in the mesocolon (retrocolic jejunostomy) is radiologically best distinguished in the oblique and lateral projections. Better estimation of the position is obtained if the colon is outlined by gas. In the antecolic anastomosis the proximal jejunal limb usually is longer than in a retrocolic anastomosis.

The anastomotic loop consists of a *proximal* (afferent) and a *distal* (efferent) *jejunal limb*. If the proximal limb coming from the duodenum leads to the lesser curvature in a right-to-left gastrojejunal anastomosis, the distal limb leaves from the greater curvature in an anisoperistaltic or antiperistaltic fashion. If the proximal limb is connected to the greater curvature of the stomach by a left-to-right anastomosis the distal jejunal limb leads away from the lesser curvature isoperistaltically.

The ligament of Treitz and the duodenal loop are the best landmarks for identification of the proximal jejunal limb. The direction of peristalsis may help to identify the type of anastomosis performed. Long proximal limbs are usually more frequently associated with postgastrectomy complications.

An oblique anastomosis with more extensive resection along the lesser curvature combined with an inferiorly located stomach will result in preferential emptying into that jejunal limb which has been attached to the greater curvature. The operation with the best functional results is a one-way gastrectomy with emptying into the distal jejunal limb. Filling of the proximal jejunal limb does not necessarily imply malfunction of the anastomosis, but distension and stasis with the late emptying of the proximal limb and duodenum indicate a pathophysiological condition [3].

After *truncal vagotomy* hypotonicity with the absence of peristalsis may persist for several days or weeks and does not have to be regarded as organic obstruction. Of diagnostic functional importance is the radiological demonstration of the *afferent* and *efferent loops* in resected stomachs. The gastric remnant usually empties the contrast medium rapidly through the efferent limb. Small amounts of contrast medium may reach the afferent loop, but usually are emptied rapidly via the efferent limb. If the contrast medium predominantly reaches a dilated afferent loop, the anastomosis of the afferent loop has been made too low.

Barium – diluted by duodenal juice – may remain in the dilated afferent loop, thus a functional delay of emptying of the afferent loop may exist without any organic stenosis. More difficult is the demonstration of an afferent loop syndrome with organic stenosis of the afferent limb, because contrast medium will not reach the afferent loop. If the afferent loop does not show up despite changing the patient's position during fluoroscopy, this has to be considered as strong evidence for a functional stenosis of the afferent loop. Postoperative functional changes, such as the afferent loop syndrome, hypotonicity due to vagotomy, dumping, and stenosis at the efferent limb of the anastomosis, may be demonstrated by radiology more clearly than by gastroscopy, which seems superior in detecting morphological alterations of the mucosa, such as ulcers, cancer, postoperative reflux gastritis or polypoid lesions as well as organic stenosis.

Early postoperative complaints often require an immediate diagnostic approach: intubation, plain abdominal X-ray, upper GI series sometimes with absorbable contrast medium to detect the acute atony of the stomach, adhesions, volvulus and obstruction. Routine X-ray after gastric surgery has been widely abandoned in favour of gastroscopy, which should be performed routinely 2–3 weeks postoperatively. Recurrent ulcers after gastric surgery mostly will be detected by X-ray if located in the jejunum, but ulcers close to the anastomosis are more accurately detected by gastroscopy. The recurrent peptic ulcer in the operated stomach is more readily detected by X-ray in an anterior-posterior or oblique diameter, with the patient upright.

The radiologist is primarily responsible for the diagnosis of *bezoars* in the gastric remnant. They present as mottled, movable filling defects within the barium-filled gastric pouch. With the patient in the upright position they float, in an iceberg-like fashion, in the barium column with a small arcuate edge of the mass protruding above the level of the barium. If sufficiently large, the barium column may split as it enters the stomach, flowing over the surface of the bezoar. The filling defect is usually sponge-like, as the barium becomes enmeshed in or adherent to the surface of the bezoar. It may be helpful to let the patient drink carbonated beverages following the barium suspension. The bezoar than stands out in excellent contrast furnished by the enmeshed and adherent barium against the water and air density of the gastric content [4].

On delayed roentgenograms the bezoar may be identified by the entrapped barium.

References

1. Ogilvie, H.: Gastrectomy: human experiment. Lancet 2, 377–379 (1947)
2. Burhenne, H.J.: Roentgen anatomy and terminology of gastric surgery. Amer. J. Roentgenol. 91, 731–744 (1964)
3 Frommhold, W., Herzer, R.: Röntgenuntersuchung des Magens. In: Handbuch der Inneren Medizin, Band 3, 183–322 (Demling, L., ed.). Berlin: Springer-Verlag 1974
4. Rogers, L.F., Davis, E.K., Harle, T.S.: Phytobezoar formation and food boli following gastric surgery. Amer. J. Roentgenol. 119, 280–290 (1973)

4 Postoperative Endoscopy

Patients commonly examined endoscopically after operation are those who have had gastric resection with either gastrojejunostomy or gastroduodenostomy or simple gastrojejunostomy and pyloroplasty. The creation of a surgical anastomosis or pyloroplasty may result in sufficient distortion to render X-ray interpretation of morphology difficult and may create special problems in identifying small or superficial ulcerations. Thus gastroscopy, which can be considered like other endoscopic gastrointestinal procedures as an extension of the physical diagnostic principle of inspection, should be superior in general to the indirect X-ray method in the operated stomach. Even larger ulcerations may escape detection in the postoperative stomach. Most ulcerations occur at the anastomosis or within a few centimetres of the stoma, usually on the duodenal or jejunal site, but may be present, too, several centimetres distal. Modern flexible fibre-optical endoscopes have little difficulty in visualisation of these lesions, especially when instruments with both a side view and a forward-viewing device are used.

Gastroscopy is superior to conventional X-ray examination after gastric surgery in cases of:

> Acute haemorrhage
> Gastric stump cancer
> Anastomotic ulceration
> Reflux gastritis/oesophagitis
> Bezoars
> Retained sutures
> Foreign-body ulceration
> Outlet obstruction.

The adequacy of the gastric outlet can be readily determined and the existence of obstruction often can be recognised. Partial obstruction may be due to an unusually small stoma or subsequent scarring and distortion caused by recurrent ulceration or severe gastritis, with production of enlarged oedematous hyperaemic folds. These might permit passage of the endoscope, but not permit adequate emptying of a meal. Following vagotomy and gastric resection, emptying may be poor and food bezoars may form even in the presence of a widely patent stoma and the absence of an organic obstruction.

In the process of making an anastomosis or in closing a portion of the resected stomach, an exuberant collection of tissue, called a plication defect, may remain within the lumen. Occasionally this pseudopolypoid conglomeration must be differentiated from neoplasms by endscopy. However, adenomatous polyps may develop on either side of a gastrojejunostomy stoma. These polyps may even be responsible for upper gastro-intestinal bleeding.

Quite often retained sutures may be detected by gastroscopy. They are usually innocent, but they may cause foreign-body ulceration.

One of the most important uses of upper gastro-intestinal endoscopy is the early identification of the source of bleeding of the upper gastro-intestinal tract.

Endoscopy is preferred to X-ray because it may identify lesions which are too superficial or too small to be accurately diagnosed radiologically.

Another important indication for upper gastro-intestinal endoscopy is the detection of gastric remnant carcinoma. Since carcinoma may develop in the operated stomach with increasing frequency seven or more years after gastric surgery, yearly gastroscopic controls seem justified. This lesion can be readily identified by gastroscopy.

Some degree of postoperative gastritis is often present after an anastomotic procedure. Gastritis may be severe and can be associated with pain and bilious vomiting. Most often it is associated with low or absent gastric acid secretion, which has given rise to the term postoperative reflux gastritis. This severe gastritis is believed to be due to reflux of bile and duodenal content (lysolecithin?) into the stomach. The diagnosis of postoperative reflux gastritis could be made in the past much more easily and frequently owing to endoscopy and the histology of the biopsy samples.

The incidence of perforation, either of the pharyngo-oesophageal area or of the stomach, in the course of gastroscopy with rigid instruments varied from 0.01%–0.16%, whereas the incidence with fibre-optical flexible endoscopes is estimated at 0.003%. Additional rare hazards induced by endoscopy include reaction to topical pharyngeal anaesthesia and respiratory arrest, especially in the elderly, associated with the intravenous administration of premedications. Cardiac arrest is rare, but electrocardiographic changes during endoscopy may occur.

5 Gastric Secretory Analysis

The rationale of nearly all surgical procedures in the treatment of peptic ulcer disease is the reduction of gastric acid secretion. The importance of acid secretion in the development of ulceration can be clearly demonstrated by the fact that after simple gastro-enterostomy all ulcers in the duodenum will heal, since acid is kept away from the ulceration.

Postoperative acid secretory studies indicate the effectiveness of the procedure in reducing acid secretion. Two acid secretory studies are clinically used: the pentagastrin test and the insulin test. Food-stimulated acid secretion (intragastric titration) is used at the moment in experimental clinical studies but is not likely to achieve general clinical importance because of its technical expenditure.

5.1 Pentagastrin Test

The synthetic pentapeptide of human gastrin G-17 has been widely used as stimulus in gastric secretory studies and has largely replaced histamine or Histalog. Pentagastrin is used at a dosage of 6 µg/kg body weight subcutaneously. The secretory analysis is performed by continuous suction; a basal period of 1 h is followed by a stimulatory period of 120–150 min. The results of acid secretion are expressed as basal acid output (BAO), maximal acid output (MAO) or peak acid output (PAO). However, at the moment the calculation of these parameters is not yet internationally standardised, so that it is difficult to compare values reported in the literature. However, the generally used stimulation of gastric acid secretion with 6 μg pentagastrin/kg body weight does not result in maximal acid secretion in all patients, since the individual sensitivity against pentagastrin varies. We were able to demonstrate that an intravenous dose response curve with pentagastrin shows an MAO about 30% higher than with subcutaneous application [1]. Therefore it is doubtful that particular high-risk groups for recurrent ulcerations can be discriminated on the basis of secretory parameters.

5.1.1 Gastric Secretion after Billroth I and Billroth II Resection

In both Billroth I and Billroth II resection, reduction of gastric acid secretion is achieved by removal of the gastrin cell area (antrum) and partial resection of parietal cells. There is a direct correlation between the amount of stomach resected and the reduction of acid secretion, as shown by Myren et al. [2] (Table 10).

The threshold of acid secretion for the development of recurrent ulceration is unknown. Obviously, a large individual variance exists for the sensitivity of the jejunum to acid; certainly, patients with high postoperative MAO develop peptic jejunal ulcers more often, but the majority of patients with peptic jejunal ulcers have an MAO below 20 mEq/h.

Although Billroth I gastrectomy of the same extent results in a similar reduction of acid secretion to that after Billroth II resection, Billroth I has a significantly higher recurrence rate [4]. The cause of ulceration developing in the duodenal mucosa even after antrectomy with consequent hyposecretion is unknown, but it has to be pointed out that compared to Billroth II patients, postprandial gastrin output is increased [5], which may result in an increased postprandial food-stimulated acid secretion.

Table 10. Effect of extent of distal gastric resection (Billroth II) on BAO and MAO (Myren et al. [2] according to Baron [3])

Operation	Mean weight of stomach removed (g)	n	BAO % reduction	MAO % reduction
Billroth II $^1/_3$	105	36	77	67
Billroth II $^2/_3$	230	44	87	93

Table 11. Effect of different types of vagotomy on BAO and MAO in duodenal ulcer patients 1 year and more after operation

Authors	Type of vagotomy	Drainage[a]	n	Reduction in acid secretion (%)	
				BAO	MAO
Kennedy et al. [6]	TV	PP	204		61
	TV	GE	200		65
Jordan and Condon [7]	TV	PP or GE	98	76	77
	TV	B I or B II	102	99	95
Jordan [8]	SGV	B I or B II	47	97	92
Johnston [9]	TV	PP	67	78	49[b]
	SGV	PP	158	79	52[b]
	SPV	without	80	82	56[b]
Kronborg and Madsen [10]	SGV	PP	50		57[b]
	SPV	without	50		61[b]
Zumtobel [11]	SPV	without	289	60	45[b]

[a] PP, pyloroplasty; GE, gastro-enterostomy
[b] Peak acid output

5.1.2 Gastric Secretion after Vagotomy

All types of vagotomy (TV, SGV, SPV) result in a significant reduction of BAO and MAO. In Table 11 a number of representative studies for the different types of vagotomy are listed. The reduction of acid secretion seems to be less after SPV than after the more extensive vagal denervation procedures.

It is not totally clear if the risk of recurrences after vagotomy is increased in patients with high preoperative values. While Clark et al. [12] found no difference, Kronborg [13] reported that 2% of patients with a preoperative MAO below 46 mEq/h developed a recurrent ulcer after TV, whereas in patients with a MAO above 46 mEq the ulceration recurred in 17%. In the same study it could be demonstrated that the per cent reduction did not correlate with recurrences. This finding indicates that at least TV may be less effective in patients with high preoperative acid output; if by this type of operation acid secretion is not decreased below 15 mEq/h, a high recurrence rate may occur.

5.1.3 Acid Secretion in Zollinger-Ellison Syndrome

Demonstration of an extremely elevated basal acid secretion is suggestive of a Zollinger-Ellison syndrome (ZES). The following parameters seem to be of diagnostic value: BAO above 15 mEq/h in a nonresected stomach or 5 mEq/h in a resected stomach; and quotient of basal to stimulated secretion above 0.6. However, several studies on acid secretion in ZES have demonstrated that at least in such an unrefined form these parameters are not valid.

Table 12. Interpretation of the insulin test

A.	Qualitative criteria (change in acidity)	
	1) Hollander [14] (1946)	Increase of 20 mval/l during first 2 h
	2) Ross and Kay [15] (1964)	As 1), but differentiation of early (0–45 min) and late positive (45–120 min)
	3) Johnston et al. [16] (1967)	As 2), except early positive = 0–16 min, late positive = 60–120 min
B.	Quantitative criteria (acid secretory capacity)	
	1) Waddell [17] (1957)	Volume increase over basal
	2) Bachrach [18] (1962)	Increase 1 mval/h over basal, or BAO higher than 2 mval/h
	3) Hubel [19] (1966)	Comparison of PAO after insulin pre- and postoperatively
	4) Bitsch et al [20] (1966)	Acid secretion during 1st and 2nd hours higher than BAO
	5) Bank et al. [21] (1967)	Acid secretion after insulin 2 mval/h higher than BAO
	6) Bachrach and Bachrach [22] (1967)	BAO higher than 0.25 mval/h, increase after insulin of 0.25 mval/h
	7) Stempien et al. [23] (1968)	0 5 mval/2 h over BAO

5.2 Insulin Test

In the follow-up period of vagotomised patients, mainly after the development of recurrent ulcerations, a test is needed which will indicate the completeness of the vagotomy. By insulin-induced hypoglycaemia the central vagal nuclei are activated, which in intact peripheral vagus results in a stimulation of acid secretion. However, it has been shown that not only cholinergic, but also adrenergic reflexes, which may be blocked by beta-receptor inhibiting agents, and other, so-called peptidergic fibres play a role in insulin-induced acid secretion. Despite these restrictions the insulin test cannot at the moment be replaced by other methods in examining the completeness of a vagotomy.

The interpretation of the insulin test leads to several difficulties, since different criteria are used by different groups. In Table 12 the most important criteria are listed and differentiated according to both qualitative criteria (changes in acidity) and quantitative criteria (changes in acid secretory capacity).

The evidence of the different criteria is small if BAO is used in the calculations, since there are severe technical problems involved in measuring this value exactly [24]. On the other hand, the work of Faber, Hobsley et al. [25, 26], who corrected their secretory data for sex and body weight, demonstrates that using these criteria a group of patients with a high risk of recurrences may be found. Furthermore, it has been known for some time that a positive insulin test, according to the Hollander criteria [14], results in a low reduction rate after pentagastrin or histamine stimulation. The best discriminatory evidence according to recurrences and reduction of acid secretion is given by an insulin test performed 7–10 days after operation, as pointed out by Johnston [9].

6 Endocrine Provocation Tests

The antral hormone gastrin is of special importance in recurrent ulcerations after gastric surgery. In the last few years several forms of hypergastrinaemia have been found; the differential diagnosis embraces the following:

1) Zollinger-Ellison syndrome
2) Antral G-cell hyperplasia
3) Retained antrum after Billroth II resection
4) Pyloric stenosis
5) Pernicious anaemia, atrophic gastritis, gastric carcinoma
6) Vagotomy
7) Chronic renal insufficiency
8) Short-bowel syndrome
9) Phaeochromocytoma.

In postgastrectomy and postvagotomy syndromes, hypergastrinaemia after vagotomy or retained gastric antrum has to be differentiated from ZES or antral G-cell hyperplasia. Since, as pointed out earlier, gastric analysis will fail in many patients to differentiate these diseases and, on the other hand, patients with ZES will have relatively low basal serum gastrin levels, several endocrine provocation tests have been developed in recent years to make the differentiation possible. Three provocation tests have to be discussed: the calcium infusion test, the secretin test, and the glucagon test.

6.1 Calcium Infusion Test

Passaro et al. [27] have shown that exogenous calcium causes a release of gastrin from Zollinger-Ellison tumours (gastrinomas). Calcium^{++} is infused for 3–4 h at a dosage of 4–5 mg/kg body weight/h or given as a bolus injection (5 mg Ca^{++}/kg body weight, i.v.). While normal subjects and duodenal ulcer patients during hypercalcaemia show only a small release of gastrin, patients with a retained antrum after gastric resection release amounts of gastrin comparable to those in ZES. This test does not therefore allow differentiation between the different forms of hypergastrinaemia.

6.2 Secretin Test

Isenberg et al. [28] and Thompson et al. [29] demonstrated that injection of secretin in patients with gastrinomas causes an abrupt increase in serum gastrin levels. These findings led to the development of the secretin test. Secretin (natural or synthetic) is injected at a dosage of 1 unit/kg body weight, i.v. During the first 15 min after secretin administration patients with ZES show an abrupt elevation of basal serum gastrin concentrations, which return to normal

Table 13. Serum gastrin levels in Zollinger-Ellison syndrome during provocation tests

Increase over basal (%)	Calcium infusion ($n=49$)	Secretin injection ($n=47$)	Glucagon injection ($n=33$)
0– 20	2	5	3
20– 50	9	6	7
50–100	15	16	8
100–200	23	20	15

after 30–45 min. This increase in serum gastrin levels is not found in normal subjects, duodenal ulcer patients or patients with other forms of hypergastrinaemia. However, Arnold and Creutzfeldt [30] were able to show that in two patients with G-cell hyperplasia of the gastric antrum a small but definite increase in serum gastrin occurred after secretin injection.

6.3 Glucagon Test

Similar results to those of the secretin test are produced by the injection of glucagon (30 mg/kg body weight, i.v.), which is structurally similar to secretin [31]. Here also, an increase of basal serum gastrin levels is observed during the first 15 min after injection of glucagon. A survey of the results of the different provocation tests in histologically verified ZES is given in Table 13. These results show that in a certain percentage of patients the increase of basal serum gastrin concentrations is minute. Therefore, in patients with suspected ZES but without a clear provocation test, it is necessary to repeat the test or to perform all three listed tests in order to reduce the danger of missing a ZES.

References

1. Becker, H.D.: Progress in diagnosis of gastric function. Ztschr. Gastroent. *16*, 118 (1978)
2. Myren, J., Gjeruldsen, S., Tretheim, B.: Gastric secretion before and after graded partial gastrectomy for duodenal ulcer. Scand. J Gastroent. *1*, 132 (1966)
3. Baron, J.H.: The rationale of the different operations for peptic ulcer. In: Cox, A.G., Alexander-Williams, J.: Vagotomy on trial. Heinemann Broks, London p. 7–36 (1973)
4. Mathieson, A.J.M.: The Billroth I recurrent ulcer. Brit. J. Surg. *50*, 251 (1962)
5. Becker, H.D., Reeder, D.D., Thompson, J.C.: Effect of truncal vagotomy with pyloroplasty or with antrectomy on food stimulated gastrin values in patients with duodenal ulcer. Surgery *74*, 580 (1973)
6. Kennedy, T., Mac Kay, C., Bedi, B.S., Kay A.W.: Truncal vagotomy and drainage for chronic duodenal ulcer disease: a controlled trial. Brit. med. J. *2*, 71 (1973)
7. Jordan, P.H., Condon, R.E.: A prospective evaluation of vagotomy-pyloroplasty and vagotomy-antrectomy for treatment of duodenal ulcer. Ann. Surg. *172*, 547 (1970)
8. Jordan, P.H.: A prospective study of parietal cell vagotomy and selective vagotomy-antrectomy for treatment of duodenal ulcer. Ann. Surg. *183*, 619 (1976)
9. Johnston, D.: Highly selective vagotomy. Progr. Surg. *14*, 1 (1975)
10. Kronborg, O., Madsen, P.: A controlled, randomized trial of highly selective vagotomy versus selective vagotomy and pyloroplasty in the treatment of duodenal ulcer. Gut *16*, 268 (1975)

11. Zumtobel, V., Engelke, B., Marrie, A., Mühe, E.: Proximale selektive Vagotomie. Langenbeck's Arch. Chir. *345*, 223 (1977)
12. Clark, C.G., Murray, J.G., Slessov, I.M., Wyllie, J.H.: Complete vagotomy and its consequences following-up of 146 patients. Brit. med. J. *2*, 900 (1964)
13. Kronborg, O.: Influence of the number of parietal cells on risk of recurrence after truncal vagotomy and drainage for duodenal ulcer. Scand. J. Gastroent. *7*, 423 (1972)
14. Hollander, F.: The insulin test for the presence of intact nerve fibres after vagal operations for peptic ulcer. Gastroenerology *7*, 607 (1946)
15. Ross, B., Kay, A.W., The insulin test after vagotomy. Gastroenterology *46*, 379 (1964)
16. Johnston, D., Thomas, D.G., Checketts, R.G., Duthie, H.L.: An assessment of postoperative testing for completeness of vagotomy. Brit. J. Surg. *54*, 831 (1967)
17. Waddell, W.R.: The acid secretory response to histamine and insulin hypoglycemia after various operations on the stomach. Surgery *42*, 652 (1974)
18. Bachrach, W.H.: Laboratory criteria for the completeness of vagotomy. Amer. J. Dig. Dis. *7*, 1071 (1962)
19. Hubel, K.A.: Insulin-induced gastric acid secretion in young men. Gastroenterology *50*, 24 (1966)
20. Bitsch, V., Christiansen, P.M., Faber, V., Rodbro, P.· Gastric secretory patterns before and after vagotomy. Lancet *1*, 1288 (1966)
21. Bank, S., Marks, I.N., Louw, J.H.. Histamine- and insulin-stimulated gastric acid secretion after selective and truncal vagotomy Gut *8*, 36 (1967)
22. Bachrach, W.H., Bachrach, L.B.: Reevaluation of the Hollander-test. Ann. N.Y. Acad. Sci. *140*, 915 (1967)
23. Stempien, S.J., Lee, E.R., Dagradi, A.E.: Clinical appraisal of insulin gastric analysis. Amer. J. Dig. Dis. *13*, 21 (1968)
24 Faber, R.G., Hobsley, M.. Basal gastric secretion: reproducibility and relationship with duodenal ulceration. Gut *18*, 57 (1976)
25 Faber, R.G, Russell, R.C.G., Parkin, J.V., Whitfield, P., Hobsley, M.: The predictive accuracy of the postvagotomy insulin test: a new interpretation. Gut *16*, 337 (1975)
26. Maybury, N.K., Faber, R.G., Hobsley, M.: Postvagotomy insulin test: improved predictability of ulcer recurrence after corrections for height and collection errors. Gut *18*, 449 (1977)
27. Passaro, E., Basso, N., Walsh, J.H.: Calcium challenge in the Zollinger-Ellison-syndrome. Surgery *72*, 60 (1972)
28 Isenberg, J.I , Walsh, J.H., Passaro, E., Moore, E.W., Grossman, M.I.: Unusual effects of secretin on serum gastrin, serum calcium and gastric acid secretion in a patient with suspected Zollinger-Ellison-syndrome. Gastroenterology *62*, 626 (1972)
29 Thompson, J.C., Reeder, D.D., Bunchman, H.H., Becker, H.D., Brandt, E.N.: Effect of secretin on circulating gastrin. Ann. Surg. *176*, 384 (1972)
30 Arnold, R., Creutzfeldt, W.: Praeoperative Untersuchungen beim Recidivulcus im operierten Magen. Dtsch. med. Wschr. *102*, 1684 (1977)
31. Becker, H.D., Reeder, D.D., Thompson, J.C.: Effect of glucagon on circulating gastrin. Gastroenterology *65*, 28 (1973)

7 Gastric Emptying

7.1 Mechanism and Regulation

The stomach stores food through the operation of a process usually called receptive relaxation. It mixes and delivers food to the bowel by the process of antral peristalsis.

Gastric emptying is related to antral, duodenal and pyloric activity. The rate of emptying of liquids depends on the pressure gradient between stomach and duodenum [1]. Food entering the stomach is initially accommodated in the fundus and body of the stomach. Pressure studies have shown that regular slow contractions push the contents towards the antrum [2]. The response to food by the body and distal stomach is much more vigorous and is characterised by a peristaltic wave which begins in the body and sweeps towards the pylorus to terminate in the distal antrum [3]. The less vigorous waves fade out in the antrum, but the more active ones result in strong segmental contraction of the antrum, which in turn is co-ordinated with duodenal muscular activity [4, 5]. It is known that fluid empties differently from solids [6]. The rate of emptying is influenced by the pH [7] and osmolarity [8, 9] of the food, a regulation requiring duodenal receptors. The volume of food in addition seems to modify the rate of emptying. Another determining factor seems to be the nutritive density of a meal. The greater the nutritive density, the less the volume transferred to the duodenum in 30 min [10]. Hormones also affect gastric emptying: gastrin and secretin delay emptying, but have opposing effects on antral motor activity.

The most important methods of measuring gastric emptying are (1) intubation tests, (2) radiological tests and (3) isotopic tests [11].

In order to avoid repeated intubations and the time disadvantage of the serial test meal, George [12] described a method using double sampling of the stomach contents. A liquid meal with a proper marker is administered and only small samples are withdrawn at regular intervals. By knowing the concentration and the volume of the marker in the original meal and the withdrawn samples it is possible to calculate the volumes of the meal left in the stomach. Modifications have been made using a radio-isotope as a marker. The double sampling method has proved reliable and popular, particularly as it has clinical applications, but the main disadvantage is that it is suitable for liquid meals only. More recently Meeroff et al. [13] described an intubation method which simultaneously allowed studies of gastric emptying and measurement of intestinal absorption and digestion. Radiological methods cannot be considered to give quantitative data on gastric emptying. Fluid barium is unphysiological and fails to reproduce the effects of solid foods. Enteric-coated barium sulphate granules added to a meal have been used [14]. The disadvantage of all radiological methods is that they only measure the total emptying time, i.e. time taken for all the food-barium mixture to leave the stomach, and cannot provide any information during the 2–6 h it may take for the stomach to empty.

7.2 Isotope Tests

The opportunity of studying gastric emptying of solid food was provided by the unique approach of Griffith et al. [15] using food labelled with a radioactive substance. After administration of the labelled test meal, the rate of emptying is obtained by a scanning detector measuring the change in activity over the stomach area. The method requires some sophistication of equipment, but the actual technique is simple and has the considerable advantage of being non-invasive. There are, however, some disadvantages:

1) There is the radiation hazard.
2) Isolated measurement of radioactivity over the stomach only is not possible; radioactivity in the small intestine may interfere with radioactivity recorded over the area of interest.
3) A final problem exists with the choice of isotopes and their affinity to be adsorbed to the chosen meal. The marker attached to solid food particles may be readily dissolved in the acid of gastric juice and the majority of the label might then be in the liquid phase.

This latter important problem has been overcome by two groups: MacGregor et al. [16–18] incorporated ^{99m}Tc into the matrix of chicken liver, and Heading et al. [19, 20] used ^{99m}Tc-tagged pieces of filter paper. A comparison of these two methods was presented by Güller [21] who found that the use of the pieces of filter paper in clinical studies to simulate a solid test meal appears to be justified. In agreement with Heading [19, 20], Güller et al. [21] found a linear pattern of gastric emptying with the filter paper technique, but pieces of filter paper emptied faster than did ^{198}Au-tagged liver. Another kind of useful marker for measurement of solid food seems to be ^{57}Co-cyanocobalamine-tagged calf liver, which has the advantage over ^{99m}Tc labelling of chicken liver that the half-life is longer and one liver may be used for studies over several days [22]. A different approach to measuring the emptying rate of solids and liquids has been introduced by Malagelada et al. [23]. As a marker of the solid phase he incubated uncooked meat with ^{51}Cr(Cl)$_3$. The labelled meat was then thoroughly mixed with 80 g fresh ground meat and cooked before serving it with the rest of the meal. The authors claimed that the radioactive label was firmly attached to the meat.

7.3 Gastric Emptying after Gastric Surgery

Studies of gastric emptying have shown that liquid test meals are emptied rapidly from the stomach of patients with subtotal gastrectomy or with truncal vagotomy and pyloroplasty [1, 16, 17]. This rapid gastric emptying markedly altered the ratio between the rate at which the meal entered the gut and the rate at which biliary or pancreatic secretion entered the bowel during the period when most of the liquid meal left the stomach. Digestive disturbances due to a decrease in concentration of biliary or pancreatic secretions may result, despite normal secretory capacity of the pancreas, in subtotal gastrectomy [17, 24]. As liquid test meals are not typical of normal food, these results cannot necessarily be applied to conditions of a solid test meal. Indeed, several groups have demonstrated that the stomach empties liquid and solid food in different ways [20, 25–27]. Whereas gastric emptying of liquid meals shows an exponential pattern, emptying of solids has been described mostly to occur linearly (Fig. 7). Until the last decade it was not possible to quantitate movement of solid particles from the stomach. The introduction of isotopic methods by Griffith et al. in 1966 [15] was the basis for studies of gastric emptying of solid food. Combining external γ-radiation counting with isotopic labelling of food has been the method used more recently for quantitating rates of gastric emptying of solid food [12, 14, 28–32] (Table 14).

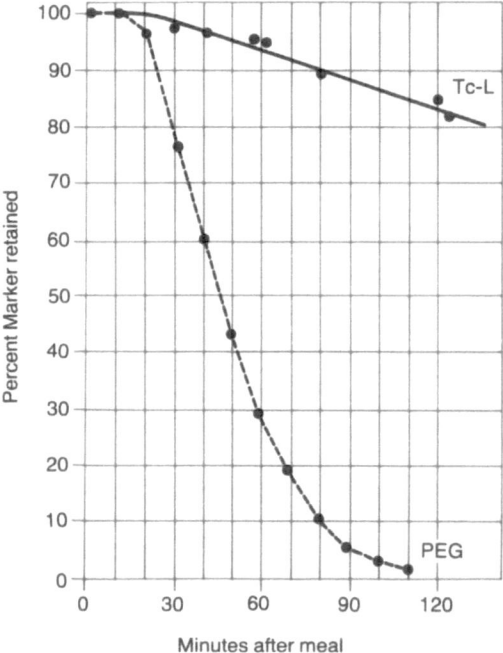

Fig. 7. Simultaneous gastric emptying of a liquid (●– – –● = water and polyethylene glycol ((PEG) labelled) and a solid (●———● = chicken liver tagged with ^{99}Tc) meal. The meal consisted of 400 ml water containing PEG and 8 oz hamburger in which ^{99}Tc-tagged chicken liver (Tc-L) was mixed. The solid meal (Tc-L) was emptied in a linear pattern (slope = − 11.1%/h) after a lag phase of 30 min, while the liquid (PEG) moved in an exponential pattern. Adapted from [18]

The results have been disputed, since in most studies the isotopic markers adsorbed to the surface of solid foods readily dissociated, apparently mixed with the liquid part of the meals, and thus would not be considered to behave like real solid particles. Studies of gastric emptying of solid food particles seem to be much more relevant to the question of what happens to gastric emptying after gastric surgery.

Results of studies of gastric emptying in patients with vagotomy and pyloroplasty are presented in Table 14 and show the conflicting results [12, 28–33]. For the emptying of a solid meal with ^{99m}Tc-tagged liver [16] in normals, a linear pattern of emptying versus time was obtained, at a mean rate of 27.96%/h. A liquid test meal was emptied considerably faster (36.9%/h).

Patients with a subtotal gastrectomy (Billroth I and Billroth II gastrectomy) showed up to three phases in their emptying pattern, which, overall, was approximately exponential with a half-time of 23.3 min (Fig. 8). The rapid gastric emptying in patients with subtotal gastrectomy has been observed, too, by Buckler [33] and Heading [19] using a meal consisting of mashed potatoes and cornflakes. Patients with truncal vagotomy and pyloroplasty (TV and P) could be divided into two groups: those with slow emptying, with a linear pattern (17.64%/h), and those with rapid emptying, with an exponential pattern (half-time

Table 14. Studies of gastric emptying of solid food in V&P subjects[a] (MacGregor et al. [16])

Reference No.	Method	Subjects studied	Time after surgery	Position of subjects	Emptying pattern in V&P's	Emptying rate
[33]	Radio-opaque spheres mixed with mashed potatoes	26 V&P's	Not specified	Not specified	Delayed vs. normal	Delayed
[28]	$^{51}Cr_2O_3$ adsorbed to eggs + porridge + milk	16 V&P's	>9 wk postop. vs. preop.	Sitting at 90°	Biphasic with exponential late phase; 40% emptied in 1st 10 min postop. vs. 12.5% preop.	Rapid
[29]	^{129}Cs adsorbed to zirconium PO_4 + eggs, toast, and milk	V&P's; 10 controls	14 1–4 wk; 9 1–4 mo; 7 1–3 yr	Supine	Linear-exponential; variable slowing, 1–16 wk; normal at 1–3 yr	Normal
[30]	$^{51}Cr_2O_3$ adsorbed to milk, bread, + porridge	10 V&P's; 10 controls	15 days	Supine	Linear, delayed in 6/10	Delayed
[12]	^{129}Cs adsorbed to zirconium PO_4 resin + eggs, toast, + milk	V&P's; 17 controls	10–22 days; 4–6 mo	Supine	Exponential; grossly delayed 10–22 days postop; slightly delayed at 4–6 mo	Normal-delayed
[31]	$^{51}Cr_2O_3$ adsorbed to milk + porridge + bread	5 V&P's; 10 controls	<3 mo	Supine or erect (standing)	Exponential; posture did not affect emptying in normal subjects but lying slowed emptying in V&P's, standing – normal lying – delayed	Normal-delayed
[32]	$^{51}Cr_2O_3$ adsorbed to eggs + cornflakes + milk	10 vagotomy, unspecified, drainage, 5 controls	5–<2 wk; 5–>3 mo	Supine	Exponential; normal in 3/5 } in both vago-delayed in 2/5 } tomy groups Mean $t_{1/2}$ increased	Normal-delayed

[a] V&P, vagotomy and pyloroplasty

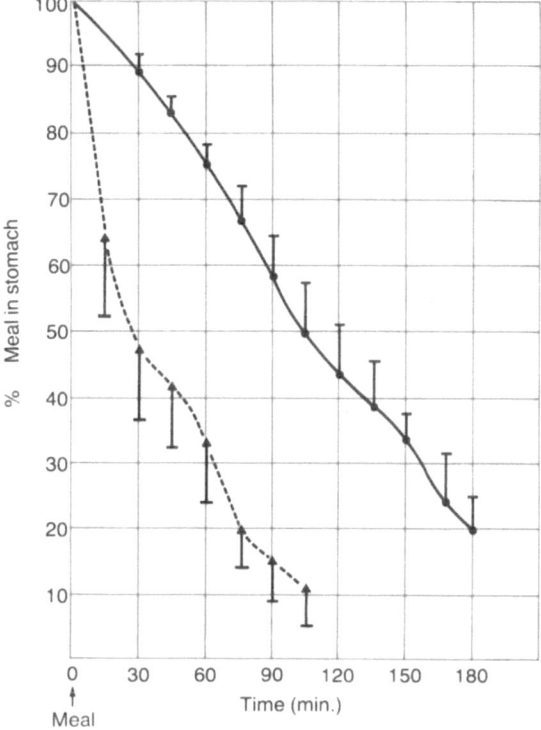

Fig. 8. Gastric emptying, measured as percentage of radioactivity remaining in the stomach versus time, in normal subjects (●) and combined subtotal gastrectomy groups (▲) (Billroth I and Billroth II resections). Normals emptied in a linear pattern, whereas patients with subtotal gastrectomy displayed an initial precipitous emptying followed by a smooth non-linear curve. Adapted from [16]

17.7 min; Fig. 9). The results showed that patients with TV and P as a group emptied solid food at an initially faster and then slightly slower rate than normal subjects. Comparing emptying rates of solids and liquids, the authors found that the slow emptying pattern of solids in some of the TV and P patients contrasted with the abnormally rapid emptying of liquid meals, stressing the disparity of emptying of solid and liquid meals [18, 19].

Using the less accurate method of measuring gastric emptying by a food-barium meal, Wilkinson and Johnston [34] compared the effects of truncal, selective and highly selective vagotomy with respect to preoperative measurements. Truncal and selective vagotomy resulted in faster and more complete emptying of the food barium meal, but highly selective vagotomy did not change the emptying pattern significantly, compared with preoperative measurements. Hinder and Kelly [22] compared in dogs the emptying rate of liver tagged with [57]Co-cyanocobalamine, either diced into 1-cm cubes or homogenized. They found that homogenization of the liver accelerated its emptying. About 45% of the homogenized liver had emptied by 1 h, compared to only 20% when the liver was given in cubes (Fig. 10). Indigestible 7-mm spheres were nearly all retained,

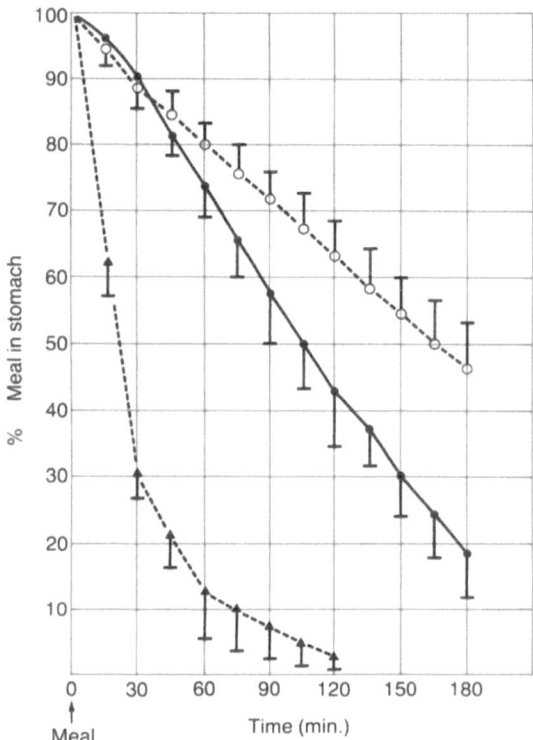

Fig. 9. Gastric emptying of solid food (^{99m}Tc-tagged chicken liver) in normals (●), and in patients with vagotomy and pyloroplasty (V + P) having slow (○) or fast emptying (▲). Patients with V + P, as a group, empty solid food at an initially faster and then slightly slower rate than normal subjects. The slowed emptying patterns of solid meals in some of the V + P patients contrasted with the abnormally rapid emptying of liquid meals in the very same patients. Adapted from [16]

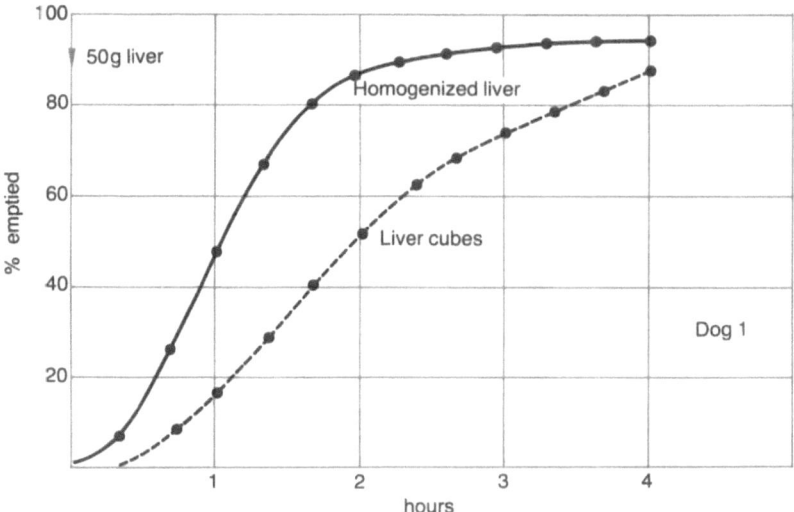

Fig. 10. Gastric emptying from dog stomach of ^{57}Co-cyanocobalamine-tagged liver in cubes or homogenized. Homogenized liver emptied faster than liver in 1-cm cubes. Adapted from [22]

whereas the liver and dextrose solution was emptied. They concluded that the stomach empties liquids, but retains solids for reduction to a smaller size, after which they are discharged at the same rate as the liquid then present in the stomach.

References

1. Nelson, T.S., Kohatsu, S.: The stomach as a pump. Rendic. rom. Gastroent. *3*, 65–70 (1971)
2. Lind, J.F., Duthie, H.L., Schlegel, J.F., Code, C.F.: Motility of the gastric fundus. Amer. J. Physiol. *201*, 197–202 (1964)
3. Smith, A.M.W., Code, C.F., Schlegel, J.F.: Simultaneous cineradiographic and kymographic studies of human gastric antral motility. J. Applied Physiol. *11*, 12–16 (1957)
4. Alvarez, W.C., Mahoney, L.J.: The relations between gastric and duodenal peristalsis. Amer. J. Physiol. *64*, 371–386 (1923)
5. Carlson, H.C., Code, C.F., Nelson, R.A.: Motor activity of the canine gastroduodenal junction: a cineradiographic, pressure and electric study. Am. J. Dig. Dis. *11*, 155–172 (1966)
6. Sheiner, H.J.: Gastric emptying tests in man. Gut *16*, 235–247 (1975)
7. Hunt, J.N., Knox, M.T.: The regulation of gastric emptying of meals containing citric acid and salts of citric acid. J. Physiol. (London) *163*, 34–45 (1962)
8. Gershon-Cohen, J., Shay, H., Fels, S.S.: Experimental studies on gastric physiology in man. IV. The influence of osmotic pressure changes of salt and sugar solutions on pyloric action and gastric emptying in normal and operated stomachs. Am. J. Roentgenol. *40*, 335–343 (1938)
9. Hunt, J.N.: The duodenal regulation of gastric emptying. Gastroenterology *45*, 149–156 (1963)
10. Hunt, J.N., Stubbs, D.F: The volume and energy content of a meal as determinant of gastric emptying. J. Physiol. *245*, 209–225 (1975)
11. Güller, R.: Magenentleerung. Z. Gastroenterologie *15*, 185–191 (1977)
12. George, J.D.: New clinical method for measuring the rate of gastric emptying: the double sampling testmeal. Gut *9*, 237–242 (1968)
13. Meeroff, J C., Go, V.L.W., Phillips, S.F.: Gastric emptying of liquids in man: quantification by duodenal recovery marker. Mayo Clin. Proc. *48*, 728–732 (1973)
14. Horton, R.E., Ross, G.M., Darling, G.H: Determination of the emptying time of the stomach by the use of enteric coated barium granules. Brit. Med. J. *1*, 1537 (1965)
15. Griffith, G.H., Owen, G.M., Kirkman, S., Shields, R.: Measurement of rate of gastric emptying using chromium 51. Lancet *I*, 1244–1245 (1966)
16. MacGregor, I.L., Martin, P., Meyer, J.H.: Gastric emptying of solid food in normal man and after gastrectomy and truncal vagotomy with pyloroplasty. Gastroenterology *72*, 206–211 (1977)
17. MacGregor, I., Parent, J., Meyer, J.H.: Gastric emptying of liquid meals and pancreatic and biliary secretion after subtotal gastrectomy or truncal vagotomy and pyloroplasty in man. Gastroenterology *72*, 195–205 (1977)
18. Meyer, J.H, MacGregor, I.L., Gueller, R., et al.: ^{99}Tc-tagged chicken liver as a marker of solid food in the human stomach Am. J. Dig Dis. *21*, 296–304 (1976)
19. Heading, R.C., Tothill, P., McLoughlin, G.P., et al.: Gastric emptying rate measurement in man: a double isotope scanning technique for simultaneous study of liquid and solid components of a meal. Gastroenterology *71*, 45–50 (1976)
20. Heading, R C., Tothill, R , McLaughlin, R., Sherman, D J.C. Gastric emptying rate measurement in man: A method for simultaneous study of solid and liquid phases. Gut *15*, 841 (1974)
21. Güller, R., Nemec, H.W, Kyle, L., Friedrich, R.: Zur Messung der Magenentleerung solider Nahrung Schweiz. Med. Wschr *107*, 442–446 (1977)
22. Hinder, R.A., Kelly, K.A : Canine gastric emptying of solids and liquids. Am. J. Physiol. *233* 335–340 (1977)
23. Malagelada, J.R : Quantification of gastric solid-liquid discrimination during digestion of ordinary meals Gastroenterology *72*, 1264–1267 (1977)

24. Tympner, F., Rösch, W., Domschke, W., Demling, L.: The function of the exocrine pancreas after exogenous and endogenous stimulation in Billroth II patients. Acta Hepato-Gastroenterol. *23*, 444–448 (1976)
25. Clarke, R.J., Alexander-Williams, J.: The effect of preserving antral innervation and of pyloroplasty on gastric emptying after vagotomy in man. Gut *14*, 300–307 (1973)
26. Cooke, A.R.: Control of gastric emptying and motility. Gastroenterology *68*, 804–816 (1975)
27. Dozois, R.R., Kelly, K.A., Code, C.F.: Effect of distal antrectomy on gastric emptying of liquids and solids. Gastroenterology *61*, 675–681 (1971)
28. Colmer, M.R., Owen, G.M., Shields, R.: Pattern of gastric emptying after vagotomy and pyloroplasty. Br. Med. J. *2*, 448–450 (1973)
29. Cowley, D.J., Vernon, P., Jones, T., et al : Gastric emptying of solid meals after truncal vagotomy and pyloroplasty in human subjects Gut *13*, 176–181 (1972)
30. Hancock, B.D., Bowen-Jones, E., Dixon, R., et al.: The effect of metoclopramide on gastric emptying of solid meals. Gut *15*, 462–467 (1972)
31. Hancock, B.D., Bowen-Jones, E., Dixon, R., et al : The effect of posture on the gastric emptying of solid meals in normal subjects and patients after vagotomy Br J Surg. *61*, 945–949 (1974)
32. Harvey, R F., Mackie, D.B., Brown, N.J.G., et al.: Measurement of gastric emptying time with a gamma camera. Lancet *I*, 16–18 (1970)
33. Buckler, K.G : Effects of gastric surgery upon gastric emptying in cases of peptic ulceration. Gut *8*, 137–147 (1967)

8 Measurement of Reflux

Bile vomiting has been reported as a complication of all types of operations for peptic ulcer disease [1, 2]. Most authors have reported bilious vomiting in about 10% of patients, studied after various surgical procedures [3, 4]. Considerable variation does, however, exist between the different series, probably because assessment of reflux was performed in different, often subjective ways. In order to establish the existence of duodenogastric reflux, which causes postoperative gastritis with its symptoms of epigastric discomfort, an objective test for reflux is necessary. Several methods of measuring duodenogastric reflux have been described (Table 15).

Assessment of reflux has been made radiologically [5] or endoscopically [6], but both methods are subjective and require a tube or a gastroscope, which may themselves cause reflux. Another method introduced by Wormsley [7] used aspiration from the stomach of a marker infused into the duodenum as the parameter for reflux. This method again required a tube. Tubeless methods have been introduced by Faber et al. [8], who measured in gastric aspirates the appearance of bromsulphthalein or indocyanine green excreted into bile by the liver. A disadvantage of this method is that bromsulphthalein will obey hepatic excretion kinetics and thus lead to inconstant concentrations of bromsulphthalein in bile [9]. The same will hold for indocyanine green, which is difficult to measure in bile [8]. Thus, naturally occurring duodenal markers in gastric aspirates were sought. Bilirubin is a natural marker and has been used to quantitate reflux, but it is broken down by gastric acid and thus may give unreliable results [10]. Similarly, trypsin is inactivated by acid [11]. Sodium is unsuitable as well, since

Table 15. Methods of quantitating duodenogastric reflux

---

1) Radiology
   Disadvantage subjective

2) Endoscopy
   Disadvantage subjective

3) Gastric aspiration of markers infused into the duodenum
   Disadvantage requires tube

4) Aspiration of bromsulphthalein and indocyanine green
   Disadvantage inconstant biliary secretion and difficulties of measurement

5) Aspiration of bilirubin
   Disadvantage broken down by gastric acids

6) Aspiration of sodium
   Disadvantage present in stomach

7) Aspiration of labelled bile acids after intravenous injection

8) Aspiration of bile acids from fasting or postprandial samples

---

it occurs in both duodenal and gastric juice and also since it may diffuse across the gastric mucosal barrier [12].

Bile acids are not normally found in the stomach, but their concentration may be increased in patients with gastric ulcer [10]. Bile acids are not attacked by gastric acid, but conjugated bile acids may be deconjugated by bacteria in the stasis syndrome. Rhodes et al. [13] measured ^{14}C-labelled chenodeoxycholic acid in gastric aspirates, and Black et al. [10] measured bile acids enzymatically. Both authors found higher concentrations of bile acids in gastric aspirates from patients with gastric ulcer, compared to controls. The greatest difference of bile acid reflux between ulcer patients and controls was observed on examination of postprandial samples. Black [10], however, found a better discrimination in fasting samples. In a recent study, Hoare et al. [14] evaluated measurement of bile acids in gastric aspirates as a test for duodenogastric reflux after gastric surgery. They measured bile acid concentration and the amount of bile acids aspirated over 30 min. Reflux was noted radiologically and endoscopically in 18 of the 20 symptomatic patients. Better discrimination of symptomatic from asymptomatic patients was achieved by measuring fasting bile reflux than mean bile acid concentrations. Fasting bile reflux was below 120 μmol/h in all 20 asymptomatic patients, whereas reflux of more than 120 μmol/h was present in 17 of the 22 symptomatic patients and in all who had complained of bilious vomiting and regurgitation.

References

1. Kennedy, T., Connell, A.M., Love, A.H.G., et al.: Selective or truncal vagotomy? Five year results of a double-blind, randomized, controlled trial. Brit. J. Surg. *60*, 944–948 (1973)
2. Amdrup, E., Jensen, H.E, Johnston, D., et al.: Clinical results of parietal cell vagotomy (highly selective vagotomy) two to four years after operation. Ann. Surg. *180*, 279–284 (1974).
3. Capper, W.M., Welbourn, R B.: Early postcibal symptoms following gastrectomy. Aetiological factors, treatment and prevention. Brit. J Surg. *43*, 24–35 (1955)

4 Griffiths, J.M.T.. The features and course of bile vomiting following gastric surgery. Brit. J. Surg. *61*, 617–622 (1964)
5. Capper, W.M., Airth, G.R., Kilby, J.O.: A test for pyloric regurgitation. Lancet *II*, 621–623 (1966)
6. Eckstam, E.E., Scudamore, H.H., Fencil, W.J., et al.: Bile reflux gastritis. Results of surgical therapy with Roux-en-Y gastrojejunostomy. Wisc. Med. J. *73*, 75–78 (1974)
7. Wormsley, K.G.: Aspects of duodeno-gastric reflux in man. Gut *13*, 243–250 (1972)
8 Faber, R.G., Russell, R.C.G., Royston, C.M.S., et al.: Duodenal reflux during insulin-stimulated secretion. Gut *15*, 880–884 (1974)
9. Wirts, C.W., Cantarow, A.. A study of the excretion of bromsulphthalein in the bile Am. J. Dig. Dis. *9*, 101–106 (1942)
10. Black, R.B., Roberts, G., Rhodes, J.: The effect of healing on bile reflux in gastric ulcer. Gut *12*, 552–558 (1971)
11. Khayat, M.H., Christophe, J.: In vitro inactivation of pancreatic enzymes in washings of the rat small intestine. Am. J. Physiol. *217*, 923–929 (1969)
12. Ivey, K.J., DenBesten, L., Clifton, J.A.: Effect of bile salts on ionic movement across the human gastric mucosa. Gastroenterology *59*, 683–690 (1970)
13 Rhodes, J., Barnardo, D.E., Philips, S.F., et al.: Increased reflux of bile into the stomach in patients with gastric ulcer. Gastroenterology *57*, 241–252 (1969)
14 Hoare, A.M., McLeish, A., Thompson, H., et al.: Selection of patients for bile division surgery: use of bile acid measurements in fasting gastric aspirates. Gut *19*, 163–165 (1978)

9 Laboratory Tests for Malabsorption

Laboratory tests commonly used to evaluate malabsorption are given in Table 16. Long-standing malabsorption, with loss of weight and chronic diarrhoea, is usually combined with several pathological routine laboratory parameters which result from decreased absorption of several important nutrients. These pathological parameters (i.e. decreased cholesterol, decreased serum iron, decreased serum folate, anaemia, hypoproteinaemia) may give information about the consequences of long-standing postoperative malabsorption, but do not give any information on the dynamics of absorption, i.e. they cannot be considered as functional tests.

9.1 Absorptive Function Tests

Dynamic tests available to evaluate the capacity of absorptive function are either direct or indirect (Fig. 11). Direct tests measure intake and output of substances administered orally (e.g. faecal fat excretion compared to fat intake). The direct method is of actual importance only for the measurement of faecal fat balance by the method of van de Kamer [1]. All other useful functional absorptive tests are indirect: after oral administration of an absorbable substance, its appearance in blood, breath or urine is measured. To obtain proper information on the absorption step, it is important to use a substrate which is not metabolised to any great extent during its passage, after absorption up to its appearance in blood, urine or breath. Functional tests measuring the appearance of substances in urine are dependent to a great extent on optimal co-operation from the patient.

Table 16. Laboratory tests to evaluate malabsorption

	Normal values	Changes in malabsorption
Blood		
Hemoglobin	14–17 g/100 ml	Diminished, esp. in iron deficiency
Erythrocytes	4.2–5.6 millions	Diminished, esp. in folic acid and vitamin B_{12} deficiency
HB_E	28–32 pg/red cell	Decreased in iron deficiency, elevated in folic acid and/or vitamin B_{12} deficiency
Serum		
Albumin	4.0–5.0 g/100 ml	Diminished
Carotin	0.06–0.4 mg/100 ml	Diminished
Calcium	9.0–10.5 mg/100 ml	Diminished
Cholesterol	150–250 mg/100 ml	Diminished
Potassium	3.5–4.7 mEq/litre	Diminished
Magnesium	1.7–2.0 mEq/litre	Diminished
Vitamin B_{12}	100–700 pg/ml	Diminished in bacterial overgrowth and tropical sprue
Folic acid	5–21 ng/ml	Diminished, particularly in small-bowel disease
Iron	65–175 µg/100 ml	Diminished
Plasma		
Prothrombin time	Control value	Prolonged
Tolerance tests		
D-Xylose test (25 g)	Urinary excretion 4.5 g/5 h Serum: >25–30 mg/100 ml after 1 h	Diminished, particularly in small-bowel disease such as coeliac disease or bacterial overgrowth, normal in pancreatic insufficiency
D-Glucose (100 g)	35 mg over fasting level	"Flat curve" in sprue, small-bowel diseases and monosaccharide malabsorption
Lactose (50 g in adults or 2 g/kg in children)	Rise in blood glucose of >20 mg/100 ml over fasting level	Low or flat curve in lactase deficiency
Sucrose (100 g)	Rise in blood glucose of >20 mg/100 ml over fasting level	Flat curve in small-bowel disease such as coeliac disease or primary sucrase-isomaltase deficiency
Faecal fat		
Chemical determination on a 80–100 g fat intake daily	<7 g/24 h	Increased
Miscellaneous		
5-hydroxyindolacetic acid (urinary excretion)	1.7–8.0 mg/24 h	Increased (9–20 mg) in spruce, 30–600 mg in metastatic carcinoid syndrome
Bile acid breath test (^{14}C-glycocholate breath test)	Minimal exhalation of $^{14}CO_2$/4–8 h	Increased exhalation of $^{14}CO_2$ in bacterial overgrowth or in ileal dysfunction

After Beeson, P.B. and McDermott, W. (eds) Textbook of Medicine, 14th edition, Philadelphia: W.B. Saunders 1975

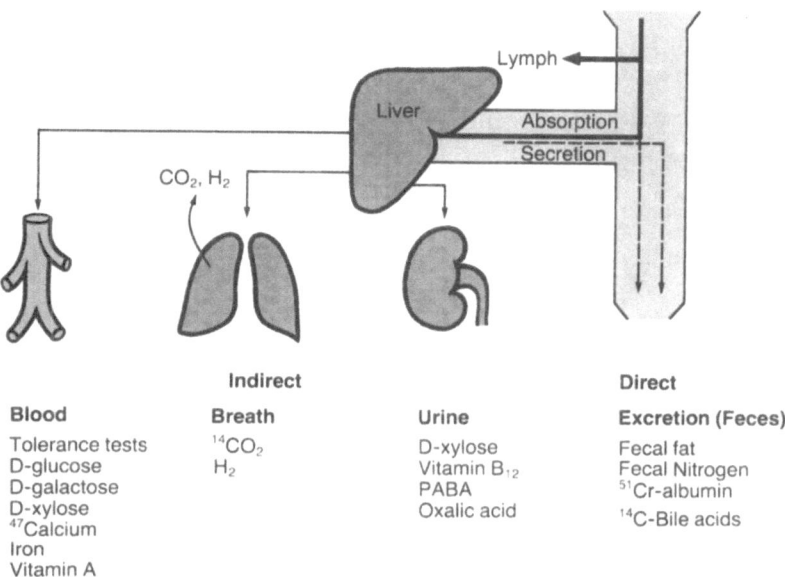

<table>
<tr><td></td><td colspan="2">Indirect</td><td>Direct</td></tr>
</table>

Blood	Breath	Urine	Excretion (Feces)
Tolerance tests	$^{14}CO_2$	D-xylose	Fecal fat
D-glucose	H_2	Vitamin B_{12}	Fecal Nitrogen
D-galactose		PABA	^{51}Cr-albumin
D-xylose		Oxalic acid	^{14}C-Bile acids
$^{47}Calcium$			
Iron			
Vitamin A			

Fig. 11. Tests for evaluation of intestinal absorptive capacity

9.1.1 Upper Small Intestine

Carbohydrates, proteins and fats, as well as minerals and vitamins (with the exception of vitamin B_{12}), are absorbed in the upper small intestine (Fig. 12). The most important test for measuring absorptive function of the upper small intestine is the D-xylose test, which is superior to the oral glucose tolerance test. D-Xylose is absorbed in the small intestine by the same transport system as D-glucose. However, in contrast to D-glucose, absorption of D-xylose is comparatively sluggish. This fact makes D-xylose particularly suitable for an absorption test, since a dose of D-xylose must be exposed to a larger part of the gut, in order to be absorbed, than the same dose of D-glucose. It can therefore give better information on the absorptive capacity of a greater part of the intestine than could be the case when D-glucose was administered. In addition, D-xylose has the advantage that it can hardly be metabolised. Therefore measurements of D-xylose in blood and urine can give proper information on the absorptive capacity of the upper small intestine for carbohydrates.

Faecal fat excretion can be considered an important parameter, too, for measuring the function of the upper small intestine. The vitamin A tolerance test is less helpful for establishing a diagnosis of fat malabsorption than measurement of faecal fat excretion. A static parameter (β-carotin) can be used as a screening test for the existence of fat malabsorption. A decrease of β-carotin ($< 50 \mu g/100$ ml) signifies a deficiency of this fat-soluble vitamin due to long-standing malabsorption.

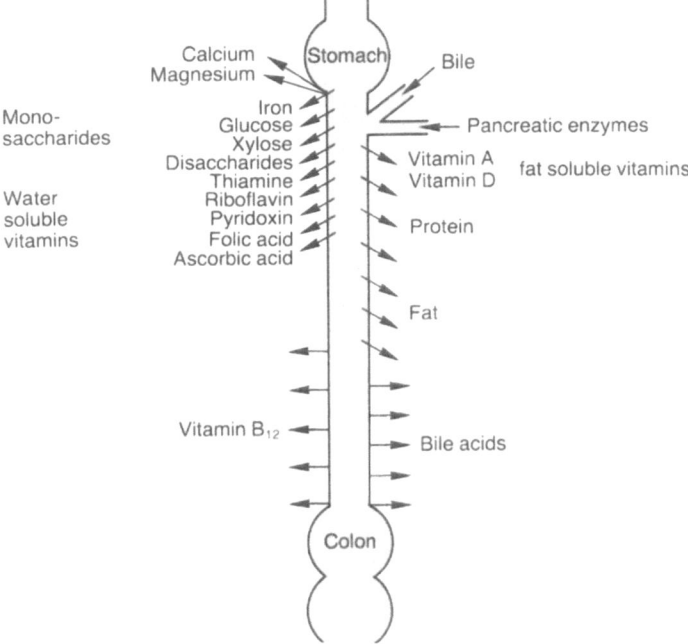

Fig. 12. Nutrient absorption and its location along the small intestine

9.1.1.1 Oral Glucose Tolerance Test

The oral glucose tolerance test is usually not very helpful for measuring absorptive capacity for carbohydrates, since postprandial increases of blood glucose are not only dependent on the absorptive capacity, but are also considerably influenced by endogenous insulin secretion. Oral glucose tolerance tests, with determination of blood glucose over 3–4 h at 30-min intervals, are helpful for establishing a diagnosis of late postprandial hypoglycaemia (late dumping syndrome), especially when insulin is determined simultaneously.

9.1.1.2 D-Xylose Test

The D-xylose test, performed with oral administration of 25 g D-xylose and measurement of D-xylose concentration in blood after 1 and 2 h and urine D-xylose excretion over 5 h, is the most useful test for measuring absorptive function of the upper small intestine. D-Xylose is the ideal substrate for measuring carbohydrate absorption because (1) it is water-soluble, (2) it can be absorbed without prior hydrolysis, (3) it is hardly metabolisable, and (4) it is not normally present in blood and urine. About 40% of the D-xylose absorbed can, however, be metabolised by an as yet unknown mechanism. The normal excretion value for the 25-g dose is 17%. Values between 12% and 17% are considered borderline. The absolute amount of D-xylose excreted in urine after administration of 25 g is 4.5–7.5 g. False positive and false negative results are possible, especially in the case of renal dysfunction or in the presence of ascites, which may lead to a false positive result when D-xylose is measured in the urine alone. An increase of blood D-xylose levels above 25–30 mg/100 ml after 1 or 2 h signifies a normal absorptive capacity for carbohydrates. If steatorrhoea exists, the D-xylose test may help to differentiate between maldigestion and malabsorption of the upper small intestine.

Bacteria are able to metabolise D-xylose [2]. A pathological D-xylose test may therefore be present in the bacterial overgrowth syndrome (i.e. afferent-loop syndrome). Normalisation of a pathological D-xylose test after a 1 week's course of treatment with antibiotics can be considered indirect proof of bacterial overgrowth of the small intestine. In patients with gastrectomy or truncal vagotomy, D-xylose absorption may be impaired owing to reduced intestinal transit time, bacterial overgrowth or a decreased absorptive capacity.

9.1.1.3 Lactose Tolerance Test

A deficiency of disaccharidases (e.g. lactase) can be the cause of osmotic diarrhoea. The most common deficiency of disaccharidases is inborn or acquired lactase deficiency, which leads to intolerance after oral ingestion of milk. Lactase deficiency as the cause of diarrhoea can well be observed in patients after gastric resections. Lactose intolerance can easily be detected by an oral lactose tolerance test [3, 4] (Table 17). In the oral lactose tolerance test, 50 g lactose is administered in 400 ml water. Blood glucose measurements are performed every 30 min for 2 h. An increase of blood glucose of less than 20 mg/100 ml above the blood glucose value before administration of lactose can be considered proof of the existence of lactose intolerance, especially when the patient in addition complains of flatulence and diarrhoea. More accurate is the direct determination of the disaccharidases (lactase) in a fresh small-bowel biopsy specimen [5] or the hydrogen (H_2) exhalation test, which can be combined with the oral lactose tolerance test [4, 6]. In the hydrogen breath test, hydrogen (H_2) is measured every 30 min after administration of lactose (50 g in adults, 1–2 g/kg in children). An increased breath excretion of hydrogen after oral ingestion of lactose signifies the consequence of lactose malabsorption due to lactose intolerance: when lactose not absorbed in the small intestine reaches the colon it is metabolised by colonic bacteria to hydrogen, which can immediately be detected in the breath.

Table 17. Diagnostic tests for detection of lactase deficiency

---

Lactose tolerance test (see below)
Direct measurement of lactase in fresh small-bowel biopsy specimen
Hydrogen breath test after oral administration of 50 g lactose
^{14}C-lactose breath test

Lactose tolerance test
50 g lactose is given orally
Blood glucose (or galactose) is measured before administration and after 30, 60, 90 and 120 min:
Rise in blood glucose < 20 mg/100 ml – lactose intolerance
Rise in blood glucose > 20 mg/100 ml – lactose intolerance excluded

---

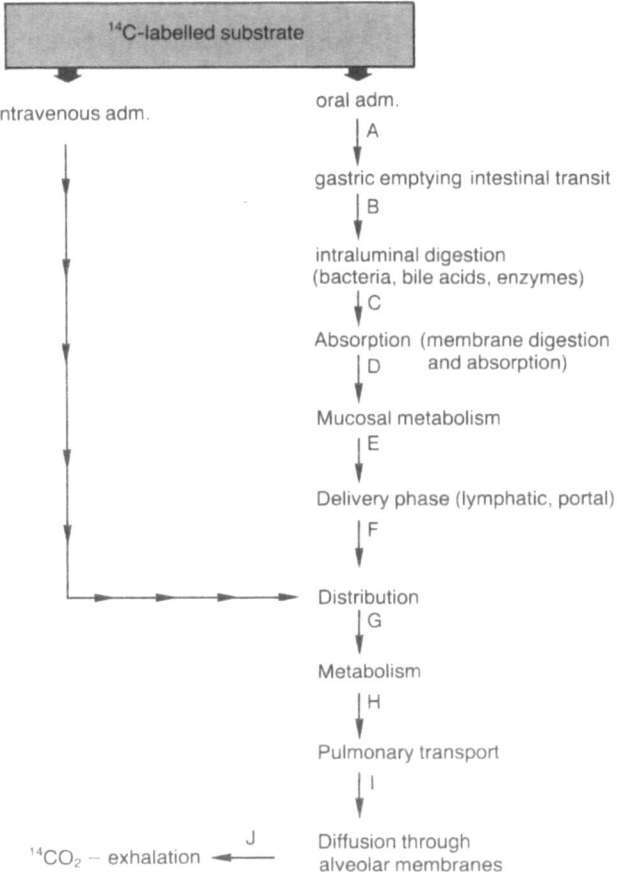

Fig. 13. Metabolic steps of labelled substrates between oral administration and appearance in breath If one step is rate-limiting the breath test with measurement of $^{14}CO_2$ in breath can be used as a quantitative test for this parcicular step (e.g. bile acid deconjugation, absorption)

9.1.1.4 Faecal Fat Excretion

Evaluation of faecal fat excretion by Sudan III staining of a faecal specimen cannot be considered a quantitative test of fat malabsorption. Since faecal fat excretion from the intake of 100 g fat normally amounts to 7 g, microscopic staining of the stool gives a high number of false positive as well as false negative results for the diagnosis of steatorrhoea. Faecal fat excretion can be used as a valuable parameter only when fat intake is sufficient (usually at least 70–100 g). The method of van de Kamer [1] can still be considered the standard one for measurement of faecal fat excretion. It has to be borne in mind, however, that this method will miss fatty acids of a chain-length of less than ten carbon atoms. This is important if faecal fat excretion is measured in patients whose normal dietary fat is replaced by medium-chain triglycerides. Several other tests have been tried for the replacement of the faecal fat analysis: e.g. the ^{131}I-triolein test and the ^{14}C-tripalmitate breath test [6]. The results are not, however, very promising.

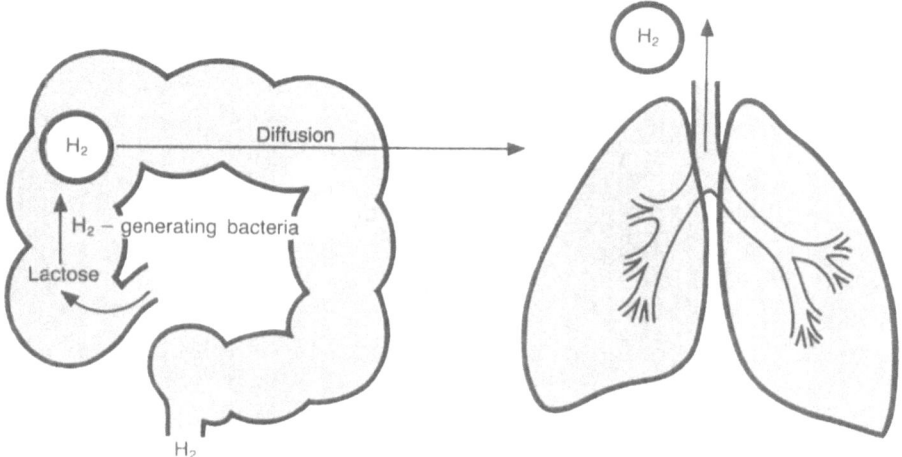

Fig. 14. Principle of H_2 breath test as a test for carbohydrate malabsorption. Unabsorbed carbohydrates arriving in the colon will be metabolised by bacteria to hydrogen, which will diffuse through the wall and can be readily detected in breath

9.1.1.5 Breath Tests

Breath tests have been used with increasing frequency in recent years for the measurement of intestinal absorptive function. The advantage of breath tests is their simplicity and non-invasive character. Of importance are two different types of test. In the first type, ^{14}C-labelled substrates are orally administered and their appearance in blood or breath ($^{14}CO_2$) is measured. The absorption step has to be the rate-limiting step between oral application and appearance in blood or breath for a labelled substrate to be used for an absorptive function test (Fig. 13) [6]. The second diagnostically useful breath test measures the appearance of hydrogen in the breath. Since animal cells are not able to metabolise substrates to hydrogen, appearance of hydrogen in the breath in humans has to be caused by bacteria (Fig. 14). An increased exhalation of hydrogen in the breath signifies therefore that bacteria have been offered substrate for generation of hydrogen. An increase of hydrogen concentration in breath after oral administration of lactose can thus be considered a safe diagnostic parameter for the existence of lactose intolerance [4, 6]. Increased hydrogen values after oral administration of glucose indicate either that the passage of glucose into the colon was increased (glucose malabsorption) or that bacterial overgrowth existed in the upper small intestine, leading to early metabolism of glucose to hydrogen in the upper small intestine. The hydrogen breath test after oral administration of carbohydrates can therefore be used as a simple, non-invasive diagnostic test to detect carbohydrate malabsorption.

Measurements of hydrogen exhalation can also be used to measure intestinal transit time (passage from mouth to caecum), if 10 or 15 g lactulose are administered as a non-absorbable substrate [7] (Fig. 15). The time elapsing after oral administration of lactulose up to the earliest rise in hydrogen concentration

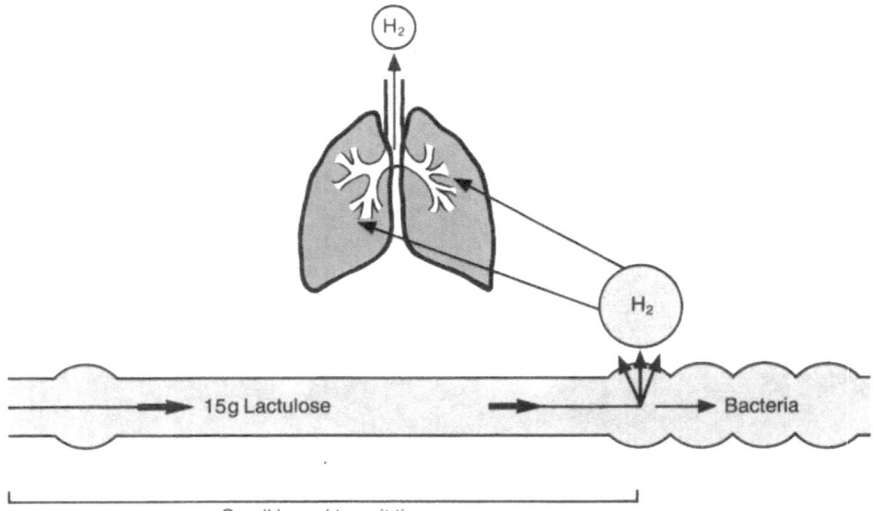

Fig. 15. H_2 breath test for measurement of small-intestinal transit time. Orally administered non-digestible lactulose will be metabolised by bacteria in the colon to H_2, which can be readily detected in breath. The time elapsing until the first H_2 peak can be detected is the small-bowel transit time

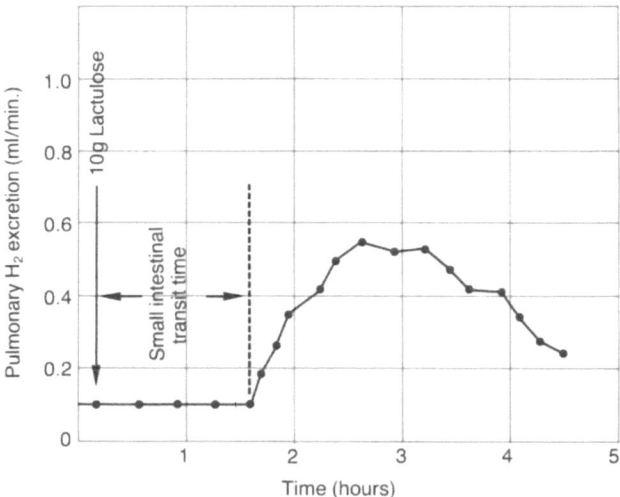

Fig. 16. Pulmonary hydrogen (H_2) excretion by a healthy subject after ingestion of 10 g of lactulose. The time interval between lactulose ingestion and the earliest detectable rise in pulmonary H_2 excretion is considered to represent the small-intestinal transit time for the test meal

signifies the time of passage of the substrate from mouth to caecum, where fermentation to hydrogen by bacteria takes place (Fig. 16).

The diagnostically most helpful test is the ^{14}C-glycocholate breath test, for the detection of increased bacterial deconjugation of bile acids in the bacterial overgrowth syndrome [6, 8, 9]. This test will be described in Chapt. 2.7.3.2. Further breath tests used to quantitate absorption by measurement of $^{14}CO_2$

in breath have been described, but are less useful (the ^{14}C-tripalmitate breath test, the ^{14}C-triolein breath test, the ^{14}C-lactose test). The ^{14}C-lactose test is an accurate test for detecting lactase deficiency, but the hydrogen breath test seems more sensitive and in addition has no radiation hazard.

9.1.1.6 Small-Bowel Biopsy

As part of the diagnostic investigation of diarrhoea and malabsorption after gastric surgery, it will be necessary to perform a small-bowel biopsy. Hydraulic bowel biopsy devices allow one to obtain specimens from several locations in the small intestine [9, 11]. This may increase the diagnostic accuracy. It also makes it possible to carry out enzymatic measurement simultaneously with morphological examination of the mucosa. The biopsy specimen obtained from the jejunum by a small-bowel biopsy capsule is larger than specimens obtained with forceps during gastroscopy of a patient with gastric resection (i.e. Billroth II resection).

Flattening of the villi may indicate a sprue-like syndrome, which could exist or appear even after gastric surgery. Decrease of enzymes, whether isolated (lactase deficiency) or generalised (sprue), can be detected by measuring the activity of small-bowel biopsy enzymes.

9.1.2 Ileum

Two specific transport systems exist in the lower part of the small intestine: absorption of the intrinsic factor – vitamin B_{12} complex and of bile acids. The function of the ileum cannot be acquired by the jejunum in cases of resection. Ileal resection or dysfunction therefore leads to vitamin B_{12} malabsorption and to malabsorption of bile acids, with consequent cholereic enteropathy. After gastric resection a decreased production of gastric intrinsic factor may lead to vitamin B_{12} malabsorption, since ileal receptors will not accept free vitamin B_{12}. In truncal vagotomy, dilatation of the gall bladder and decreased intestinal transit time will diminish ileal contact of bile acids and therefore result in bile acid malabsorption, with consequent watery, explosive diarrhoea.

The function of the lower part of the small intestine may be assessed by
(1) the Schilling test [11, 12],
(2) the ^{14}C-glycocholate breath test [6, 8, 9],
(3) determination of ^{14}C in faeces after oral administration of ^{14}C-labelled bile acids [8, 9], and
(4) enzymatic determination of bile acids in faeces [13].

Since the Schilling test can be abnormal either owing to a lack of intrinsic factor or owing to a decrease in absorptive sites in the ileum, differentiation between these two conditions can be achieved by performing the Schilling test both with and without intrinsic factor. The ^{14}C-glycocholate breath test can be positive in ileal dysfunction and in bacterial overgrowth of the upper small intestine.

9.1.2.1 Schilling Test

Serum vitamin B_{12} determination can be used as an indicator of the storage of vitamin B_{12}. Direct information on the intestine's absorptive capacity for vitamin B_{12} cannot, however, be obtained by determination of serum vitamin B_{12} levels. The standard method of evaluating vitamin B_{12} absorption is the Schilling test [11, 12]. In the standard procedure, 0.5–1 µCi radioactively labelled vitamin B_{12} is administered orally. Two hours later a flushing dose of 1,000 µg non-labelled vitamin B_{12} is administered intramuscularly. Urine is collected for 24 or 48 h and the amount of radioactivity excreted in urine is measured over that period of time. A pathological Schilling test (urinary excretion of less than 7% of the orally ingested labelled vitamin B_{12}) may be due to

(1) lack of intrinsic factor (i.e. total gastrectomy),
(2) metabolic alteration of the intrinsic factor-vitamin B_{12} complex by bacteria (i.e. afferent-loop syndrome),
(3) decreased absorption of the intrinsic factor-vitamin B_{12} complex,
(4) lack of absorptive capacity of the ileum (ileal dysfunction), or
(5) lack of receptors.

Normalisation of a pathological Schilling test after administration of hog intrinsic factor establishes the diagnosis of a lack of intrinsic factor, which may be the case in total gastrectomy or extensive gastric resection. Normalisation of a pathological Schilling test after treatment with antibiotics can be considered proof of the presence of bacterial overgrowth of the small intestine.

9.1.2.2 ^{14}C-Glycocholate Breath Test

The ^{14}C-glycocholate breath test has to be considered a very helpful new test for detecting bacterial overgrowth after gastric surgery. Direct determination of the amount of bacteria present in the upper small intestine after intubation of the duodenum or jejunum is an invasive method which sometimes even does not give reliable results owing to contamination of the tube by bacteria from the pharynx. The ^{14}C-glycocholate breath test is a quantitative test for the detection of bacterial deconjugation of bile acids. Since bile acids can be deconjugated by bacteria only and deconjugation is the limiting factor for the appearance of ^{14}CO$_2$ from ^{14}C-glycocholate, an increased deconjugation of bile acids signifies an increased bacterial enzymatic activity. In the glycocholate breath test, 5 µCi ^{14}C-glycocholate [6, 8, 9] is orally administered (Fig. 17). Normally the tracer amount of ^{14}C-glycocholate mixes with the endogenously secreted bile acids and remains within the enterohepatic circulation, less than 10% reaching the colon through circulation. In bacterial overgrowth of the upper small intestine, bile acids are deconjugated by bacteria, the ^{14}C-glycine moiety is liberated from the conjugated bile acid, and the glycine may also be decarboxylated by bacterial enzymes, yielding ^{14}CO$_2$ in the lumen of the gut. ^{14}C-glycine or ^{14}CO$_2$ liberated from ^{14}C-glycocholate leaves the lumen of the gut and can appear after metabolism (^{14}C-glycine → ^{14}CO$_2$) or by direct exhalation (^{14}CO$_2$) in breath. The exhaled specific activity of ^{14}CO$_2$ can be measured simply by direct exhalation of expired air into a liquid scintillation vial containing a trapping solution of 1 ml 1 M hyamine hydroxide, 2 ml methanol, and 2 drops phenolphthalein in alcohol. Change from violet to colourless indicates that 1 mmol CO_2 has been neutralised by 1 mmol hyamine hydroxide. Discontinuous measurements of ^{14}CO$_2$ exhalation are performed up to 6 h. An increased exhalation of ^{14}CO$_2$ indicates an increased deconjugation of bile acids. Since an increased decon-

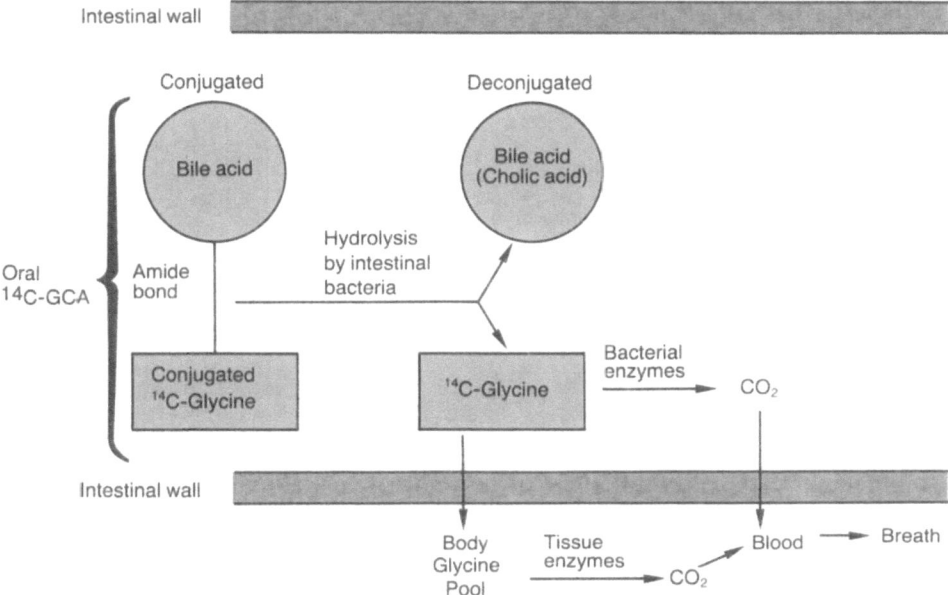

Fig. 17. Principle of the ¹⁴C-glycocholic acid breath test. Orally ingested ¹⁴C-glycocholic acid (¹⁴C-GCA) mixes with bile acids from bile, passes to the upper small intestine, is reabsorbed in the ileum and remains within the enterohepatic circulation. Only a minor percentage per passage will be deconjugated by bacteria in the colon. In the case of bacterial overgrowth of the upper small intestine, deconjugation to cholic acid and ¹⁴C-glycine will take place. Bacterial enzymes may even be able to produce decarboxylation of glycine, liberating ¹⁴CO₂. ¹⁴C-glycine and ¹⁴CO₂ can readily be absorbed from the gut. After final decarboxylation of glycine, an increased specific activity of ¹⁴CO₂ can be detected in breath. In ileal dysfunction, increased bacterial deconjugation takes place in the colon. An increased exhalation of ¹⁴CO₂ after administration of ¹⁴C-glycocholic acid demonstrates that an increased deconjugation of the conjugated bile acid has taken place. Since only bacteria are able to deconjugate bile acids, an increased specific activity of ¹⁴CO₂ in breath signifies increased bacterial deconjugation

jugation of bile acids may be due either to bacterial overgrowth of the small intestine or to bacteria in the colon in cases of bile acid malabsorption (i.e. ileal resection), a positive breath test signifies only an increased deconjugation of bile acids. The test is not able to give exact information on where the deconjugation occurs, i.e. whether in the small or the large intestine. Early maxima of exhalation (1–3 h) indicate increased deconjugation by bacteria in the upper small intestine, whereas exhalation maxima 3–5 h after oral ingestion are found more frequently in bile acid malabsorption. An exact differentiation is possible by simultaneous measurement of the appearance of ¹⁴C in faeces (Table 18). An increased faecal excretion of bile acids indicates bile acid malabsorption. The ¹⁴C-glycocholate breath test was originally designed to measure deconjugation of bile acids due to bile acid malabsorption, its main diagnostic value nowadays, however, is in the detection of bacterial overgrowth of the upper small intestine [6, 8, 9].

Table 18. Interpretation of the ^{14}C-glycocholate breath test

	^{14}C breath test	^{14}C in faeces
Normal absorption and normal intestinal flora	Low	Low
Normal absorption, no intestinal flora	Trace	Low
Bacterial overgrowth of the small intestine (e.g. afferent-loop syndrome)	High	Low
Malabsorption of bile acids (e.g. after ileal resection) with low bacterial activity in colon	Trace	High
Malabsorption of bile acids with normal bacterial activity	High	High

9.2 Measurement of Enteric Loss of Protein

Hypo-albuminaemia in the absence of liver disease or albuminuria and with sufficient protein intake may be induced by increased enteric loss of protein. An increased loss of protein can be detected most exactly by measurement of faecal excretion of ^{51}Cr (96-h stool collection) after intravenous administration of ^{51}Cr-albumin [13]. Normally between 5 and 25 ml of plasma or less than 1% of the plasma albumin pool is excreted via the gastrointestinal tract.

References

1 van de Kamer, J.H., Ten Bokkel Hiunnik, H., Weijers, H A.: Rapid method for the determination of fat in feces. J. Biol Chem. *177*, 347 (1949)
2 Donaldson, R.M Small bowel bacterial overgrowth Adv Intern Med. *67*, 1250 (1974)
3. Caspary, W F Kohlenhydratresorption und Malabsorption Leber Magen Darm 7, 150 (1977)
4 Newcomer, A.D., Thomas, P J., McGill, D.B. et al.: Prospective comparison of indirect methods for detecting lactase deficiency New Engl. J. Med *293*, 1232 (1975)
5. Dahlqvist, A.: Method for assay of intestinal disaccharidases Anal Biochem. 7, 18–25 (1964)
6 Caspary, W F Breath tests. In: Clinics in Gastroenterology. R I Russell, ed, London W.B. Saunders 1978
7. Bond, H., Levitt, M D. Investigation of small bowel transit time in man utilizing pulmonary hydrogen (H$_2$) measurement. J. Lab. Clin Med. *85*, 546 (1975)
8. Fromm, H, Hofmann, A F Breath test for altered bile acid metabolism Lancet *II*, 621 (1971)
9. Thaysen, E.H.. Diagnostic value of the ^{14}C-cholylglycine breath test. In Clinics in Gastroenterology Vol 6 No. 1, 227, London. W.B. Saunders 1977
10 Brandborg, L.L., Rubin, C.E., Quinton, W B.. A multipurpose instrument for suction biopsy at the esophagus, stomach, small bowel and colon. Gastroenterology 37, 1 (1959)
11 Sleisenger, M.H., Brandborg, L.L. Malabsorption. Philadelphia-London-Toronto: W.B. Saunders Comp. 1977
12 Schilling, R.F . Intrinsic factor studies. II The effect of gastric juice on the urinary excretion of radioactivity after the oral administration of radioactive vitamin B$_{12}$. J Lab. Clin. Med. *42*, 860 (1965)
13 Waldmann, T.A.: Gastrointestinal protein loss demonstrated by ^{51}Cr-labelled albumin. Lancet *II*, 121 (1961)

Part III
Postgastrectomy Syndromes

Symptoms may occur both after gastric resection and after vagal denervation. The symptoms may be attributed specifically to either resection or vagotomy, or they may occur after both types of operation. Syndromes occurring more frequently after gastric resection are described in this chapter, whereas typical postvagotomy symptoms are discussed in Chap. 3.2.

10 Dumping

10.1 History and Definition

Clinically it is difficult to define what is meant by dumping, but it is generally agreed that in its full form the dumping syndrome consists of both gastro-intestinal and cardiovascular or vasomotor symptoms.

The unpleasant postprandial symptoms called the dumping syndrome may in fact occur whenever a stoma is created between the stomach and the small intestine. In 1913 Hertz [1] called attention to the phenomenon of "too rapid emptying of the stomach after gastrectomy" associated with "excessive distension of the jejunum" and symptoms of fullness, nausea, diarrhoea and tachycardia. He observed rapid transit of a bismuth meal from the stomach and attributed the symptoms to exaggerated jejunal distension. He treated his patients by telling them to lie down for 30 min after meals and suggested to the surgeons that they make the stomas smaller. The term "dumping" of the stomach's contents into the jejunum was first used by Andrews [2] in 1920 ("dumping stomach") and by Mix [3] in 1922 ("dumping following gastrojejunostomy"). Thereafter the term dumping came into common use for the description of this constellation of symptoms.

The troublesome symptoms of the dumping syndrome usually occur 10–20 min after a meal. "Early dumping" and "late dumping" have to be differentiated. The two syndromes show somewhat similar symptoms, but in late dumping the symptoms occur 90–120 min after meals and are due to postprandial hypoglycaemia.

Table 19. Symptoms of the dumping syndrome in 87 cases.
[Fenger, H.J.: Clinical and experimental studies of dumping disposition. Acta Chirurg. Scand. (Suppl.) *371*, 1 (1967)]

	n	%
Nausea	49	56
Sensation of warmth	40	46
Changes in arterial blood pressure exceeding 300 mm Hg	30	34
Eructations	29	33
Pronounced perspiration	28	32
Epigastric fullness	20	23
Vomiting	14	16
Palpitations	12	14
Dyspnoea	7	8
Abdominal pulse	4	5

10.2 Early Dumping

10.2.1 Symptoms

The symptoms and their frequency are indicated in Table 19. The sequence of occurrence of the symptoms is important. Vasomotor and cardiovascular symptoms usually predominate, sometimes to the complete exclusion of gastro-intestinal symptoms. Within 5–10 min after eating, the patient experiences a feeling of fullness in the epigastrium. Then a characteristic flush occurs, followed by pallor, sweating and a feeling of weakness. Usually 20–30 min after eating, when vasomotor symptoms are already no longer present, gastro-intestinal symptoms with nausea, vomiting and diarrhoea may predominate.

Many patients will note that particular foods will precipitate an attack: liquid meals with a high carbohydrate content are usually responsible. Symptoms occur most seriously after breakfast, less seriously after lunch, and most patients will have least symptoms after an evening meal. There is a close parallel between the severity of the dumping syndrome and the degree of weight loss and malnutrition exhibited by the patient. Since the patient feels better when he does not eat, he avoids eating and thus may lose weight considerably.

10.2.2 Incidence

The early dumping syndrome occurs most frequently after gastric resections. Harvey et al. [4] found that dumping occurred in one-third of 666 patients who had had subtotal gastrectomy for duodenal ulcer. The dumping symptoms persisted in 13% of the patients. An even higher percentage was reported by Muir [5], who found that 75% of 124 patients with subtotal gastrectomy experienced dumping symptoms to some extent; 15 patients were unable to resume work for 5 months.

High incidences of dumping were observed, too, by Jordan et al. [6] (65 of 141 patients, i.e. 46%) and Hastings et al. [7] (two–thirds of 343 patients). The persistence of the disturbances for 2 years or more was reported to be 20% [7]. The incidence seems to depend on the amount of stomach resected; patients with total gastrectomy will have more frequent dumping symptoms than patients with less extensive amounts of stomach resected.

The dumping syndrome will occur less frequently in patients with a Billroth I gastrectomy than with a Billroth II resection [8, 9]. This difference seems to disappear if more extensive resection is performed in the Billroth I operation. Thus Fischer and Jordan [10] found dumping in 47 of 93 patients (51%) with 75% gastrectomy and Billroth I anastomosis. A direct comparison, however, between the kinds of operation with respect to incidence of dumping cannot be made on the basis of these studies, since there were no controlled trials comparing the two methods as performed at the same hospital by the same surgeons.

Early postprandial dumping seems to be less frequent after vagotomy and a drainage procedure. The incidence was reported to be 15% (of 443 cases) after truncal vagotomy and pyloroplasty [11]; the follow-up 7 years later showed a spontaneous tendency towards recovery, since only 4% (10 of 257 cases) where still experiencing dumping symptoms [12]. The Leeds/York trial reported early dumping in 21.5% of patients with subtotal gastrectomy, 17.9% in truncal vagotomy and gastro-enterostomy, but only 8.6% in truncal vagotomy and antrectomy. Truncal vagotomy and pyloroplasty was complicated in 11.9% with early dumping; the least incidence (0.9%) was found in proximal gastric vagotomy [13].

10.2.3 Natural Course

Although dumping syndrome occurs frequently, with sometimes intense suffering, in most cases appropriate dieting will result in partial or complete relief of symptoms. A careful follow-up examination of 42 out of 58 patients known to

Table 20. Change in degree of suffering among patients initially presenting severe suffering during the years. (After Chaimoff, Ch., and Dintsman, M., 1972)

Years	Complaint-free	Slight suffering
Up to 3 years	2	—
From 5 years on	3	1
From 7 to 12 years	9	6
No. of patients	14	7
(% of total)	(50%)	(25%)

Follow-up was performed on 42 patients of 58 known to have dumping syndrome after partial gastrectomy, at least 10 years earlier. 28 of the 42 patients had severe suffering, 14 had slight dumping symptoms.

have had dumping syndrome after partial gastrectomy 10 years earlier revealed that two–thirds of the sufferers had become symptom-free, half of them in about 5 years, the other half needing 7–12 years. One–sixth had slight symptoms of dumping, and in another one–sixth the symptoms continued unchanged [40] (Table 20).

10.2.4 Aetiology

Hypertonic Solutions and Distension. Symptoms of the dumping syndrome were originally attributed to jejunal distension [1]. Indeed, part of the symptoms can be reproduced by jejunal distension of the gastric remnant or by distension of the jejunum with a balloon [5, 14]. Vasomotor symptoms, however, usually preceding gastro-intestinal symptoms, are not sufficiently explained by distension alone.

Machella [15, 16] postulated that in order to induce dumping a meal should have the following two characteristics: (1) osmolality > 3,000 mosmol, (2) adequate amount of fluid accompanying ingested food. He was able to reproduce some of the dumping symptoms by distending the proximal jejunum with a bollon. But not everybody agrees that distension of the efferent jejunum is necessary for induction of dumping [17].

Plasma Volume. A number of investigators regarded the hypovolaemic phase during dumping as responsible for the vasomotor symptoms. Roberts et al. [18] detected a decrease in plasma volume as early as 10 min after feeding (maximal decrease at 30–40 min), with an associated rise in haematocrit. The massive reduction in plasma volume varied between 400 and 800 ml. The observation that there is a sharp fall in blood volume in the early postprandial dumping syndrome has been confirmed by Hinshaw et al. [19] and Peddie et al. [20].

Hypertonic solutions induced a fall in plasma volume not only in subtotal gastrectomy, but also in patients who had vagotomy with a drainage procedure. Thomson et al. [21] found that patients with dumping symptoms had a greater rate of percentage fall of plasma volume (mean $\pm 0.46\%$ per min) than post-operative patients without such symptoms (0.15% per min) (Fig. 18). Since there was a significant inverse relationship between the hydrogen-ion concentrations of the gastric juice in the basal state and in the stimulated state, they concluded that the occurrence of the dumping syndrome after vagotomy with a drainage procedure is related to the hydrogen-ion concentration of the gastric juice.

Le Quesne et al. [22] postulated, too, that the symptoms are brought about by a decrease of plasma volume during the dumping syndrome and suggested that rapid infusion of a plasma expander should control postcibal symptoms. However, later work of Butz [23] showed that the dumping syndrome still occurred in susceptible patients even if the blood volume was maintained by infusion of a plasma expander.

Thus the early postprandial dumping syndrome is not merely another example of hypovolaemic shock, although the symptoms and signs are sometimes similar. Another difference between postprandial hypovolaemia and hypovolaemia induced by phlebotomy was in addition reported: whereas in nearly all hypo-

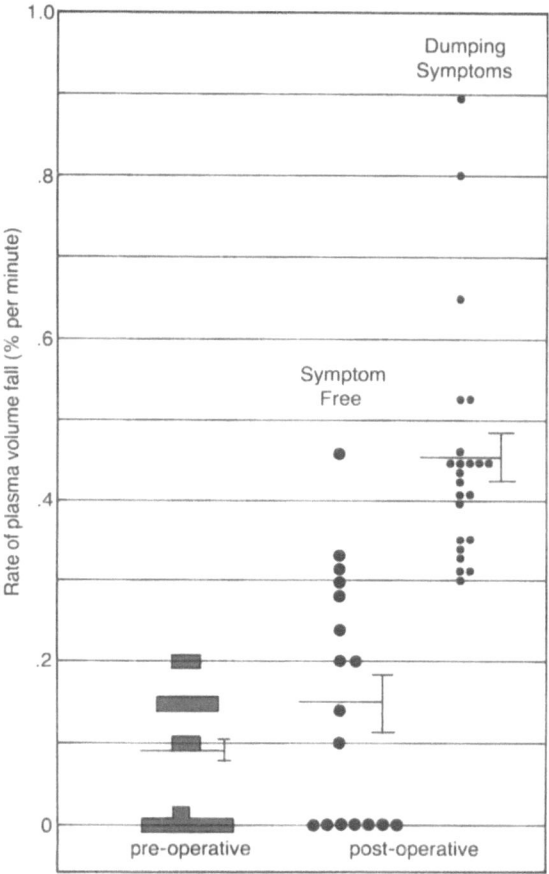

Fig. 18. Results of a dumping provocation test (ingestion of 200 ml of a 50% glucose solution) in 40 patients before and after vagotomy (truncal 18, selective 22) on the rate of percentage fall in plasma volume. Patients with dumping had a significantly greater rate of percentage fall in plasma volume (mean = 0 46% per minute) than those postoperative patients without dumping symptoms (mean = 0 15%). (After Thomson, J P.S., et al., 1974)

volaemic dumpers a rise in blood pressure – mostly systolic – was observed, leading to an increased amplitude of blood pressure, phlebotomy performed in non-dumpers did not result in changed blood pressure values [24].

Humoral Hypothesis. An alternative explanation of the vasomotor signs and symptoms was that hormones released from the distended gut wall were responsible for the peripheral effects.

The possible role of serotonin (5-hydroxytryptamine) was first suggested by Bulbring [25], and a humoral theory was later proposed by Johnson and Jesseph in 1961 [26] to explain the vasomotor symptoms in the postprandial dumping syndrome.

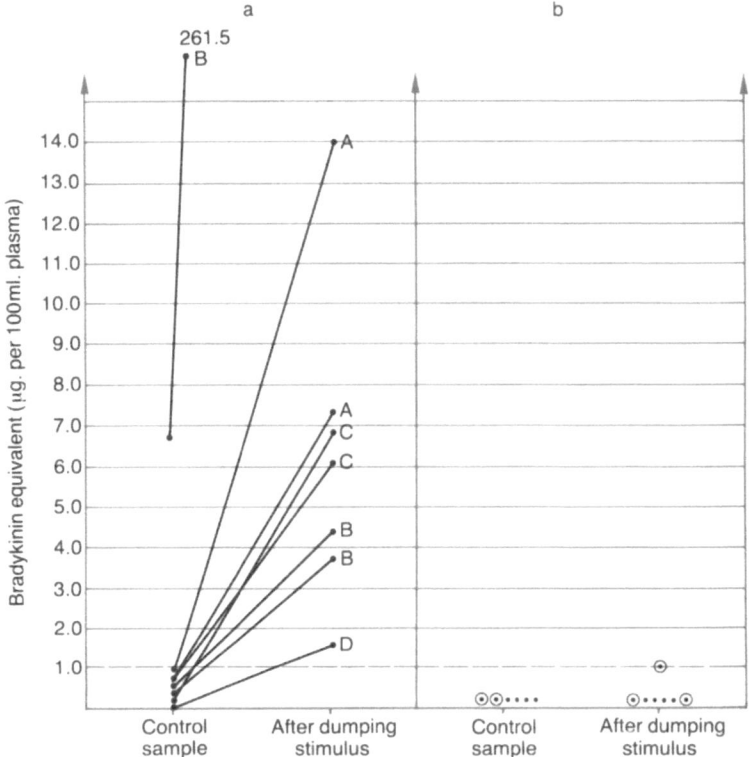

Fig. 19. Levels of venous free-plasma-kının measured before and at the height of vasomotor symptoms of the dumping syndrome. a) Levels in dumping patients A–D, dumping provoked by ingestion of 250 ml hypertonic glucose. b) Levels in dumping patients A–C (●) after ingesting 250 ml hypotonic saccharın placebo and in healthy controls E–H (○), after ingesting 250 ml of hypertonic glucose. (After Zeitlın, I.J., and Smıth, A.N., 1966)

The latter authors pointed out that the subjective symptoms actually begin before changes in the blood volume, haematocrit, electrolyte levels and electro-cardiogram can be measured. They were able to show in dogs [26] that instillation of hypertonic glucose into a mesenteric vein resulted in peripheral circulatory changes similar to those seen in human postgastrectomy dumpers. Peripheral circulatory changes were observed by digital plethysmography [27]. Evidence that serotonin might be responsible for the vasomotor changes observed in early dumping emerged from studies in which patients with early postprandial vasomotor and gastro-intestinal symptoms were challenged with hyperosmolar glucose solutions. The majority of patients responded with increases in digital pulse volume and amplitude. Administration of pharmacological agents known to inhibit some effects of serotonin [28] resulted in a reduction of the plethysmographic changes. It was also observed that there was marked overall improvement of symptoms [28, 29].

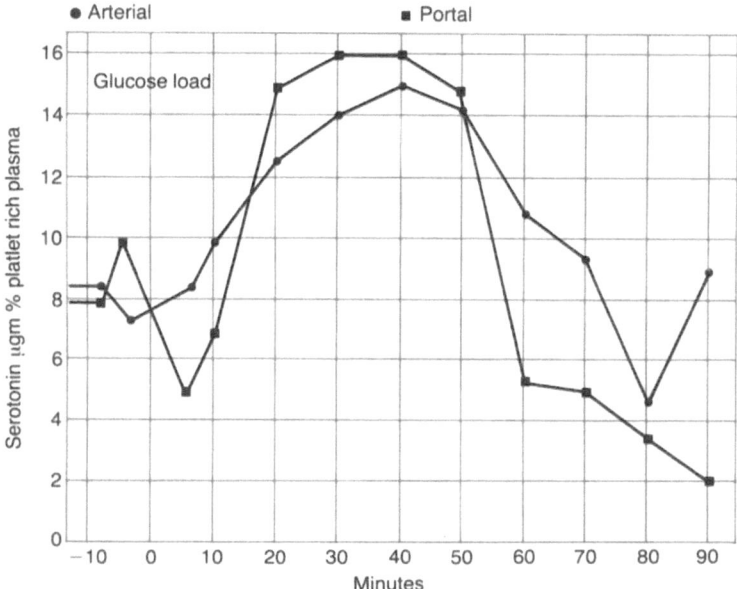

Fig. 20. Time course of portal and arterial serotonin levels in response to a dumping stimulus (150 ml of 50% glucose) in conscious dogs. After MacDonald et al., 1969

Drapanas et al. [30] were able to show increased levels of serotonin in circulating blood after hypertonic stimulation of the proximal intestine, and Peskin and Miller [31] produced the same kind of changes in animals and seemed convinced that serotonin plays a major role in initiating basal vascular changes in dumping. Further confirmation was supplied by Silver et al. [32], who compared blood levels of serotonin and urinary levels of hydroxyindolacetic acid at rest and after a 75-g glucose load, in normal patients and gastrectomized patients with and without dumping. They found that after glucose ingestion the serotonin levels increased significantly in patients with moderately severe dumping but remained the same in normal subjects and in gastrectomized patients without the dumping syndrome. Other workers, however, have failed to show a correlation between blood serotonin levels and occurrence of the dumping syndrome [33–35].

Serotonin, a strong constrictor of gastro-intestinal and bronchial smooth muscle, has been found to induce gastro-intestinal symptoms of nausea, cramps and diarrhoea, but it did not reproduce the characteristic initial flush which is also observed in the carcinoid syndrome. It is indeed difficult to attribute the gastro-intestinal symptoms to serotonin, which is so effectively cleared from the blood stream by the lungs.

Zeitlin and Smith [35] suggested that the humoral agent responsible for dumping is a plasma kinin. They observed in the human a release of a bradykinin-like polypeptide into the circulation (Fig. 19) and a concomitant fall in plasma levels of the corresponding kininogen. Increased kinin levels after gastric surgery have been observed by others, too [36].

In a later study Mac Donald et al. [37] studied simultaneously the release of serotonin and kinins following hypertonic dumping challenge in unanaesthetized dogs. Portal serotonin showed a mean peak increase of 101% over controls (Fig. 20). The increase in serotonin concentration began 15 min after the dumping stimulus. Arterial levels of TAME esterase (p-tosyl-l-arginine methyl ester) as an indicator of protease (kallikrein) activity showed a sustained rise. Portal brady-kinin increases and decreases of bradykininogen were observed immediately following the dumping stimulus. Thus it was concluded that bradykinin may be responsible for the early vasomotor symptoms, whereas serotonin could cause the more delayed gastro-intestinal responses.

High levels of glucagon-like immunoreactivity (GLI) after orally administered glucose have been reported in the dumping syndrome by Bloom et al. [38]. In order to decide whether the GLI responses were due to release of pancreatic glucagon or to the gut GLI, O'Connor et al. [39] studied GLI responses in 20 dumpers following 50 g glucose given orally using two antibodies in the glucagon RIA (radio-immunoassay) so as to allow them to discriminate between gut GLI and pancreatic glucagon. Gut GLI rose in dumpers no matter whether the meal was glucose, fat or protein and the rise exceeded that of control subjects. Abnormalities were observed for pancreatic glucagon, too: pancreatic glucagon paradoxically rose after glucose administration in 7 of 15 dumpers, while it was suppressed in controls. It remains undecided whether the abnormalities of pancreatic glucagon in gut GLI release in dumpers reflect a compensatory change or a causative influence of the various features of dumping, including gastric emptying, diarrhoea and hypoglycaemia. Since the gut harbours numerous endocrine cells releasing several hormones, both defined and not yet defined, it may well be that in the future we will find other hormones responsible for the changes occurring in the dumping syndrome.

10.2.5 Medical Treatment

One-half or more of patients recovering from gastric resection suffer in some measure from unpleasant symptoms of the early postprandial dumping syndrome. Symptoms do disappear within weeks or months in many patients, most likely owing to intestinal adaptive changes and the dietary regimen the patient may follow in order to prevent symptoms [40].

Diet. The treatment should be largely, in fact almost exclusively, dietary. Simple dietary rules to prevent early dumping are given in Table 21.

The empiric observation has been that free carbohydrates (disaccharides or free monosaccharides) in liquid form will precipitate symptoms. Since liquids empty faster even from a resected stomach than solids, one of the basic rules of an anti-dumping diet is to take meals without liquids. Patients have to take breakfast therefore without the often customary orange juice and coffee or tea with sugar. They may take liquids 1 h after breakfast or the other meals. They should have six to eight meals a day and should lie down if possible for 20–30 min after completion of each meal.

Table 21. Principles of an antidumping diet

1. No fluids of any kind during meals
2. Avoid concentrated sweets such as:
   sugar, jelly, cake, pie, pudding, candy
3. Meals should be eaten slowly
4. Plan six meals a day
5. Diet low in carbohydrates, high in protein
6. Starch and glycogen should replace disaccharides and free sugars

Drugs. Several drugs have been used in the management of the early dumping syndrome, but have not been very helpful in most cases. Serotonin antagonists such as cyproheptadine (Periactin) and methyl-*d*-lysergic acid (Sansert) have been effective in preventing vasomotor symptoms. On theoretical grounds anticholinergic drugs should be helpful in delaying gastric emptying. Banthine and Dactil have been reported to be the most effective anticholinergics in inhibiting hypermotility. Recently, addition of carbohydrate gelling agents (i.e. guar gum, pectin) has been suggested to be of benefit in postgastrectomy patients [41] (Fig. 21). Further clinical trials with this kind of treatment are to be expected. In particular, long-term studies will have to show whether patients will accept the palatability of carbohydrate gelling agents as food additives. First in vitro studies in rat intestine have shown that carbohydrate gelling agents such as guar will reduce carbohydrate and amino acid absorption and possibly also final oligosaccharide digestion at the level of the brush border membrane of mucosal epithelial cells (Table 22).

Other agents retarding gastric emptying and intestinal absorption have been reported to be beneficial in preventing symptoms of the dumping syndrome: biguanides [42–44] and prenylamine [45]. Both drugs directly interfere with active transport of sugars and amino acids and have been reported to be effective in preventing symptoms of the late as well as the early dumping syndrome. Since biguanides will completely disappear in the future, a trial with prenylamine seems justified, but consistent dietary treatment seems to be sufficient in most cases.

Table 22. Possible beneficial effects of carbohydrate gelling agents

Retarding gastric emptying
Retarding pancreatic digestion
Retarding terminal membrane digestion
Retarding absorption of final digestive products
Retarding release of gastro-intestinal hormones

10.2.6 Surgical Treatment

Although the majority of patients with dumping symptoms show an improvement by medical or dietary measures, 2%–5% of dumping patients do not respond to conservative treatment and have to undergo surgery. However, before a surgical

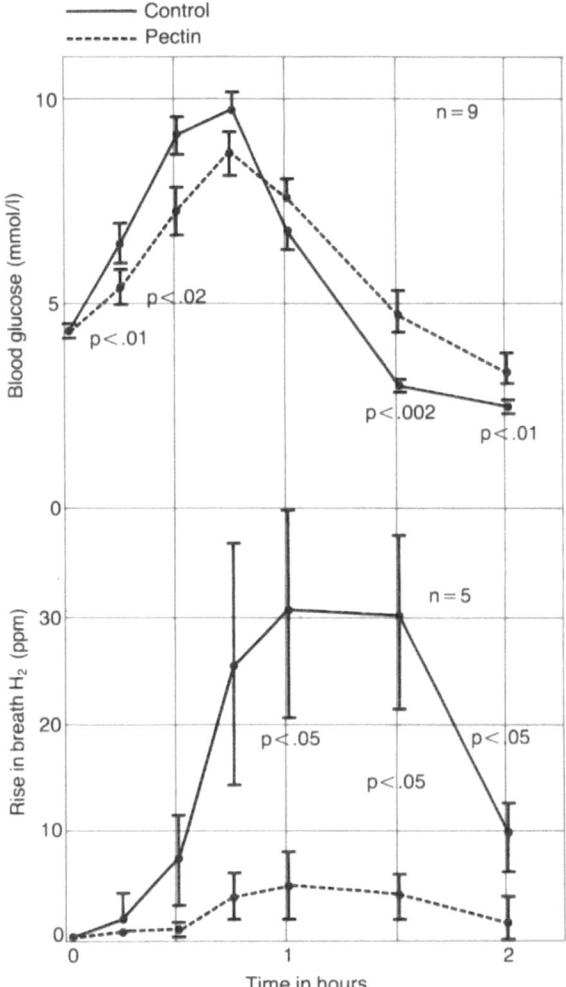

Fig. 21. Blood glucose concentration in nine patients *(upper graph)* and breath hydrogen concentration in five patients *(lower graph)* during 2-h period after a glucose drink alone (●——●) or a glucose drink with pectin (●----●). Pectin reduced postprandial glycaemia and prevented rise in breath hydrogen, an indicator of glucose appearance in the colon due to small-intestinal glucose malabsorption. (After Jenkins et al., 1977)

procedure is recommended, an exact diagnosis has to be made, which should include psychiatric examination. The different surgical procedures used can be summarised as follows:

a) Narrowing the gastrojejunal stoma
b) Reconstruction of the duodenal passage in Billroth II resection
c) Interposition of an intestinal segment between stomach and duodenum
d) Creation of a pouch as an additional reservoir.

Several operative procedures have been developed; however, an exact comparison of the different methods is not possible at the moment because of the lack of controlled studies [46].

a) Narrowing the Gastrojejunal Stoma. Narrowing of the gastrojejunal anastomosis has been proposed by several authors [47, 48]; there seems to exist a certain correlation between the diameter of the gastrojejunostomy and the incidence of dumping symptoms [48, 49]. On the other hand, Kennedy et al. [50] could not confirm the finding that the diameter of the stoma is of clinical importance, since it will enlarge during the postoperative period, so that the diameter of the jejunum represents the real diameter of the gastric outlet.

b) Reconstruction of the Duodenal Passage. The restoration of the duodenal passage by conversion of a Billroth II gastrojejunostomy to a Billroth I gastro-duodenostomy results in a significant improvement of dumping symptoms in a high percentage of patients [51–54]. Woodward and Bushkin [55] reported excellent or good results in eight of 11 patients, and only one patient showed unchanged symptoms. Furthermore, it has been known for some time that patients with a Billroth I anastomosis have a much lower frequency of dumping symptoms than patients with a Billroth II anastomosis [52]. Other authors, however, doubt the efficiency of reconstruction of the duodenal passage in treating early dumping symptoms [56]. The pathophysiological rationale of this type of operation is that osmoreceptors of the duodenum regulate gastric emptying, so that the duodenal passage is necessary for an osmotic equilibrium to be reached.

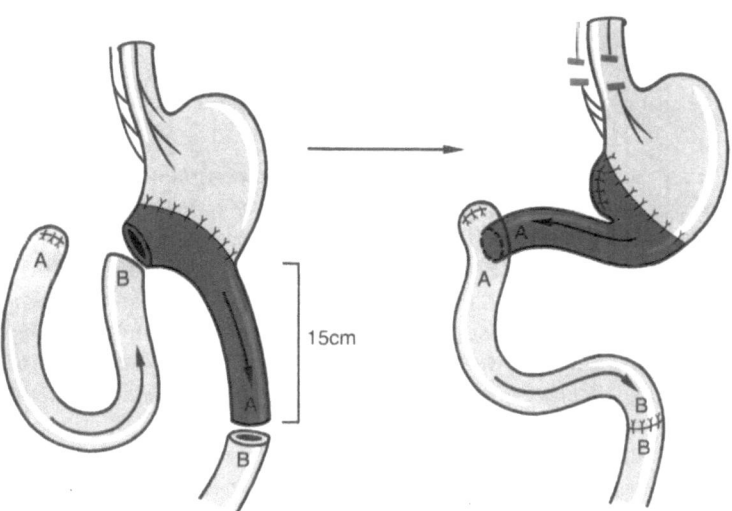

Fig. 22. Reconstruction of the duodenal passage after Billroth II resection (Henley-Soupault modification of Biebl procedure)

Table 23. Results of isoperistaltic jejunal interposition in severe dumping syndrome

Authors	Number of patients	Postoperative follow-up (years)	Results (%)		
			Excellent or good	Fair	Poor
Sawyers and Herrington [64]	10	2–9	20	30	50
Alexander-Williams [65]	10	2–3	60	20	20
Nygaard and Fretheim [66]	26	—	59	36	5
Fenger et al. [61]	30	—	20	—	—
Own results	18	2–3	50	33	17

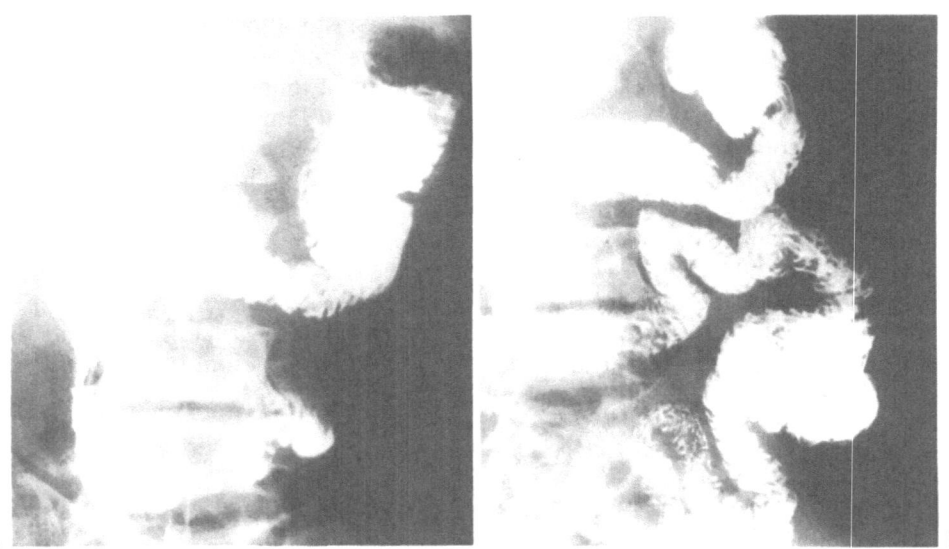

Fig. 23a, b. Isoperistaltic jejunal interposition in patient with dumping symptoms

c) Interposition of an Intestinal Segment. Most authors recommend the interposition of a small-bowel loop for restoration of the duodenal passage, according to the procedure of Biebl [57] (Fig. 22). The length of an isoperistaltic interposed loop is of great importance and should be between 15 and 20 cm. The anastomosis to the duodenum should be terminolateral, since the preparation of the duodenal stump a long time after primary surgery may cause severe technical problems. According to Hedenstedt [58] the operation has to be combined with a vagotomy, since otherwise ulcerations in the interposed small-bowel segment will occur.

The results of isoperistaltic jejunal interposition in the treatment of dumping syndrome vary widely, as is shown in Table 23. In half of our 18 patients we achieved excellent results, but 17% showed no change in symptoms. However, this procedure should always be used in patients with symptoms of more than one postgastrectomy syndrome, e.g. dumping syndrome plus afferent-loop syn-

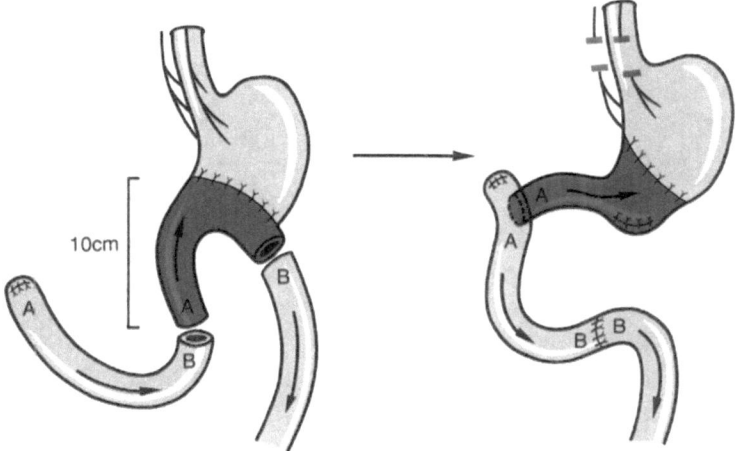

Fig. 24. Anisoperistaltic reconstruction of the duodenal passage after Billroth II resection (Poth procedure)

Table 24. Results of anisoperistaltic jejunal interposition in severe dumping syndrome

Authors	Number of patients	Postoperative follow-up (years)	Results (%)		
			Excellent or good	Fair	Poor
Sawyers and Herrington [64]	28	0.5–11	92	4	4
Alexander-Williams [65]	6	2–3	100	—	—
Fink et al. [67]	11	—	—	100	—

drome. This is very common in our patients (Fig. 23). Most patients on whom we operated had bile vomiting besides early dumping symptoms, so the use of an anisoperistaltic small-bowel loop would have caused increased reflux of bile into the stomach, and subsequent symptoms.

The interposition of an antiperistaltic jejunal segment (Fig. 24) between gastric stump and duodenum has been propagated by Poth [68, 69]. According to the studies of Hammer et al. [70] and Wilms et al. [71], the interposed segment should be 6–10 cm long, since longer segments cause a disturbance of gastric emptying, and shorter segments will not induce the wanted delay in gastric emptying.

The results which have been achieved by this procedure are shown in Table 24. In patients with pure dumping symptoms an anisoperistaltic interposition seems to give better results than the isoperistaltic modification. In our own patients, however, we were not able to use this procedure since nearly all had a combination of several postgastrectomy syndromes.

d) Creation of a Pouch. For patients with a very small gastric stump who have dumping symptoms, several authors have recommended the creation of an interposed pouch of jejunal loops (Fig. 25). Poth's method [68, 72, 73] and the method

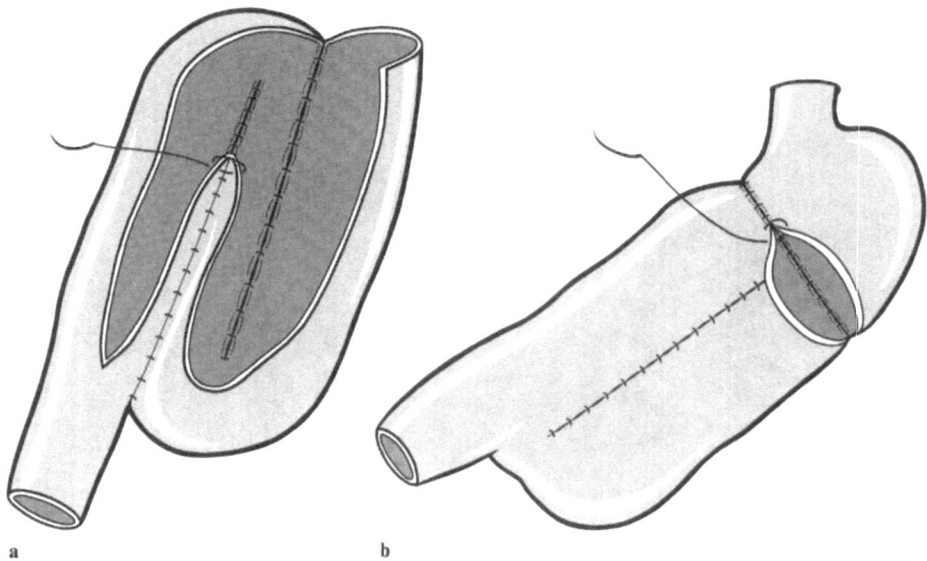

a   b

Fig. 25a, b. Creation of a gastric reservoir in the small-stomach syndrome and isoperistaltic reconstruction of the duodenal passage

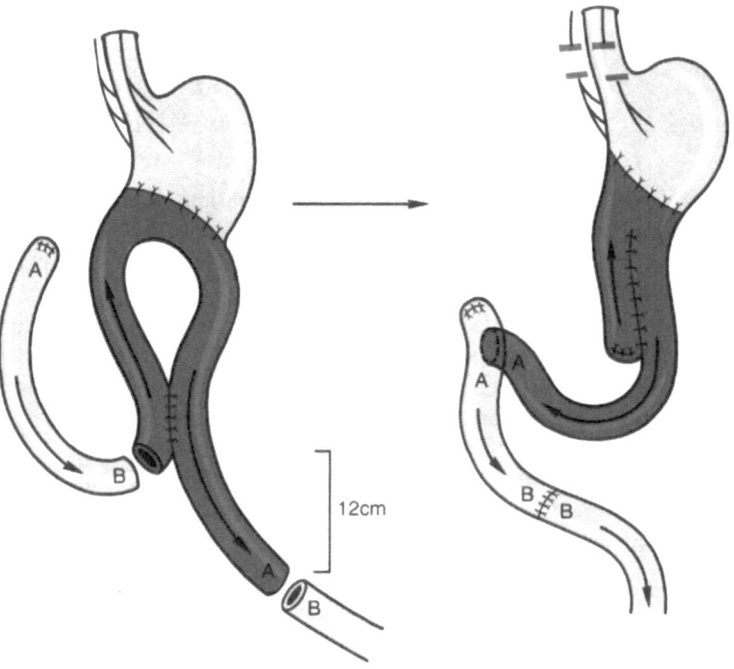

12cm

Fig. 26. Isoperistaltic reconstruction of the duodenal passage and creation of a pouch in patients with an entero-anastomosis

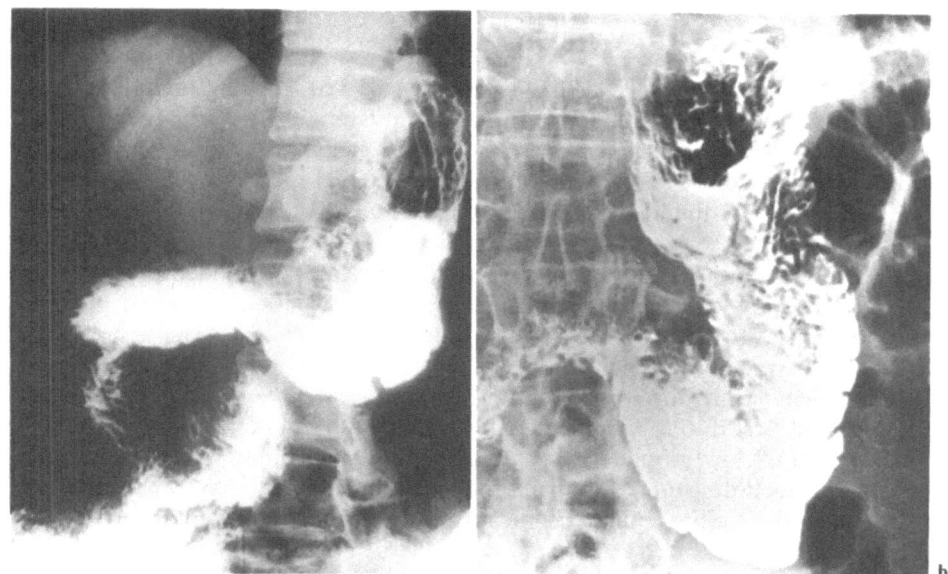

Fig. 27 a, b. Isoperistaltic jejunal interposition with creation of a gastric pouch

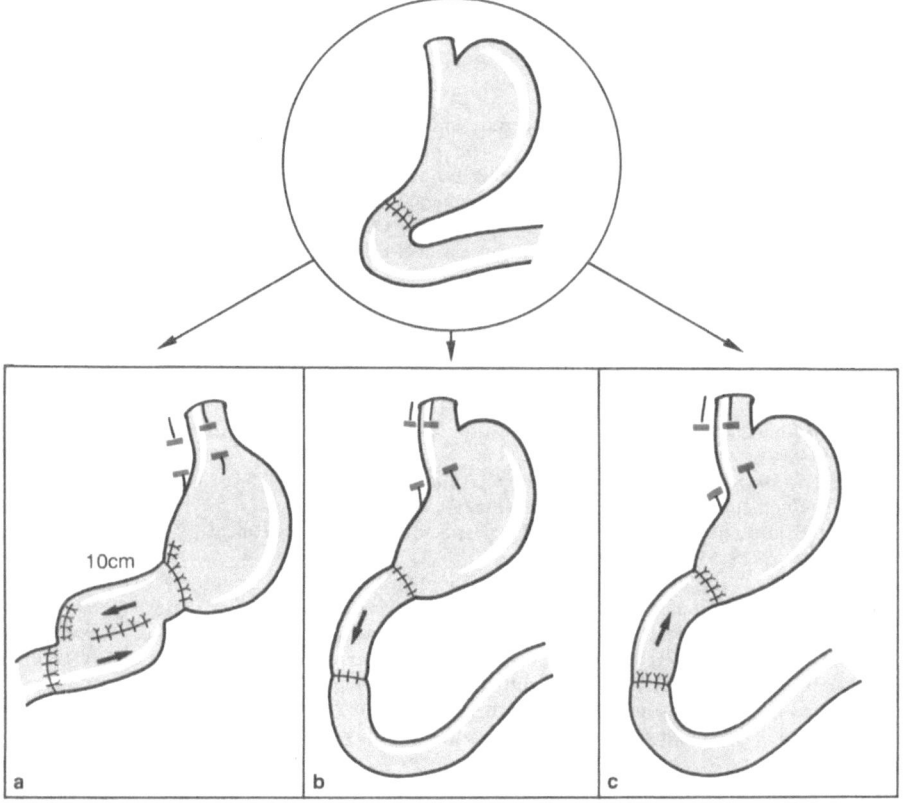

Fig. 28a–c. Surgical procedures in patients with dumping after Billroth I resection: **a** interposition of an anisoperistaltic pouch; **b** interposition of an isoperistaltic jejunal loop; **c** interposition of an anisoperistaltic loop

of Bushkin and Woodward [55] have mainly been used. Herrington and Sawyers [62] found satisfactory results in eight of 13 patients (60%). The pouch became dilated and hypertrophic after some time, which caused stasis and obstruction in some cases. In two of their 13 patients, ulcers occurred in the pouch. Woodward and Bushkin [55] found excellent or good results in three of nine patients, whereas six patients were unsatisfied.

The modification we are using is a Hunt-Lawrence-type pouch as used after total gastrectomy for reconstruction (Fig. 26). Of three patients in whom we used this procedure, two showed a good response, whereas one patient noted no change of his symptoms (Fig. 27a, b).

In patients who develop dumping symptoms after vagotomy and gastro-enterostomy, best results are achieved by removal of the gastro-enterostomy and construction of a pyloroplasty. In patients with severe dumping symptoms after Billroth I resection, either narrowing the anastomosis [55] or interposition of a 10 cm anisoperistaltic jejunal segment may be discussed [55, 62] (Fig. 28). Woodward [55] reported excellent results in six patients. Dumping syndrome after vagotomy plus pyloroplasty may be treated either by antrectomy and inter-position of an isoperistaltic segment or by reconstruction of the pylorus [74].

References

1. Hertz, A.F.: The cause and treatment of certain unfavourable after effects of gastroenterostomy. Ann. Surg. 58, 466 (1913)
2. Andrews, E.W.: "Dumping stomach" and other results of gastrojejunostomy: operative cure by disconnecting the old stoma. Surg. Clin North America 4, 883 (1920)
3. Mix, C.L.: Dumping following gastrojejunostomy Surg. Clin. N. America 2, 617 (1922)
4. Harvey, D.D., St. John, F.B., Volk, H.: Peptic ulcer: late followup results after partial gastrectomy: analysis of failures. Ann. Surg. 138, 680 (1953)
5. Muir, A.: Postgastrectomy syndromes. Brit. J. Surgery 37, 165 (1949)
6. Jordan, G.L., Bolton, B.F., DeBakey, M.E.: Experience with gastrectomy at a Veterans Hospital. J.A.M.A. 161, 1605 (1956)
7. Hastings, N., Halsted, J.A., Woodward, E.R., Gasster, M., Hiscock, E.A.: Subtotal gastric resection for benign peptic ulcer. Arch. Surg. 76, 74 (1958)
8. Higginson, J.F., Claggett, O.T.: Gastric resection: the Shoemaker-Billroth I operation. Surgery 24, 613 (1948)
9. Ross, F.P, Meadows, E.C.: The treatment of peptic ulceration by extensive partial gastrectomy with gastroduodenostomy. Surgery 32, 426 (1952)
10. Fischer, P.B., Jordan, G.L.: The Billroth I gastrectomy for the treatment of duodenal ulcer. Ann. Surg. 24, 922 (1958)
11. Eisenberg, M.M., Woodward, E.R, Carson, T.J., Dragstedt, L.R.: Vagotomy and drainage procedure for duodenal ulcer: the results of ten year's experience. Ann. Surg. 170, 317 (1969)
12. O'Leary, J.F., Woodward, E.R., Hollenbeck, J.I, Dragstedt, L.R.: Vagotomy and drainage procedure for duodenal ulcer: the results of seventeen years' experience Ann. Surg. 183, 613 (1976)
13. Goligher, J.C., Hill, G.L., Kenny, T E., Nutter, E.: Proximal gastric vagotomy without drainage for duodenal ulcer: results after 5–8 years. Brit. J. Surg. 65, 145 (1978)
14. Capper, W M. The etiology of the early postgastrectomy syndrome. Gastroenterology 76, 319 (1950)
15. Machalla, T.E.: The mechanism of postgastrectomy dumping syndrome. Ann Surg. 130, 145 (1949)

16. Machella, T.E.: Mechanism of postgastrectomy dumping syndrome. Gastroenterology 14, 237 (1950)

17 Amdrup, E., Jorgensen, J.B.: Further investigations on the pathogenesis of the dumping syndrome with special reference to the role of distension of efferent loop. Acta chirurg. Scand. 113, 22 (1957)

18. Roberts, K E., Randall, H , Farr, H.: Acute alteration in blood volume plasma electrolytes and electrocardiogram produced by oral administration of hypertonic solutions to gastrectomized patients. Surg. Forum 4, 301 (1954)

19. Hinshaw, D.B., Joergenson, E.J., Davis, H.A., Stafford, C.E.: Peripheral blood flow and blood volume studies in the dumping syndrome. Arch. Surg. 74, 686 (1957)

20. Peddie, G H., Jordan, G L , DeBakey, M.E.: Further studies on the pathogenesis of the postgastrectomy syndrome. Ann. Surg 146, 892 (1957)

21. Thomson, J.P.S., Russell, R.C.G., Hobsley, M., Le Quesne, L.P.: The dumping syndrome and the hydrogen ion concentration of the gastric contents Gut 15, 200 (1974)

22. Le Quesne, L.P., Hobsley, M., Hand, B.H.: "The dumping syndrome" I. Factors responsible for the symptoms. Brit. Med. J. I, 141 (1960)

23. Butz, R : Dumping syndrome studied during maintenance of blood volume. Ann. Surgery 154, 225 (1961)

24. Read, R.C., Swenson, D · Blood pressure and osmolarity changes in the dumping syndrome. Surg. Gynecol. Obstetr. 112, 448 (1961)

25. Bulbring, E., Lynn, R.C. The effect of intraluminal application of 5-hydroxytryptamine and 5-hydroxytryptophan on peristalsis, the local production of 5-HT and its release in relation to intraluminal pressure and propulsive activity J. Physiol 140, 381 (1958)

26. Johnson, L.P., Jesseph, J E.: Evidence for a humoral etiology of the dumping syndrome Surg. Forum 12, 316 (1961)

27. Johnson, L.P., Sloop, R.D., Jesseph, J.E.: Plethysmographic evidence supporting the concept of a humoral etiology of the experimental dumping syndrome. J Surg. Res 2, 241 (1962)

28. Johnson, L.P., Sloop, R D., Jesseph, J.E., Harkins, H.N : Serotonin antagonists in experimental and clinical "dumping" Ann. Surg. 165, 537 (1962)

29 Jesseph, J.E.: Serotonin and dumping syndrome. Surgery 63, 536 (1968)

30. Drapanas, T., McDonald, J.C , Stewart, J.D.: Serotonin release following instillation of hypertonic glucose into the proximal intestine. Ann Surg. 156, 528 (1962)

31. Peskin, G.W., Miller, L D.: The role of serotonin in the "dumping syndrome". Arch. Surg. 85, 701 (1962)

32. Silver, D., McGregor, F.H , Porter, J.M., Anylan, W.G. The mechanism of the dumping syndrome. Surg. Clin North Am. 46, 425 (1966)

33. Howe, C.T.: Surg Gynecol. Obstetr. 119, 92 (1964)

34. Walker, G.R., Turner, M.D , Hardie, J D.: Serotonin levels in portal vein blood in the experimental dumping syndrome. Surg. Forum 13, 241 (1962)

35. Zeitlin, I.J., Smith, A.N : 5-Hydroxyindoles and kinins in the carcinoid and dumping syndrome. Lancet II, 986 (1966)

36. Cuschieri, A., Onabanjo, O.A Kinin release after gastric surgery Brit. Med. J II, 565 (1971)

37 MacDonald, J.M., Webster, M.M., Tennyson, C H., Drapanas, T.: Serotonin and bradykinin in the dumping syndrome. Am. J Surgery 117, 204 (1969)

38. Bloom, S.R., Royston, C M.S , Thomson, J.P.S : Enteroglucagon release in the dumping syndrome Lancet II, 789 (1972)

39. O'Connor, F A , Buchanan, K.D., Trimble, E.R., Hayer, J R., Kennedy, T L Characterization of glucagon responses to different meals in the dumping syndrome. Gut 15, 348 (1974)

40. Chaimoff, C.H., Dintsman, M.. The long-term fate of patients with dumping syndrome. Arch Surgery 105, 554 (1972)

41. Jenkins, D.J A., Gassull, M.A , Leeds, A.R., Metz, G., Dilawari, J.G., Slavin, B., Blendis, J.L M.. Effect of dietary fiber on complications of gastric surgery: prevention of postprandial hypoglycemia by pectin. Gastroenterology 72, 215 (1977)

42. Gyr, K., Berger, W , Goschke, H., et al.: Postprandiale Beschwerden nach Gastrektomie und ihre Beeinflussung durch Dimethylbiguanid. Dtsch. Med. Wochenschr 95, 2421 (1970)

43. Humphreys, W.G , Parks, T.G , Buchanan, K G., Love, A H.G.. Effect of phenformin on provoked dumping in man. Gut 18, 956 (1977) (abstr.)

44. Caspary, W.F.: Biguanides and intestinal absorptive function. Acta Hepato-Gastroenterol. *24*, 473–480 (1977)
45. Slatlocky, E.: Behandlung des Dumping-Syndromes mit zuckerresorptionshemmenden Mitteln. Dtsch. Med. Wochenschr. *96*, 308 (1971)
46. Becker, H.D.: Pathogenese, Diagnostik und Therapie des Dumping-Syndroms. Chirurg *48*, 247 (1977)
47. Amdrup, E.: Surgical treatment of postgastrectomy symptoms Acta chir. Scand. *120*, 151 (1960)
48. Porter, H.W., Clarman, Z.B.: A preliminary report on the advantage of a small stoma in partial gastrectomy for ulcer. Ann. Surg. *129*, 417 (1949)
49. Salessiotis, N.A.: Gastroenteric anastomosis in Billroth II gastrectomy with maintenance of the pyloric diameter of the normal pylorus to prevent dumping syndrome. Amer. J. Surg. *129*, 656 (1975)
50. Kennedy, C.S, Reynolds, R.P., Cantor, M.O.. A study of the gastric stoma after partial gastrectomy. Surgery *22*, 41 (1947)
51. Perman, E.: The so-called dumping syndrome after gastrectomy. Acta med. Scand. *196*, 361 (1947)
52. Bohmansson, G.: Prophylaxis and therapy in late postgastrectomy complications. Acta med. Scand. *246*, 37 (1950)
53. Mathewson, C. Jr.: Conversion of Billroth II to Billroth I for the relief of postgastrectomy symptoms. Amer. J. Surg. *90*, 317 (1955)
54. Holle, F.: Spezielle Magenchirurgie. Berlin, Heidelberg, New York: Springer 1968
55. Bushkin, F.L., Woodward, E.R.: Postgastrectomy syndromes. Vol. XX. Major problems in clinical surgery. Philadelphia: W.B. Saunders 1976
56. Barg, I., Borgström, S.G., Hager, K.: The value of B II–B I conversion operation in the treatment of the postgastrectomy syndrome. Acta chir. Scand. *134*, 655 (1968)
57. Biebl, M.: „Interpositions-Billroth I" mittels ausgeschalteter Dünndarmschlinge; ein ptotisches Anastomosierungsverfahren bei Magenresektion mit Gultigkeit fur das Ulcus. Zbl. Chir. *72*, 1568 (1947)
58. Henley, F.A.: Gastrectomy with replacement. Brit. J. Surg. *40*, 118 (1952)
59. Herrington, J.L.: Utilization of small bowel segments as a gastric reservoir for control of the dumping syndrome. Amer. J. Surg. *111*, 89 (1966)
60. Poth, E.J.: The dumping syndrome and its surgical management Am. Surg. *23*, 1097 (1957)
61. Fenger, H.J., Gudmand-Höyer, E., Kallehauge, H.E., Andreassen, M.: Clinical experience with isoperistaltic interposition of a jejunal segment for the incapacitating dumping syndrome. Ann. Surg. *175*, 274 (1972)
62. Herrington, J.L., Sawyers, J.L.: Remedial operations. In: Nyhus, L.M., Wastell, C.: Surgery of the stomach and duodenum. 3. Ed. Boston: Little Brown and Company 1977
63. Hedenstedt, S: Experiences with gastric resection with transposition of the jejunum and vagotomy. Acta chir. Scand. *125*, 518 (1960)
64. Sawyers, J.L., Herrington, J.L.· Superiority of antiperistaltic jejunal segments in management of severe dumping syndrome. Ann. Surg. *278*, 311 (1973)
65. Alexander-Williams, J.: Gastric reconstructive surgery. Ann. R. College Surg. Engl. *52*, 1 (1972)
66. Nygaard, K., Frethein, B.: Jejunal transposition in treatment of postgastrectomy syndromes. Scand. J. Gastroent. *9*, 59 (1974)
67. Fink, W.J., Hucke, S.T., Gray, T.W., Thompson, B.W., Read, R.C.: Treatment of postoperative reactive hypoglycemia by a reversed intestinal segment. Am. J. Surg. *131*, 19 (1976)
68. Poth, E J.. The dumping syndrome and its surgical management. Am. Surg *23*, 1097 (1957)
69. Poth, E.J. The use of gastrointestinal reversal in surgical procedure. Amer. J. Surg. *118*, 893 (1969)
70. Hammer, J.M., Seay, P.H, Hill, E., Prust, F.H., Campbell, R.J.: The effect of antiperistaltic bowel segments in intestinal emptying time. Arch. Surg. *79*, 537 (1959)
71. Wilms, R.K, Barton, H.L., Angel, R.T., Jordan, G.L.: Reversed intestinal segments and their effect upon gastrointestinal motility, nutrition and the dumping syndrome following subtotal gastrectomy in 6 dogs. J. A. M. A. *178*, 1008 (1961)
72. Poth, E.J., Cleveland, D.R.: A functional substitution pouch for the stomach. Arch. Surg. *83*, 58 (1961)
73. Poth, E.J, Smith, L.B.: Gastric pouches, their evaluation Amer. J. Surg. *112*, 721 (1966)
74 Christiansen, T M., Hart-Hansen, O., Petersen, T.. Reconstruction of the pylorus for post-vagotomy diarrhea and dumping Brit. J. Surg. *61*, 519 (1975)

10.3 Late Dumping

The late dumping syndrome is less common after gastric resection than early dumping. But a certain group of patients with or without the early phase may have a period of weakness, hunger and sweating with onset at least 1 h, but mostly 2–3 h after a meal. The symptoms and signs of this variation of the dumping syndrome are similar to, but not identical with the vasomotor symptoms of the early postprandial dumping syndrome. The symptoms are identical with those of hypoglycaemia: the patient becomes weak, feels faint and perspires profusely. Less prominent are other vasomotor symptoms, but central nervous system signs are more common, sometimes even reaching the point of unconsciousness. The late dumper often feels hungry, but usually does not experience gastro-intestinal symptoms.

Symptoms of both late and early dumping syndromes are induced by ingestion of free sugars or easily digestible carbohydrates such as disaccharides. The late dumper in comparison with the early dumper has a better caloric intake and severe nutritional deficiencies are usually absent. The sensations of late postprandial hunger move patients to further caloric intake to relieve symptoms, and they may therefore eat more than necessary, in a similar way to patients with reactive hypoglycemia or an insulinoma, who usually are obese.

10.3.1 Pathogenesis

The pathogenesis of the late dumping syndrome was discovered earlier than that of the more common early postprandial dumping syndrome. For many years the two sets of symptoms were not clearly distinguished, although it has to be admitted that both syndromes may be present in the same patient.

Lapp and Diebold [1] reported in 1933 the rapid rise and equally rapid fall in blood glucose after ingestion of carbohydrates by postgastrectomy patients. In the same year Beckerman [2] reported on 10 patients who developed episodes of sweating, weakness, restlessness and hunger following meals rich in carbohydrates. Five of the 10 patients were found to have hypoglycaemia at the time of symptoms and two cases developed typical symptoms 2 h after meals, with blood sugar levels in the range of 50 mg/100 ml. Despite attributing the symptoms to the deleterious effect of a carbohydrate-rich meal on the mucosa of the intestine – causing a jejunitis, they recognised the beneficial effect of a low-carbohydrate diet in preventing the late dumping syndrome.

Glaessner [3] hypothesised that the symptoms of late dumping were due to hyperglycaemic shock, since he observed extremely rapid rises in blood sugar level following an orally administered 100-g glucose load. Machella [4] disproved this theory and Adlersberg and Hammerschlag [5] made the clear distinction between early and late dumping syndrome.

Muir [6] called late postprandial dumping the "hypoglycemic type" and suggested that it was due to hyperinsulinaemia following initial exaggerated hyperglycaemia. Since hyperglycaemia induced by intravenous administration of glucose was not followed by reactive hypoglycaemia, he suggested the possibility

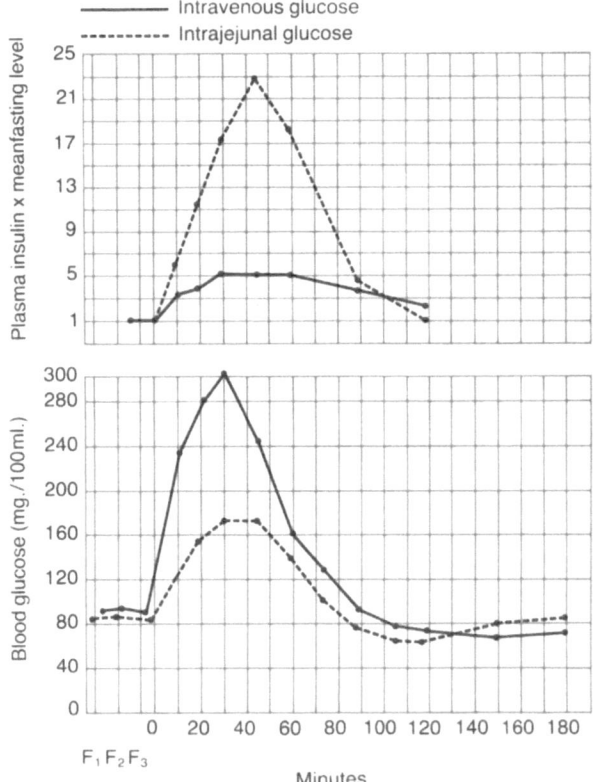

Fig. 29. Despite lower blood glucose levels after intrajejunal than intravenous administration of glucose, insulin responses are much more pronounced after intrajejunal than intravenous glucose (After Holdsworth et al., 1969)

that late dumping syndrome was due to insulin sensitivity resulting from the reduction of carbohydrate intake. Serum insulin levels in postgastrectomy patients were first measured by radio-immunoassay in 1965 by Roth and Meade [7]. Serum insulin levels at 30 and 60 min rose to three or four times those observed in normal subjects following the same glucose challenge. Holdsworth [8] found that glucose administered intravenously to postgastrectomy patients did not result in such an exaggerated output of insulin as they observed on infusing a hypertonic glucose solution into the intestine (Fig. 29). They assumed therefore that some material is released from the gut which sensitises the beta cells and finally results in exaggerated insulin release in response to hyperglycaemia.

Since glucose taken orally leads to a higher insulin response than the same amount of glucose given intravenously, it had to be assumed for normal subjects as well as gastrectomized patients that an intestinal factor was responsible for the more pronounced insulin release. Several hormones have already been considered to perform this incretin-like function: secretin, enteroglucagon and, more recently, gastric inhibitory polypeptide (GIP). Since the gut harbours a whole group of gastro-intestinal hormones which are released in response to a meal, it seems likely that with the loss of the reservoir function of the stomach, the increased amount of food – mostly, what is more, in the form of a hypertonic solution – will result in an exaggerated release of intestinal hormones. GLI, the immuno-reactivity of a material in intestinal extracts that cross-reacts with pancreatic glucagon antibodies, and which more recently has been called enteroglucagon, was found to be significantly elevated in the serum of postgastrectomy patients following an oral glucose challenge. This was later confirmed by Bloom et al. [9], who observed higher levels of serum enteroglucagon in 17 patients who had undergone vagotomy plus drainage procedure.

O'Connor et al. [10] observed, too, that a meal of glucose, fat or protein resulted in a markedly increased GLI response in dumpers, compared to controls. The release of GIP was also markedly increased in dumpers, as compared to controls.

In summary, the late dumping syndrome occurs after resection or by-pass of the normal pyloric sphincter and is due to hypoglycaemia following an exaggerated insulin release induced by rapid passage of carbohydrates into the upper intestine. The hypertonicity or rapid absorption of glucose apparently leads to an increased hormonal release from the intestine which in accord with high serum glucose levels seems to sensitise the beta cells and thus results in exaggerated insulin release. Whether enteroglucagon or some other, as yet unidentified intestinal hormone(s) are acting as "sensitisers" for exaggerated insulin release remains undetermined at the moment. Any decrease of intestinal absorption resulting in lower postprandial glucose levels will be combined with lower insulin and GIP levels.

10.3.2 Therapy

It has been shown that biguanides known to inhibit or retard intestinal glucose absorption [11] will act beneficially in postprandial reactive hypoglycaemia by smoothing the blood glucose and insulin curve following carbohydrate ingestion. It therefore seems logical that any agent producing a delay of intestinal carbo-hydrate absorption will favourably affect symptoms of the late dumping syndrome. Favourable results have been reported with biguanides [11–13] and prenylamine [14]. Carbohydrate gelling agents [15] seem to act in a similar way and may be a beneficial dietary supplement in meals for patients with the late dumping syndrome. Dietary instructions to the patients may be more important and have to be followed more strictly in the late dumping syndrome, since patients may not recognise that the symptoms they experience 2 h after a meal are in fact due to the food then eaten.

References

1. Lapp, F.W., Diebold, H.: First description of rapid rise and fall of blood glucose after subtotal gastric resection. Blutzuckerablauf in seiner Beziehung zum resezierten Magen. Klin. Wschr 12, 547 (1933)
2. Beckermann, F.: Spontaneous hypoglycemia following gastric surgery. Dtsch. Med. Wschr. 59, 683 (1933)
3 Glaessner, C.L : Disturbances in sugar metabolism after subtotal gastrectomy. Am. J Dig. Dis. 12, 157 (1945)

4. Machella, T.E : The mechanism of postgastrectomy dumping syndrome. Ann. Surg. *130*, 145 (1949)
5. Adlersberg, D., Hammerschlag, E.: Mechanism of the postgastrectomy syndrome. JAMA *139*, 429 (1949)
6 Muir, A.: Postgastrectomy syndromes. Brit. J. Surgery 37, 165 (1949)
7. Roth, D.A., Meade, R.C.. Hyperinsulinism – hypoglycemia in postgastrectomy patients. Diabetes *14*, 526 (1965)
8. Holdsworth, C.D., Turner, D., McIntyre, N.: Pathophysiology of post-gastrectomy hypoglycemia. Brit. Med. J. *4*, 257 (1969)
9. Bloom, S.R., Royston, C.M.S., Thomsen, J.P.S.: Enteroglucagon release in the dumping syndrome. Lancet *II*, 789 (1972)
10. O'Connor, F.A., Buchanan, K.D., Trimple, E.R., Hayer, J.R., Kennedy, T L. Characterization of glucagon responses to different meals in the dumping syndrome. Gut *15*, 348 (1974)
11 Caspary, W.F.: Biguanides and intestinal absorptive function. Acta Hepato-Gastroenterol. *24*, 473–480 (1977)
12. Gyr, K., Berger, W., Goschke, H., et al.. Postprandiale Beschwerden nach Gastrektomie und ihre Beeinflussung durch Dimethylbiguanid. Dtsch. Med. Wschr. *95*, 2421 (1970)
13. Humphreys, W.G., Parks, T.G., Buchanan, K.G., Love, A.H.G.: Effect of phenformin on provoked dumping in man. Gut *18*, 956 (1977) (abstr.)
14. Slatlocky, E.: Behandlung des Dumping-Syndromes mit zuckerabsorptionshemmenden Mitteln. Dtsch. Med. Wschr. *96*, 308 (1971)
15. Jenkins, D.J.A., Gassull, M.A., Leeds, A.R., Metz, G., Dilawari, J.G., Slavin, B., Blendis, J.L M.: Effect of dietary fiber on complications of gastric surgery: prevention of postprandial hypoglycemia by pectin. Gastroenterology 72, 215 (1977)

11 Afferent-Loop Syndrome

Shortly after the first gastric resection was performed, a new syndrome was described, which consisted of bile vomiting occasionally mixed with food particles, combined with upper right abdominal pain [1]. Braun [2] therefore suggested in 1893 an entero-anastomosis between the afferent and efferent jejunal loops, since he had observed an increased reflux of bile into the stomach. In the following decades several authors were able clearly to demonstrate that bile reflux into the stomach causes vomiting. The clear differentiation between the afferent-loop syndrome (ALS) and the other postgastrectomy syndromes was made by Hoffmann [3], who described the clinical picture as follows:

> Without pain, and usually in the morning after getting up or some time after meals bile-stained vomiting occurs without any food contents. There is sometimes only nausea with possibly slight regurgitation but no pyrosis. The bile vomiting sometimes occurs alone, but it is usually preceded by nausea or anorexia.

In the following years the ALS was exactly defined and described as a special type of postgastrectomy syndrome [5, 6].

The ALS can be divided into an acute form and a chronic form. The severity of symptoms allows the following classification:

1. Acute ALS
2. Chronic ALS
   a) Mild symptoms
   b) Moderate symptoms
   c) Severe symptoms.

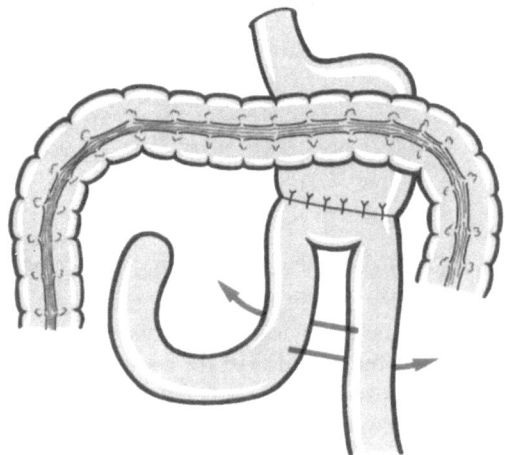

Fig. 30. Internal hernia can cause ALS after Billroth II resection

11.1 Acute ALS

The acute ALS is characterised by the total occlusion of the afferent loop after Billroth II gastrectomy or gastro-enterostomy. The occlusion causes a rapid increase in pressure in the afferent loop due to the continuing pancreatic and biliary secretion.

The first description of a patient with total occlusion of the afferent loop after partial gastrectomy was made by Goebel [6] in 1927. The day after surgery, the general condition of the patient deteriorated rapidly, showing signs of shock with tachycardia and intra-abdominal pain. The patient died 24 h later. Post-mortem examination showed an extreme dilatation of the afferent loop, with necrosis of the anterior wall of the duodenum. The total occlusion was caused by kinking of the afferent loop, which had slipped behind the gastro-enterostomy (Fig. 30). A similar patient was described by Balfour [7].

The incidence of the acute ALS after partial gastrectomy is unknown, but should be around 0.5%. The most important pathogenetic factor is mechanical obstruction, as shown in Table 25, which is based on a compilation of the world literature, covering 105 cases, by Dahlgren [8]. Internal hernias are mainly found after antecolic gastroenterostomies where in most cases the afferent loop has been fixated to the lesser curvature. In 30% of the cases this severe complication is observed in the immediate postoperative course, whereas in 20% it happens after an interval of from 3 weeks to 6 months, as described by Dahlgren [8].

The clinical picture is characterised by the acute onset of the symptoms. In a few patients, a subtotal compression of the afferent loop will occur before the total occlusion. The first symptom in most cases is severe epigastric pain with occasional vomiting and characteristically without bile admixture. The general condition of the patients deteriorates rapidly. In about one-third of patients a resistance is palpable in the epigastrium or below the right costal arch. One-third

Table 25. Pathogenetic factors in acute ALS. (Dahlgren [8])

Internal hernia	48.5%
Kinking	23.8%
Adhesions	5.7%
Anastomotic stenosis	3.8%
Others	8.5%

of the patients show icterus and hyperamylasaemia. The X-ray examination of the abdomen typically demonstrates a dense shadow in the upper abdominal part, occasionally combined with gas-fluid levels. The emptying of contrast medium from the stomach is delayed. A cholangiogram may demonstrate an obstructed choledochal duct. It may be difficult to differentiate acute ALS from pancreatitis; often laparotomy has been performed under the diagnosis of obstruction ileus.

Therapy of acute ALS depends on the intra-operative findings. In the majority of patients at laparotomy perforation of the afferent loop with extended necrosis of the wall will be found according to Dahlgren [8]. If total occlusion of the afferent loop occurs during the first 24 h after gastrectomy, a leakage of the duodenal stump has to be expected. The best results will be achieved in patients with internal hernia: after reposition of the hernia, not only should fixation of the afferent loop be carried out, but an entero-anastomosis should also be created. Altogether, the prognosis of acute ALS is poor, with a mortality of about 50%.

11.2 Chronic ALS

The clinical picture of the chronic ALS is characterised by postprandial bile vomiting of varying degree. In the mild forms, symptoms are rare and well tolerated by most patients (Fig. 31). In moderate forms, symptoms occur after food intake or during fasting. The symptoms may begin immediately after operation or up to 10 years later; they are provoked by special food components, such as fat. The volume of vomited bile varies between a few millilitres and 1 litre. At the end of the vomiting, small food particles are occasionally found. Before vomiting, patients complain of a feeling of pressure in the upper abdomen, which disappears after vomiting. In severe cases bile vomiting occurs either following food intake or independently. The volume of vomited material may amount to several litres. The general and nutritional condition is poor, and signs of steatorrhoea and hypoproteinaemia are present.

The pathogenesis of chronic ALS consists in intermittent obstruction of the afferent jejunal loop (Fig. 32a, b). At laparotomy, the mechanical factor often cannot be demonstrated. The most frequent causes of chronic ALS are compiled in Table 26.

The ALS does not only occur in patients with distal gastric resection and Billroth II anastomosis, but also after simple gastro-enterostomy, where the conditions are similar. An ALS is more frequently observed in patients without an

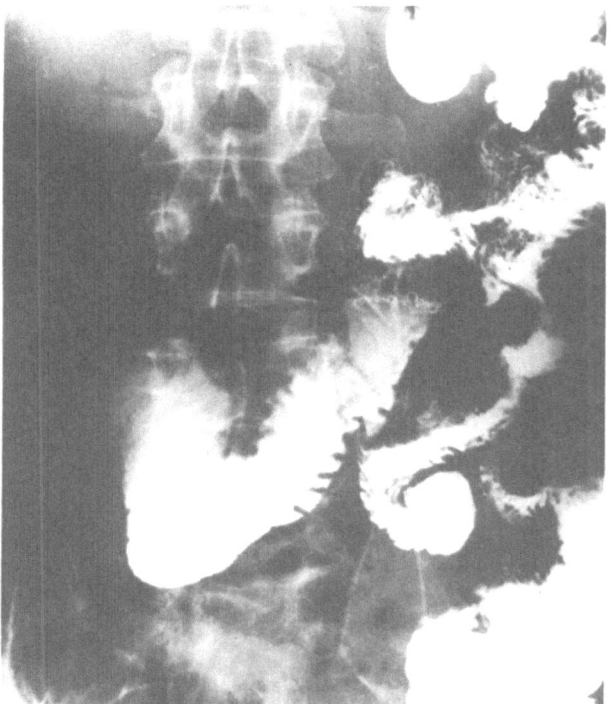

Fig. 31. X-Ray of a patient with chronic ALS

additional entero-anastomosis (Braun's anastomosis). After antecolic gastro-enterostomy a chronic ALS is more often found than after retrocolic modifications.

The severity of symptoms is strongly influenced by the underlying primary disease (duodenal ulcer, gastric ulcer, gastric tumour). On the other hand, a direct correlation between the extent of gastric resection and the incidence of bile vomiting can be documented.

The diagnosis of chronic ALS is made on the basis of the typical clinical symptoms with postprandial bile vomiting, postprandial fullness in the upper abdomen with pain radiating to the back, and disappearance of symptoms after vomiting. The X-ray examination is not helpful in most cases, only the dilatation of the duodenal loop is of diagnostic importance. Gordon [9] described a provo-cation test in which a fatty test meal is passed via a nasogastric tube into the afferent loop; under normal conditions, shortly after the meal is administered bile will appear in the efferent loop (it is detected via the nasogastric tube). In patients with ALS, upper abdominal symptoms appear; they disappear as soon as bile is found in the jejunal aspirate. Dahlgren [8] described another provocation test, in which hormonal stimulation of pancreatic and biliary secretion is used. After intravenous application of secretin and cholecystokinin (CCK-PZ), patients will have typical symptoms within a few minutes, followed by projectile vomiting. On endoscopic examination, mechanical obstruction in the anastomotic region can be seen; furthermore, it is possible to differentiate alkaline reflux gastritis (see below) by histological examinations.

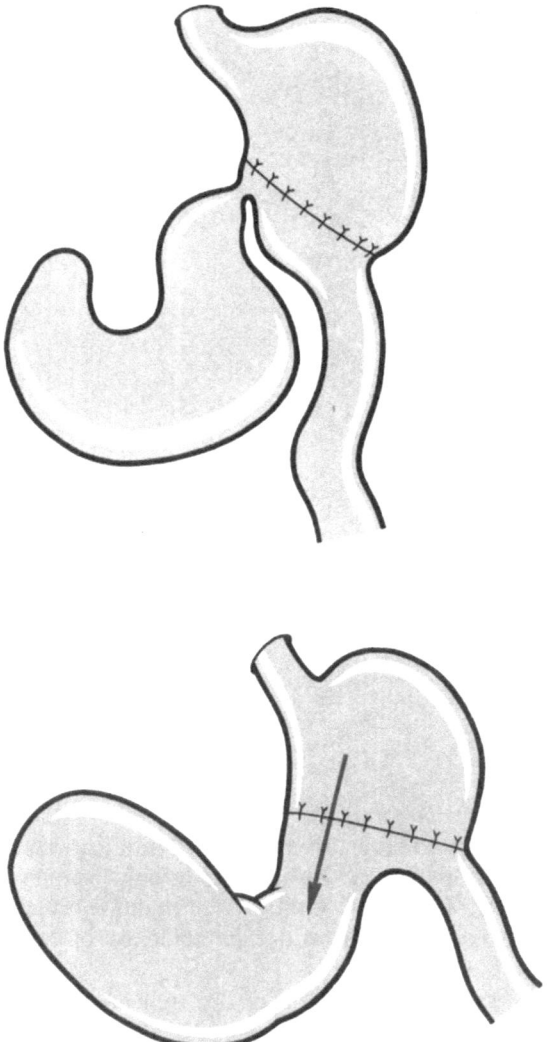

Fig. 32a, b. Pathogenetic factors in chronic ALS: **a** organic stenosis; **b** functional form

Table 26. Pathogenetic factors in chronic ALS

Internal hernia
Kinking
Inflammatory obstruction of a simple gastro-enterostomy
Adhesions
Atonia of the afferent loop
Spasms of the duodenum?
Forced contraction of the gall bladder?
Gastritis?

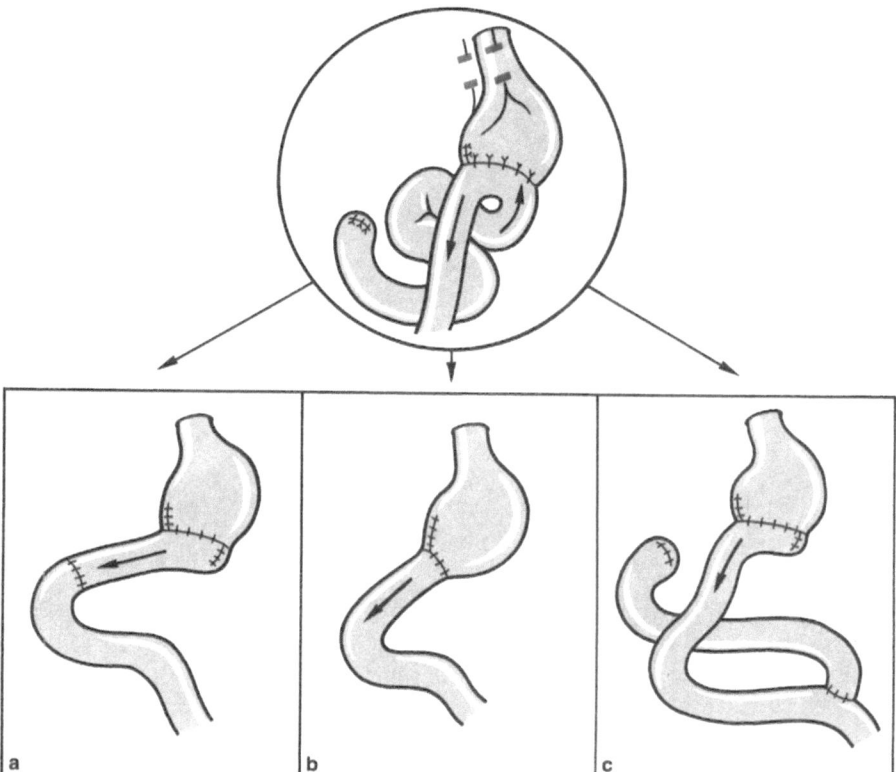

Fig. 33a–c. Therapeutic approach to chronic ALS: **a** interposition of jejunal loop; **b** Billroth I anastomosis; **c** Roux-en-Y anastomosis

11.2.1 Therapy

There is general agreement that postprandial bile vomiting will disappear in a certain percentage of patients in the first year after partial gastrectomy. Mercer [14] reported that one-third of his patients with bile vomiting became symptom-free during the first 12 months after operation.

All patients with clinically significant symptoms due to a chronic ALS should undergo surgery, unless a severe secondary disease exists. If the pre-operative diagnosis was correct, all surgical procedure which lead to a decompression of the afferent loop will reduce the patients' symptoms (Fig. 33). The different therapeutic techniques which have been used are listed in Table 27.

Table 27. Surgical procedure in chronic ALS

1) Braun's entero-anastomosis
2) Roux-en-Y anastomosis
3) Conversion of Billroth II to Billroth I
4) Removal of a simple gastro-enterostomy
5) Jejunoplasty of Wells and Welbourn

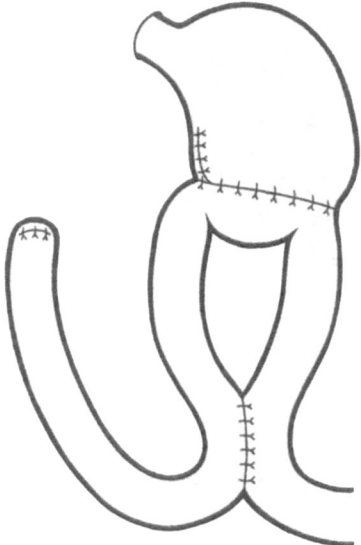

Fig. 34. Treatment of chronic ALS by Braun's entero-anastomosis

11.2.1.1 Braun's Jejunojejunal Entero-anastomosis

An entero-anastomosis between the afferent and efferent jejunal loops (Fig. 34) is a simple method with a tolerably low risk. Since Dahlgren [8] showed that only 3.3% of patients with an entero-anastomosis after Billroth II resection present chronic ALS, whereas 21.5% of patients without this modification, but otherwise given identical surgical treatment, show these symptoms, it is assumed that also in cases with existing ALS an entero-anastomosis will reduce the symptoms. According to Dahlgren [8], good results can be expected in two-thirds of patients. The best results by this method are achieved in cases with dilated afferent loop and proven mechanical obstruction of the anastomosis.

11.2.1.2 Roux-en-Y Anastomosis

Most authors agree that the Roux-en-Y anastomosis for chronic ALS (Fig. 35) gives excellent results [10, 11]. Since this method is more reliable than Braun's entero-anastomosis for keeping duodenal contents from the stomach, it is the procedure of choice in cases where chronic ALS is combined with symptoms of alkaline reflux gastritis. Compared to the jejunal interposition (see below) the operative risk is much lower. As shown in Fig. 35, the transected afferent loop should be implanted into the efferent loop about 60 cm distal to the gastrojejunal anastomosis, since with a smaller distance reflux of bile into the stomach may occur.

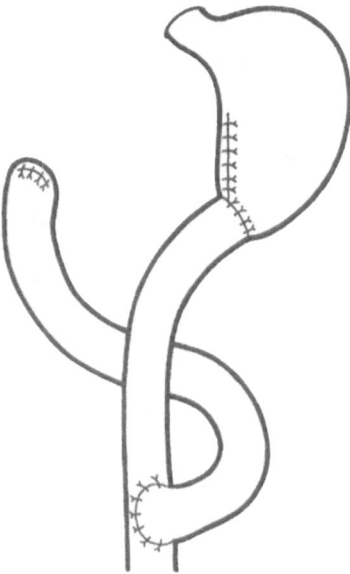

Fig. 35. Roux-en-Y anastomosis. Implantation of the afferent loop 40–60 cm distal to the gastro-jejunostomy

11.2.1.3 Conversion of Billroth II to Billroth I

The conversion of a Billroth II gastrojejunostomy to a Billroth I gastroduodeno-stomy (Fig. 22) removes the anatomical preconditions of an ALS. If the anasto-mosis between stomach and duodenum is created without interpositions of a jejunal segment, a terminolateral anastomosis is to be preferred, since the mobilisation of the duodenal stump may be technically difficult and the anasto-mosis has a higher risk of complications. In most cases, however, a jejunal inter-position procedure according to Henley-Soupault is performed; the technical details are described in Chap. 10.2.6.

Compared to the Roux-en-Y anastomosis, the Henley-Soupault procedure, which includes the restoration of the duodenal passage, does represent a much larger surgical intervention. The Henley-Soupault procedure always has to be combined with vagotomy, since otherwise ulcers will occur in the interposed jejunal segment.

11.2.1.4 Removal of a Simple Gastro-enterostomy

Simple gastro-enterostomy is only rarely used in treating peptic ulcer disease, but it is used as a drainage procedure after vagotomy. As a method for treating a chronic ALS, removal of the gastroenterostomy and performance of another drainage procedure, such as a pyloroplasty, can be recommended (Fig. 36). If a drainage procedure cannot be performed because of anatomical findings, a Billroth II resection with an additional entero-anastomosis should be performed.

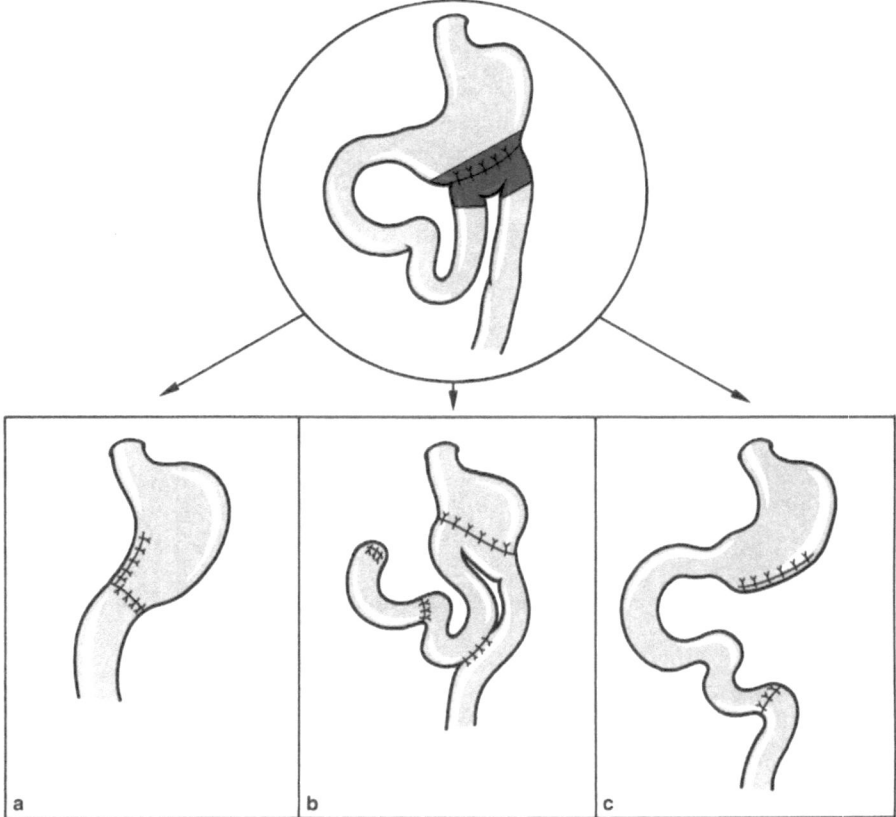

Fig. 36a–c. Removal of simple gastroenterostomy

11.2.1.5 Jejunoplasty

A jejunoplasty has been propagated by Wells and Welbourn [5]; this method originates from a procedure described by Hoag and Saunders [12] and by Steinberg [13]; however, more extensive clinical experience with this method does not exist.

References

1. Wolfler, A.: Gastroenterostomie. Zbl. Chir. 8, 705 (1881)
2. Braun, H.: Über Gastroenterostomie und gleichzeitig ausgefuhrte Enteroanastomose Arch. klin. Chir. 45, 361 (1892)
3. Hoffmann, V.: Klinische Krankheitsbilder nach Magenoperationen. Münch. med. Wschr. 86, 332 (1939)
4. Muir, A.: Postgastrectomy syndromes. Brit. J. Surg. 37, 165 (1949)
5. Wells, C.A., Welbourn, R.: Postgastrectomy syndromes. Brit. med. J. 1, 546 (1951)

6. Goebel, C.: Ileus der zuführenden Schlinge nach Magenresektion wegen Ulcus duodeni und Megaduodenum. Zbl. Chir. *54*, 2721 (1927)
7. Balfour, D.C.: Emergency complications occurring after operations on the stomach and duodenum and their treatment. Coll. Papers Mayo Clin. *25*, 58 (1959)
8. Dahlgren, S.: The afferent-loop-syndrome. Acta chir. scand. (Suppl.) *327*, 1 (1964)
9. Gordon, O.: cited by 8.
10. Bushkin, F.L., Woodward, E.R.: The afferent-loop-syndrome. In: Bushkin, F.L., Woodward, E.R.: Post-gastrectomy-syndromes. Vol. XX. Major problems in Surgery. Philadelphia: Saunders 1976
11. Fromm, D.: Complications of gastric surgery. Clin. Gastroent. monograph series. New York: Wiley 1977
12. Hoag, C.L., Saunders, J.B.: Jejunoplasty for obstruction following gastro-enterostomy or subtotal gastric resection. Surg. Gynec. Obstet. *68*, 703 (1939)
13. Steinberg, M.E.: A double jejunal gastro-jejunal anastomosis. Surg. Gynec. Obstet. *88*, 453 (1949)
14. Mercer, S.: An investigation of the results of gastric resection for peptic ulceration in 100 consecutive cases. Ulster med. J. *23*, 132 (1954).

12 Efferent-Loop Syndrome

The efferent-loop syndrome in a narrow sense refers only to obstruction of the efferent jejunal loop after gastric resection or simple gastro-enterostomy; it occurs hours or years after operation and varies greatly in symptoms and chronicity (Fig. 37). The efferent-loop obstruction is less frequent than the afferent-loop syndrome and generally occurs as a result of internal hernia [1].

Two forms can be distinguished: an acute and a chronic. In the acute form, internal hernia may be a consequence especially of technical problems to do with the anastomosis at surgery, including large intra-operative invagination at the suture line [2, 3]. The often-cited oedema of the anastomosis and cord formation immediately below the gastrojejunostomy are rare. The later-occurring forms of the efferent-loop syndrome may be caused by ulcerations in the region of anastomosis, scarred stenosis, old adhesions (Fig. 38), hernias of the efferent or the afferent or both loops, or by jejunogastric invagination [3–5].

The clinical symptoms of the acute forms of efferent-loop obstruction are characterised by abdominal cramps, which are mostly localised around the umbilicus [6]. The patients vomit large volumes of fluid which contains bile and food particles [7]. Clinical examination reveals a tympanous abdomen, but no palpable resistance [6]. Also, jejunogastric invagination (Fig. 39) is in most cases characterised by acute symptoms accompanied by blood vomiting. In this type of acute efferent-loop syndrome a mass is palpable in the upper abdomen in most cases; the diagnosis is verified by an upper GI series.

The more chronic types show attacks of vomiting, similar to the symptoms of the afferent-loop syndrome. Only the admixture of food particles or large volumes of bile may be indicative of an efferent-loop syndrome [1].

During the diagnostic procedures, signs of an upper small-bowel occlusion are found. The incarcerated small-bowel loops may cause a compression of the transverse colon, with subsequent dilatation [6]. An upper GI series often reveals

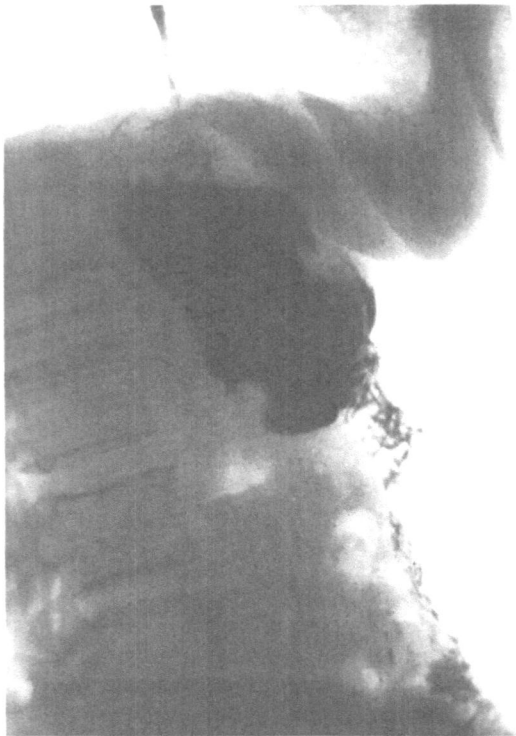

Fig. 37. X-Ray of a patient with an efferent loop syndrome 8 weeks after Billroth II resection

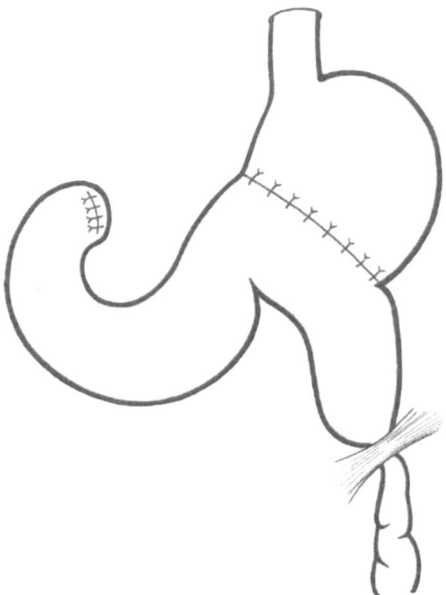

Fig. 38. Efferent-loop syndrome caused by adhesions

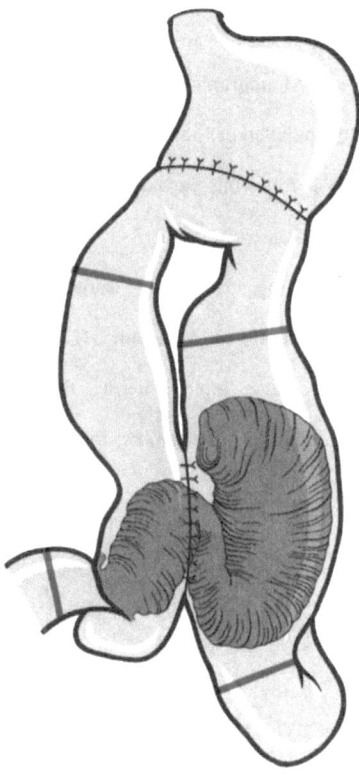

Fig. 39. Invagination of the jejunum causing afferent- and efferent-loop syndrome

delayed gastric emptying. In more chronic forms radiological diagnosis may be impossible.

Only by surgery may the efferent-loop syndrome be removed, although in cases with the acute form caused by technical problems in the anastomotic region, adopting a conservative attitude may be sensible. Immediate surgery is required in cases with jejunogastric invagination or incarceration of internal hernias. In cases where the anastomosis is not patent, reintervention should not be performed before the seventh postoperative day [8]. The surgical procedure of choice is a second antecolic gastro-enterostomy above the first, with an entero-enterostomy. Surgical interventions at the original anastomosis are unsafe.

The existence of an incarcerated internal hernia calls for repositioning and fixation of the herniated small bowel, with an additional entero-anastomosis. A jejunogastric invagination is treated in most cases by an entero-anastomosis. In chronic forms, resection of the mechanical barrier and fixation of the contorted small bowel have to be performed.

References

1. Fromm, D.: Complications of gastric surgery. Clin. Gastroent. Monograph series. New York: Wiley 1977
2. Herrington, J.L.: Experience with the surgical management of the afferent loop syndrome. Ann. Surg. *164*, 797 (1966)
3. Hibner, R., Richards, V.: Stomach or small bowel obstruction following partial gastrectomy. Report of thirty cases. Amer. J. Surg. *96*, 309 (1958)
4. Cooling, C.J.: Small bowel obstruction following antecolic partial gastrectomy Brit. J. Surg. *46*, 656 (1959)
5. Conklin, E.F., Markowitz, A.M.: Intussusception, a complication of gastric surgery. Surgery *57*, 480 (1965)
6. Rutledge, R.H.: Retroanastomotic hernias after gastrojejunal anastomoses. Ann. Surg. *177*, 547 (1973)
7 Bastable, J.R.G., Huddy, P.E.: Retro-anastomotic hernia. Eight cases of internal hernia. Brit. J. Surg. *48*, 183 (1960)
8. Nissen, R.: Eingriffe an Magen und Duodenum. In: Brandt, G., Kunz, H., Nissen, R.: Intra- und postoperative Zwischenfälle. Stuttgart: Thieme 1965

13 Postoperative Reflux Gastritis

13.1 Pathogenesis

Bile is not usually present in gastric juice, because the pylorus normally prevents reflux of duodenal contents. In some pathological conditions, however, duodenal juice with bile refluxes into the stomach or even into the oesophagus, leaving a trail of mucosal damage. One of the first observations on reflux of bile into the stomach was made by Beaumont in 1833 [1], who observed in his subject, Alex St. Martin, that "bile was seldom found in the stomach except under peculiar circumstances". In the 1940s Schindler [2] performed gastroscopy in 54 patients who had undergone gastrectomy for various reasons. Practically all had some type of gastritis. In four patients who had a normal mucosa there was a pylorus-like function of the stoma; the others had rigid open stomas. Browne and McHardy [3] noted similar changes and also emphasised the possible role of stomal dysfunction. They stated that achlorhydria was the rule.

Little attention was paid to the phenomenon of bile reflux until DuPlessis [4, 5] suggested in 1963 that reflux of bile might play an important role in the pathogenesis both of gastric ulcer and of the gastritis that often follows gastric surgery.

It was generally considered up to this time that all patients with chronic bilious vomiting had the chronic form of the afferent-loop syndrome, with intermittent obstruction of the afferent loop.

Bile regurgitation was originally considered solely part of the afferent-loop syndrome. Wells and Welbourne [6], studying 300 patients with various types of gastrectomy, described afferent-loop stasis and bile regurgitation as occurring typically in the early postprandial period. It occurred after procedures that converted the duodenum and afferent loop into a functional extension of the common bile and pancreatic ducts. Gastric resection with a gastrojejunostomy was the most common procedure leading to this clinical syndrome. They identified mechanical obstruction at the junction of the afferent loop with the gastric remnant as the cause of increased pressure and accumulation of fluid in the afferent loop. When pressure increased in the loop to a critical point, sufficient to overcome the obstruction, forceful bilious vomiting occurred, with simultaneous relief of the symptoms. The food had already passed down the efferent loop and therefore was not usually part of the projectile vomiting. The chronic afferent-loop syndrome differs from the acute form by the incompleteness of the mechanical obstruction. When pressure increases within the duodenal loop, decompression occurs through the gastric remnant. Woodward [7] has stressed that the history provides the most helpful information for diagnosis of chronic afferent-loop syndrome. The distinction between reflux gastritis and the chronic afferent-loop syndrome is important, because the various forms of bilious vomiting may require different therapeutic approaches.

Symptoms of the afferent-loop syndrome usually occur within minutes but may occur up to 1 h after eating. A dull pressure or crampy gastric pain is experienced. Projectile vomiting results in immediate relief of the symptoms. The vomit is usually voluminous and bile-stained and contains no food. Between meals, patients are often completely asymptomatic. Since eating initiates symptoms, the patients progressively restrict their food intake, and weight loss may therefore be considerable.

The English surgeon Capper [8] and Wells and Welbourne [6] observed, however, that in some of these patients no evidence of mechanical obstruction existed. They even observed abdominal distress and bilious vomiting in the absence of an afferent loop, as for example in Billroth I partial gastrectomy. It was also observed that some patients considered to suffer from the chronic afferent-loop syndrome failed to exhibit symptomatic improvement after construction of a Braun entero-anastomosis or after conversion from a Billroth II to a Billroth I reconstruction.

Capper [8] continued to study pyloric function and reflux of duodenal contents into the stomach in several clinical situations, including gastric ulcer, gastritis and gall-stone dyspepsia.

The physiologists Code and Davenport at the Mayo Clinic [9–11], with their work on the gastric mucosal barrier, prepared the scientific basis for further investigations on the mechanism of action of bile acids, the most important constituent of bile, or duodenal contents on the gastric mucosa. Several groups later showed that bile acids would induce functional changes of the gastric mucosa, such as increased H^+ back-diffusion, increased Na^+ influx, decrease in transmural potential difference and cytolysis [12]. Toye and Alexander Williams [13] showed in 1965 that drainage of the duodenal afferent-loop contents of a patient with previous Billroth II gastrectomy resulted in complete relief of the distress and vomiting he experienced before the drainage. Reinfusion of saline had no effect, but reinfusion of the drained duodenal contents rapidly produced the symptoms of vomiting once more. Thus they concluded that reflux of duodenal fluid into the gastric remnant was responsible for abdominal pain and bilious vomiting.

13.1.1 Differentiation from Chronic Afferent-Loop Syndrome

Bartlett and Burrington [14] observed that the complex of symptoms associated with bilious vomiting did not require the presence of an afferent loop. In some patients it occurred after distal gastric resection with a Billroth I anastomosis; it rarely happened after vagotomy and pyloroplasty; similar observations were reported by Mackman et al. [15]. Van Heerden et al. [16] used in 1969 the term "postoperative alkaline reflux gastritis", a term which has now been widely adopted. We consider this term misleading, however, because it is not the alkalinity that causes the condition. Experimental studies have clearly shown that bile salts increase the permeability of the gastric mucosa at neutral pH, and that in the presence of acid the mucosal alterations are greater [11, 12]. Patients had severe midepigastric pain that was usually not relieved by antacids and became worse after eating, and they lost weight. Hypochlorhydria or achlorhydria was the rule. Occult blood loss produced anaemia. This gastritis at neutral pH developed over an average of 2 years after gastric resection and 22 years after gastrojejunostomy. Chronic afferent-loop syndrome and postoperative reflux gastritis may coexist, but the pain of reflux gastritis is different in character. Although aggravated by ingestion, it tends to be continuous. It is burning rather than crushing or cramping. The vomiting is not protectile and does not relieve symptoms. In a later publication [17], van Heerden et al. categorised the clinical syndrome of postoperative reflux gastritis by the following five symptoms or diagnostic findings:

1) Pain
2) Vomiting
3) Anaemia
4) Gastric hyposecretion
5) Endoscopic evidence of peristomal gastritis.

Signs and symptoms suggesting postoperative reflux gastritis are given in Table 28. Diagnostic criteria to differentiate between chronic afferent-loop syndrome and postoperative reflux gastritis are given in Table 29.

Table 28. Signs and symptoms in 42 patients with bile reflux gastritis. (After Scudamore et al., 1973)

	n	%
Pain	42	100
Nausea and vomiting	16	38
Gas-belching	13	31
Loss of weight	10	24
Anorexia	10	24
Diarrhoea	9	21
Heartburn	7	17
Sour eructations	5	12
Dumping	4	10
Dysphagia	3	7
Anaemia or vitamin B_{12} deficiency	4	10

Table 29. Clinical differences between afferent-loop syndrome and postoperative reflux gastritis

	Afferent-loop syndrome	Reflux gastritis
Pain		
Quality	Bursting, cramping, crushing, colicky	Burning, aching
Timing	Only postcibal	Continuous, aggravated by meal
Relief by vomiting	Complete and prompt	Little or none
Bilious vomiting		
Character	Postcibal projectile	Frequently both postcibal and later, less projectile
Content	Not containing food	Often containing residue of recent meal
Malnutrition	Usual and severe	Not always, less prominent

The fundamental work of physiologists on the mechanism of action of bile acids on the gastric mucosa, in conjunction with the rapid improvement in fibre-optical endoscopy, facilitated correlation of the gross morphological appearance of the mucosa with the histology of the mucosa. It thus became possible to diagnose reflux gastritis by the classic gross appearance and the histological changes noted on biopsy.

13.1.2 Measurement of Bile Reflux

Borg [18] examined the gastric juice of a large number of patients who had had gastric surgery and noted that of patients with a Billroth II operation, 25% had unstained gastric juice, in 16% it was slightly stained and in 59% it was bile-stained; nocturnal gastric juice samples even showed a bile stain in 78% of the patients examined. In normal subjects and in subjects with Billroth I gastrectomy, all the samples were either unstained or only slightly stained.

Measuring bile acid composition in a small number of patients with and without symptoms of postoperative reflux gastritis, Gadacz and Zuidema [19] did not find significant differences of total bile acid concentrations between the symptomatic and asymptomatic patients; they did, however, observe a significant increase of secondary bile acids (i.e. deoxycholic acid) in the gastric juice of symptomatic patients (Table 30). Since the secondary bile acid deoxycholic acid is a more potent damaging agent than primary bile acids, they suggested that it might be responsible for the development of bile reflux gastritis. Secondary bile acids are formed by bacterial action from primary bile acids; thus bacterial contamination of the upper intestine could contribute to the higher concentrations of secondary bile acids in reflux gastritis.

DuPlessis [4] measured the concentration of bile acid conjugates in fasting samples from six patients who had had a partial gastrectomy. Very high concentrations were observed in some patients. Kilby [20] measured duodenal gastric reflux in 30 patients with a pyloroplasty and in 15 patients after gastric resection (Billroth I) and observed reflux in all of them. He concluded that any operation on the pylorus increased the force with which reflux occurred.

Table 30. Qualitative profile of bile acids in patients with truncal vagotomy and Billroth II gastrectomy with and without symptoms of postoperative reflux gastritis. (After Gadacz, Th.R., and Zuidema, G.D., 1978)

Group	CA	CDCA	DCA	LCA
No symptoms	33%–64%	32%–56%	3%–17%	1%–13%
	86.8%		13.2%	
Symptoms	31%–33%	16%–41%	19%–44%	6%–9%
	63.7%		36.3%	

CA cholic acid; CDCA, chenodeoxycholic acid; DCA, deoxycholic acid; LCA, lithocholic acid

Table 31. Relationship between symptoms, bilirubin concentrations, radiological reflux, endoscopy, and gastroscopic biopsy in patients 1–15 years after gastric surgery with and without dyspepsia. Group A consisted of patients with a low symptom score, Group B consisted of patients with a high symptom score. Bilirubin concentration was increased in Group B, radiological evidence of reflux was present in Group B and severe gastric hyperaemia was more frequently found in Group B. (After Keighley, M.R.B., Asquith, P., Alexander-Williams, J., 1975)

	Symptoms		P
	Group A	Group B	
Maximum Bilirubin Concentration			
< 1.0 mg/100 ml	12	3	(30 cases)
> 1.0 mg/100 ml	3	12	P < 0.01
Radiological Reflux			
Absent	13	4	(26 cases)
Present	0	9	P < 0.001
Endoscopy			
Mild hyperaemia or none	13	7	(28 cases)
Severe gastric hyperaemia	1	7	P < 0.02
Histological Grading			
Gastritis:			
(a) Chronic inflammatory cell infiltrate			
Moderate/mild	5	7	
Severe	1	5	(18 cases)
(b) Acute inflammatory cells			
Minimal/absent	3	9	
Marked	3	3	NS

Keighley et al. [21] examined three groups of about 20 patients who had had gastric surgery, i.e. patients with proximal gastric vagotomy (PGV), truncal vagotomy and pyloroplasty (TV + PP) and truncal vagotomy and antrectomy (TV + A). Reflux was assessed radiologically and by measurement of bilirubin concentration in gastric contents. Radiological evidence of reflux was observed in 12% of PGV patients, 45% of TV + PP patients and 78% TV + A patients.

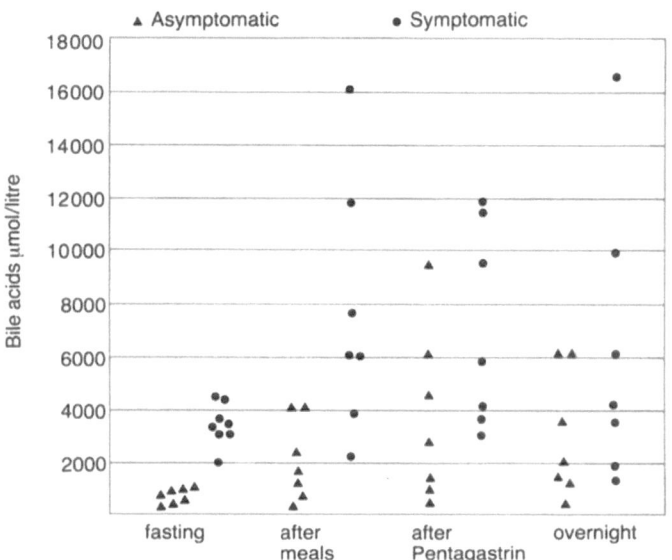

Fig. 40. Concentration of bile acids in gastric aspirates from patients fasting, after food, after penta-gastrin and overnight. The mean values of patients with and without symptoms are shown. (After Hoare et al., 1978)

The lowest concentrations of bilirubin reflecting bile reflux were observed in PGV patients. In a concomitant study they investigated possible association between duodenogastric reflux, gastritis and the symptoms of 35 patients with and without dyspepsia 1–15 years after gastric surgery. In 80% of patients with a low symptom score, bilirubin levels were less than 1 mg-%; severe endoscopic changes were observed in only one patient, and reflux in none. In contrast, in patients with a high symptom score, fluoroscopic and biochemical reflux was seen in 69% and 80% respectively, and severe mucosal hyperaemia in 50%. There was a significant correlation between symptoms, gastric hyperaemia and duodenal reflux (Table 31).

The same group of workers [22] used measurement of bile acids in fasting gastric aspirates as an objective test to quantitate bile reflux after gastric surgery. The most useful index for discriminating between symptomatic and asymptomatic patients was the amount of bile reflux in half an hour's aspiration from the fasting stomach. A "fasting bile reflux" of more than 120 µmol/h was present in 17 of the 22 symptomatic patients and in all complaining of bile regurgitation or bile vomiting. The fasting bile reflux was less than 120 µmol/h in all of the 20 asymptomatic patients (Fig. 40).

13.1.3 Experimental Results

Many attempts have been made to determine if duodenal contents are harmful to the gastric mucosa, either alone or in combination with gastric acid. The duodenal mucosa resists digestion by biliary and pancreatic juice, whereas such secretions cause damage to the skin, as seen in patients with duodenal or pancreatic fistulas. A variety of animal models have been used to study the corrosiveness of duodenal contents.

Byers and Jordan [23] anastomosed grafts from the greater curvature of the stomach to the gall bladder in dogs. No histological evidence of gastritis was found in the grafts, despite acid production and massive exposure to bile. In an experimental study in dogs, Wickbom et al. [24] diverted bile into the stomach for 4 months without producing substantial mucosal changes. In addition diversion of pancreatic juice into the stomach for 1–12 months resulted in no significant mucosal damage. Thus individual duodenal secretions produced little or no damage on contact with the gastro-intestinal mucosa.

Belowski [25] drained pure bile, pure pancreatic juice or a combination of the two into the intact stomach of dogs. Except for minimal changes around the anastomosis, gastric mucosal damage did not occur.

Sander et al. [26] studied reflux of duodenal contents into the rat stomach and did not find any changes of gastric cellular enzymatic activity. Both control and test rats showed immediate postoperative changes, such as a decrease of parietal cell mass.

Lawson [27] reported that in dogs, bile or pancreatic juice alone would cause moderate inflammatory changes around the stoma when secretions were drained into the stomach. Maximal changes occurred in antral mucosa. Combination of the two secretions would cause much more pronounced changes. The results of Lawson [27], showing that combined biliary and pancreatic secretion induced more pronounced changes in the gastric mucosa, are taken as evidence that pancreatic juice may contain an additional factor that is responsible for the histological changes of gastric mucosa seen in postoperative gastritis.

The different results by these groups may be explained in terms of the experimental procedures applied. The effect of pure bile was studied by cholecystogastrostomy to the fundus of the stomach, with ligation of the common duct; in studies on the effect of pure pancreatic secretion, a preparation was used which induced gastric hypersecretion. Lawson [28] later reported that diversion of duodenal contents from the gastric remnant by a Roux-en-Y anastomosis would reverse the mucosal changes to a normal appearance.

Menguy and Max [29] observed, in dogs, inflammatory changes in antral mucosa after prolonged exposure to bile.

Delaney et al. [30] found that bile or pancreatic juice caused minor mucosal changes in a tube made from the greater curvature of a dog's stomach. Duodenal juice, however, including biliary and pancreatic secretions resulted in more extensive gastritis.

Kirk [31] observed in rats that implantation of the bile duct into the stomach produced gastric ulcers or areas of erosion in roughly 30% of the animals.

Dragstedt et al. [32], finally, drained the full duodenal contents into the stomach of dogs and observed no histological changes in the gastric mucosa, but the portion of the jejunum adjacent to the stoma showed ulcerations.

13.1.4 Mechanisms Involved in Gastric Mucosal Damage

The normal stomach is lined with a membrane which not only protects the mucosa from ulceration, but also helps to contain secreted gastric acid within the lumen in order to facilitate initial food assimilation.

Some of the harmful consequences of bile in the stomach are due to disruption of the mucosal defence mechanism, allowing hydrogen ions to escape from the lumen, penetrate and damage the mucosa (Fig. 41).

Hollander's concept [33] of the protective action of gastric mucus was an anatomical one, in which the surface layer of mucus was continually replaced by secretions from the epithelium. This mucus layer was thought to protect the underlying mucosal cells. Bile changes the character of the gastric mucus and causes cytolysis of the epithelial cells [34]. In the intact stomach, bile strips off surface mucus and depletes the intestinal cells of their mucus content [35]. In addition to its effect on cells and mucus, bile breaks the functional barrier of the mucosal epithelial cell layer, which serves under normal conditions to resist hydrogen back-diffusion and sodium influx [11, 12].

The physiological concept of a barrier to the movement of hydrogen was established by Code at the Mayo Clinic [9] and has since been extensively investigated by Davenport [9–11]. After exposure to bile, the intact gastric mucosal membrane no longer prevents hydrogen leakage into the mucosa; an increased influx of sodium and a fall of transmural potential difference can be observed [10–12] (Fig. 42). Black, Hole and Rhodes [36] reported that the damage which follows contact with bile was related to both the concentration of bile acids and their acidity. Using three concentrations of human bile at pH 2, 4, and 8, they

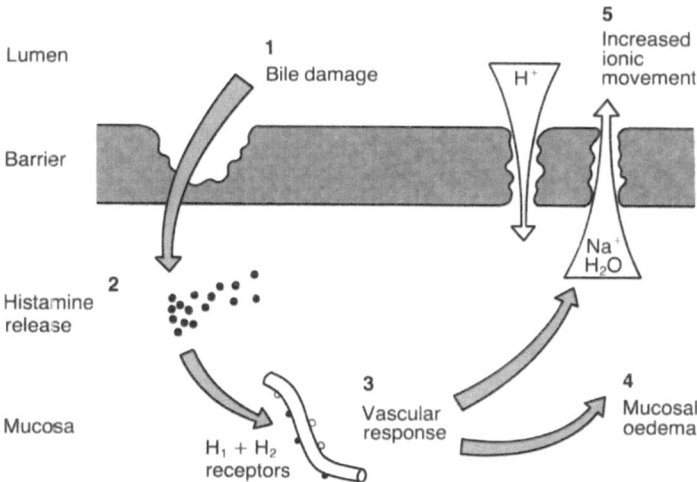

Fig. 41. Hypothetical events to explain the mechanisms involved following bile damage to the gastric mucosa. Bile acids damaging the mucosal barrier release histamine, which acts through both H_1 and H_2 receptors causing oedema and increasing ionic movement across the mucosa. The histamine may act primarily on mucosal blood vessels (After Rees, W, and Rhodes, J. [40])

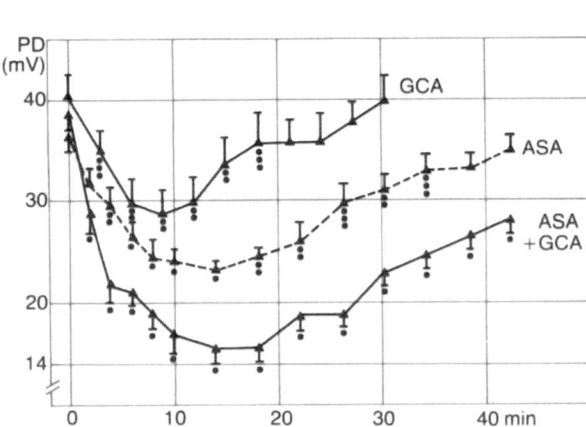

Fig. 42. Functional changes of the gastric mucosal barrier induced by the bile acid glycocholic acid (7.5 mM; GCA), acetylsalicylic acid (640 mg; ASA) and a combination of the two. Changes of transmural potential difference (PD) were recorded after intragastric instillation of GCA, ASA or both

found that damage was least at pH 8 and greatest at pH 2. These findings argue, too, against the term alkaline reflux gastritis. It is not the alkalinity which facilitates bile acid damage. More likely, bile acids induce an increased H^+ back-diffusion and thus facilitate the alkalinity. Similar results to those of Black et al. have been reported by Eastwood [37], who performed histological studies based on the appearance of surface epithelial cells. It has, however, to be admitted that the mechanism involved in damage to the mucosa by the detergent action of bile acids and the acidity of the gastric contents is not yet completely understood.

It had been claimed that histamine might play an important role for the inflammatory reactions with edema, loss of plasma protein and sometimes acute erosion of the mucosa [11, 12]. Changes in mucosal blood flow, which are difficult to measure exactly, have also been observed and seem to depend on bile acid concentration [38, 39].

Ritchie and Shearburn [39] tested recently the hypothesis that three factors are responsible for acute gastric mucosal ulcerogenesis, namely: intraluminal acid, topical bile acids capable of increasing mucosal permeability to H^+, and a concomitant gastric mucosal nutrient ischaemia. They observed that intra-arterial isoproterenol significantly protected against lesion formation induced by shock. They also observed that topical cholestyramine significantly protected against lesion formation by bile acids. Their results led to the conclusion that mitigation of both factors (topical bile acid concentration and mucosal nutrient ischaemia) achieves significant mucosal protection. We may therefore conclude that acute mucosal damage to the gastric mucosa may occur in the presence of bile acids and shock, thus showing that bile acids are important not only in the patho-genesis of postoperative reflux gastritis, but also in acute erosive gastritis.

Whether administration of H_2-receptor antagonists can prevent the increased ionic permeability which usually follows exposure of the gastric mucosa to bile acids has not yet clearly been settled. Rees et al. [40] showed that the combined use of H_1- and H_2-receptor antagonists prevented the increase in ionic permeability following exposure of a canine Heidenhain pouch to bile acids.

The following sequence of events has been suggested to be reponsible for gastric intestinal mucosal damage induced by bile acids [12] (Fig. 41). Bile acids, especially at low pH values, damage the surface epithelial cells and diffuse across the mucosa [41, 42], causing the release of histamine [43]. Histamine acting on H_1- and H_2-receptors of mucosal blood vessels increases the permeability of capillaries, leading to oedema, with increase in the flux of both hydrogen and sodium across the mucosa. Back-diffusion of hydrogen is considered an additional factor causing damage. Thus histamine may play the role of a mediator for the increased ionic permeability of the gastric mucosa induced by bile acids (Fig. 41).

13.1.5 Lysolecithin – a Pathogenetic Factor?

Since several investigators showed that duodenal juice was more injurious to the gastric mucosa than bile alone, other factors have been looked for which in conjunction with bile acids might be responsible for mucosal damage induced by reflux of duodenal contents. One of the pancreatic factors discussed is lysolecithin, which is formed in the duodenum when phospholipase A of the pancreatic juice hydrolyses lecithin in bile. This reaction is activated by bile acids and trypsin (Fig. 43). Lecithin may be further hydrolysed to glycerylcholine by phospholipase B, a reaction inhibited by bile acids.

Lysolecithin is highly toxic to cell membranes [44], has strong detergent properties, like bile acids, and was shown to damage the gastric mucosal barrier [45].

Lysolecithin has been shown to be present in gastric juice [46, 47] in patients with stress ulcers [48] or after gastric resections.

Johnson and McDermott [46] observed up to tenfold increases of lysolecithin concentrations in patients with gastric ulcer, and in four patients with two recurrent gastric ulcers after surgery with destroyed pylorus they reported more

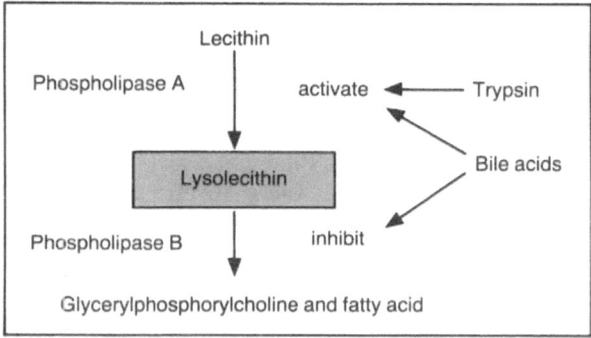

Fig. 43. Metabolic pathways of lysolecithin. (After Johnson and McDermott, 1974)

than tenfold increases of mean peak lysolecithin concentrations in the gastric juice. There are, however, no clear-cut correlations between measurements of bile acid reflux, lysolecithin concentrations and the presence of postoperative reflux gastritis.

13.2 Symptoms and Diagnosis

The diagnosis of postoperative reflux gastritis is based primarily on a thorough and careful history of the onset and course of the illness, confirmed by endoscopic appearance and histopathological study of the gastric mucosa. The two basic complaints of the patients are the same as those of patients with chronic afferent-loop syndrome, namely upper abdominal pain and bilious vomiting. It has also to be remembered that the two syndromes may coexist.

The quality of the pain is different. Whereas the chronic afferent-loop syndrome patient complaints of crushing, bursting, cramping or colicky pain, the reflux gastritis patient complaints of a burning distress or pain. Pain may be similar to previous duodenal ulcer pain, but it is not relieved by antacids and is aggravated by food intake.

Reflux gastritis patients have more persistent and often continuous pain, aggravated by food intake. Their weight loss is, however, mostly less pronounced than that of patients with chronic afferent-loop syndrome. The bilious vomiting is also different. The patient with postoperative reflux gastritis vomits frequently, unpredictably and at any time, even at night, and the vomit usually contains considerable amounts of the previously ingested meal, whereas postcibal projectile vomiting not containing food is typical for the chronic afferent-loop syndrome.

Fluoroscopic examination may give information on the presence of an afferent-loop syndrome or gastric emptying. A basal gastric acid analysis or a stimulatory gastric analysis may be difficult to perform because of the heavy bile-staining of the aspirates in patients with reflux gastritis. These patients, however, usually have basal anacidity and only minimal response to stimulation.

The most important diagnostic step in confirming the diagnosis of reflux gastritis is a gastroscopy combined with mucosal biopsy. The gross appearance of the mucosa in the body of the stomach or the gastric remnant is characteristic in patients with reflux gastritis. In contrast to the afferent-loop syndrome, in which mucosal changes are confined to the peristomal regions, a diffuse process is noted in reflux gastritis. Frequent suctioning may be necessary to obtain optimal vision, owing to heavy bile-stained reflux into the gastric remnant. The mucosa is erythematous and friable and bleeds readily on contact with the endoscope. Superficial erosions may be seen with interdispersed areas of atrophy, allowing one to see submucosal blood vessels. Microscopic examinations of biopsy specimens will reveal the following pathological findings: absence of parietal chief cells, ulcerations of superficial mucosa, haemorrhage and atrophy, and chronic inflammation with cell infiltrates of lymphocytes.

13.3 Medical Treatment

Medical treatment of postoperative reflux gastritis has been tried, but it is not considered very successful. Even dietary means, which are so important in the treatment of the dumping syndrome, are mostly without any effect. A logical therapeutical approach would be to use binding agents for bile acids. Cholestyramine has therefore been used by several groups. Scudamore et al. [49] reported successful results with cholestyramine (Table 32), but others were disappointed by this kind of treatment. A recent randomized, double-blind trial on the effect of cholestyramine on the symptoms of reflux gastritis in 16 patients showed no differences in frequency of abdominal pain, nausea, vomiting and bitter taste compared to the placebo period [50]. Several possible explanations have been offered for the therapeutical failure of cholestyramine in reflux gastritis: the dose used (3×4 g$= 12$ g) might not have been large enough, or the presence of the resin in the stomach might have been too short to protect the gastric mucosa from bile acids. A low intragastric pH [51] and perhaps other unknown factors might interfere with the binding of cholestyramine and bile salts. Our observations on the effect of bile acids in the normal stomach have shown that 5 or 7.5 mM glycocholic acid or taurocholic acid markedly reduced transmural potential difference. Simultaneous administration of cholestyramine (4 g) was not able significantly to reduce changes in potential difference evoked by glycocholic acid (Fig. 44), but simultaneous administration of a potent antacid containing magnesium and aluminium hydroxides did reduce the drop in transmural potential difference induced by the glycocholic acid (Fig. 45), the transmural potential difference being taken as a parameter for the integrity of the gastric mucosal barrier. The experimental design for the measurement of transmural gastric potential difference is shown in Fig. 46. Antacids containing aluminium hydroxide have potent bile acid binding properties [51a]. It was concluded that the binding properties of cholestyramine are too weak at the low pH of gastric juice. Whether reduced acidity in reflux gastritis might account for better binding of bile acids to cholestyramine has not yet been established. It seems that the most likely explanation for the

Table 32. Results of medical treatment of bile reflux gastritis with cholestyramine. (After Scudamore et al., 1973)

Condition		Number of patients
Incomplete information		8
Ulcer treatment, sedation		5
Good results	0	
Fair results	2	
Poor results	3	
Cholestyramine treatment		20
Good results	10	
Fair results	4	
Poor results	6	

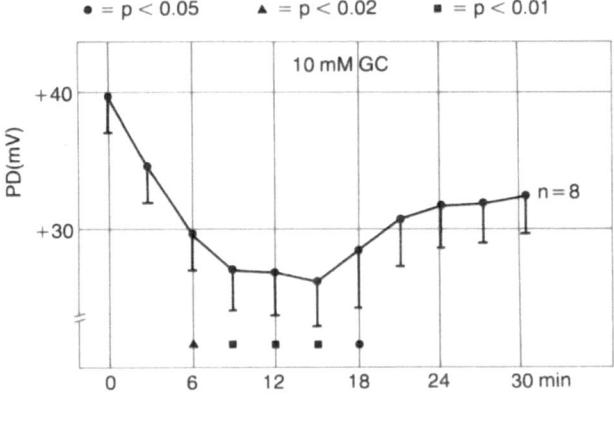

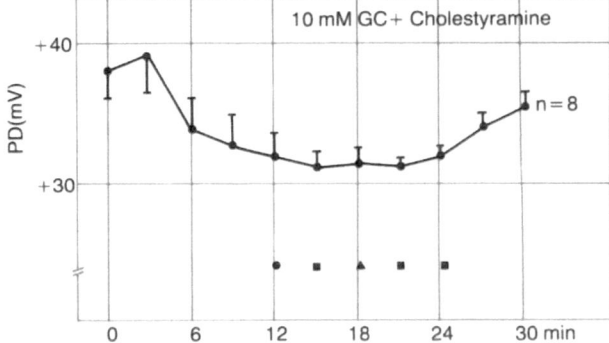

Fig. 44. Time course of intragastric transmural potential difference (PD) after instillation of 100 ml of 10 mM glycocholic acid (GCA) alone or together with 4 g cholestyramine. PD is still significantly reduced in the presence of cholestyramine. Ordinate: PD (serosa: positive) in mV. Given are means ± SEM, $n = 8$

failure of treatment of reflux gastritis with cholestyramine is that cholestyramine was given only three times per day, whereas reflux occurs continuously. It may be that larger doses, more frequently administered, different time schedules, longer treatment periods and possibly additional antacids (Fig. 47), might be effective, but constipation, which often occurs after only 12 or 16 g of treatment with cholestyramine, may limit patient compliance with such regimens.

Total parenteral nutrition has been advocated, even as a diagnostic procedure [52]. If anaemia is present, substitution of iron and/or vitamin B_{12} is indicated. One of the side-effects of cholestyramine treatment due to increased elimination of bile acids is hypocholesterinaemia and deficiency of fat-soluble vitamins (vitamins A, D, E. K), which should be supplemented parenterally if long-term treatment with cholestyramine is performed. Since cholestyramine may interfere with the absorption of other drugs (i.e. digitoxin) careful consideration has to be given to the dose of other drugs which are urgently necessary.

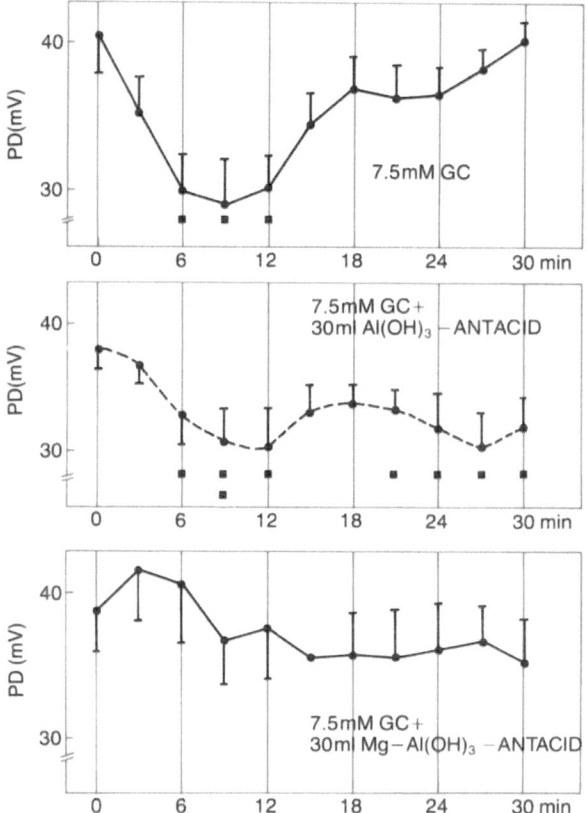

Fig. 45. Time course of transmural potential difference (PD) after intragastric instillation of 100 ml 7.5 mM glycocholic acid (GCA) plus 30 ml water (upper graph) and after administration of 100 ml 7.5 mM GCA with either 30 ml of a liquid antacid (Aludrox) containing $Al(OH)_3$ (*middle graph*) or 30 ml of a liquid antacid (Maaloxan) containing $Mg(OH)_2$ and $Al(OH)_3$ (*lower graph*). The potent antacid containing $Mg(OH)_2$ and $Al(OH)_3$ prevents the GCA-induced drop of transmural PD. Ordinate: PD (serosa: positive) in mV. $*p = <0.05$, $**p = <0.02$

13.4 Surgical Treatment

Careful consideration has been given to the patients' symptoms and their duration. A certain percentage with symptoms of reflux gastritis will spontaneously improve. Patients who have lost weight or who are incapacitated by their symptoms and patients showing bleeding and/or microcytic anaemia should be considered for operation.

Two surgical approaches are possible. In the Henley-Soupault procedure (Fig. 48), an isoperistaltic jejunal loop is interposed between stomach and duodenum, thereby increasing the distance involved in reflux to the stomach. The interposed jejunal segment should be 25 cm long. In the Roux-en-Y procedure, the bile is diverted from the stomach (Fig. 49). For this operation to be effective,

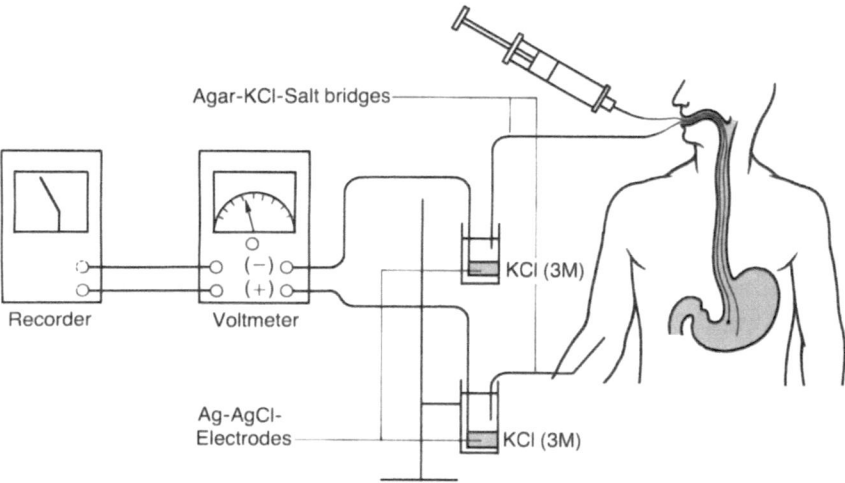

Fig. 46. Experimental design for measurement of gastric transmural potential difference in humans. A biluminal tube is placed into the fundus of the stomach. One tube is used for intragastric instillation, the other one is filled with 3M KCl and 1.5% agar and serves as a luminal electrode. The peripheral electrode consists of a butterfly filled with 3M KCl and 1.5% agar placed in a peripheral vein. Both salt bridges are connected via KCl-containing beakers with silver/silver chloride electrodes to a voltmeter and recorder

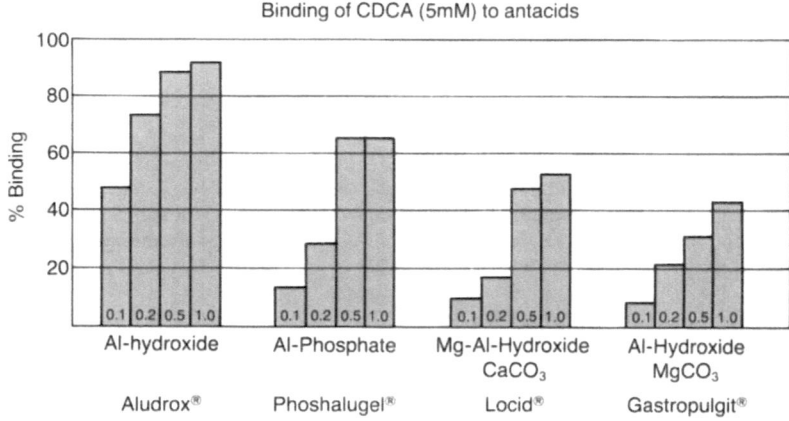

Fig. 47. Binding of chenodeoxycholic acid (CDCA) in vitro to various aluminium-containing commercial German antacids. Binding of 5 mM CDCA was measured in a volume of 5 ml which contained 0 1–1.0 ml of the commercial liquid antacids

the length of jejunum from stomach to the Roux-en-Y anastomosis should be at least 60 cm.

The Henley-Soupault procedure is more difficult and risky than the Roux-en-Y (see Sect. 3.1.4.2b and c). Most groups seem to prefer the Roux-en-Y procedure, which has given good-to-excellent results in 125 of 135 patients (92.6%), if the operative results of several groups are taken together (Table 33).

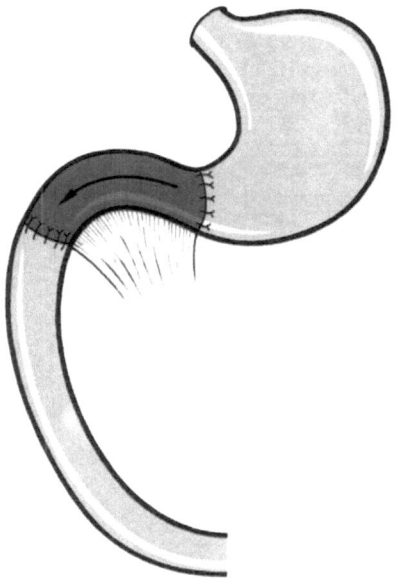

Fig. 48. Interposition of an isoperistaltic loop in the treatment of reflux gastritis

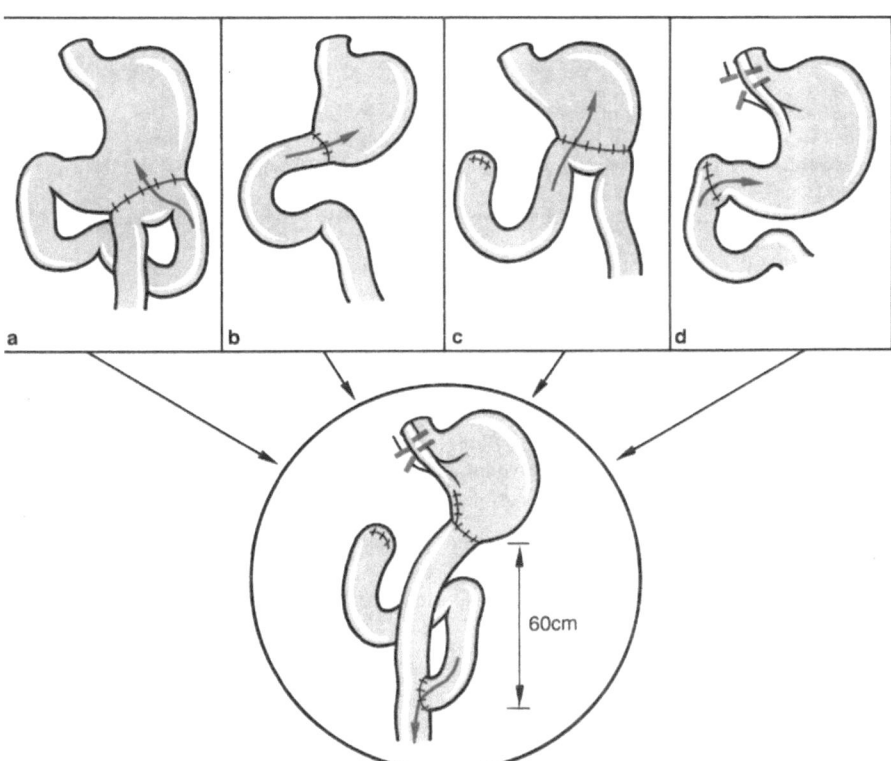

Fig. 49 a–d. Roux-en-Y anastomosis in the treatment of alkaline reflux gastritis

Table 33. Surgical treatment of postoperative alkaline reflux gastritis. Comparison of results using the jejunal loop interposition or the Roux-en-Y duodenal diversion in the treatment of alkaline reflux gastritis

	Results good to excellent	
	Jejunal loop	Roux-en-Y
Van Heerden et al. [16]	6/12 (50%)	26/31 (84%)
Herrington et al. [53]	18/20 (90%)	27/27 (100%)
Drapanas and Bethea [54]	3/ 3 (100%)	14/15 (93%)
Joseph et al. [55]	—	11/11 (100%)
Bushkin and Woodward [56]	4/10 (40%)	24/25 (96%)
Coppinger et al. [57]	—	23/26 (88%)
Totals	31/45 (69%)	125/135 (93%)

References

1. Beaumont, W.: Experiments and observations on the gastric juice and the physiology of digestion. 2nd Edition New York: Dover
2. Schindler, R.: Gastroscopic observations in resected stomachs. Am. J. Dig. Dis. 7, 505 (1940)
3. Brown, D.C., McHardy, G.: Postgastrectomy gastritis. Ann. int. Med. 20, 789 (1944)
4. du Plessis, D.J.: The importance of the pyloric antrum in peptic ulceration. South African J. Surgery 1, 3–11 (1963)
5. du Plessis, D.J.: Pathogenesis of gastric ulceration. Lancet I, 974 (1965)
6. Wells, C.A., Welbourne, R.: Postgastrectomy syndromes. Brit. Med. J. 1, 546 (1951)
7. Woodward, E.R.: The pathophysiology of the afferent loop syndrome. Surg. Clin, North Amer. 46, 411 (1966)
8. Capper, W.M., Butler, T.J.A.: A clinical study of the early postgastrectomy syndrome. Brit. Med. J. 2, 265 (1951)
9. Davenport, H.W., Warner, H.A., Code, C.F.: Functional significance of the gastric mucosal barrier to sodium. Gastroenterology 47, 142 (1964)
10. Davenport, H.W.: Destruction of the gastric mucosal barrier by detergents and urea. Gastroenterology 54, 175 (1968)
11. Davenport, H.W.: The gastric mucosal barrier. Digestion 5, 162 (1972)
12. Rees, W., Rhodes, J.: Bile reflux in gastroesophageal disease. In: Clinics in Gastroenterology; G. Paumgartner, ed., Vol. 6, 179 (1977)
13. Toye, D.K.M., Alexander-Williams, J.A : Post-gastrectomy bile vomiting. Lancet II, 524 (1965)
14. Bartlett, M.K., Burrington, J.D.: Bilious vomiting after gastric surgery. Arch. Surg. 79, 34 (1968)
15. Mackman, S., Lemmer, K.E., Morrissey, J.F.: Postoperative reflux alkali gastritis and esophagitis. Am. J. Surg. 121, 694 (1971)
16. van Heerden, J.A., Priestley, J.A., Farrow, G.M., Phillips, S.F.: Postoperative reflux gastritis – surgical implications. Am. J. Surg. 118, 427 (1969)
17. van Heerden, J.A., Phillips, S.F., Adson, M.A., McIllrath, D.C.: Postoperative reflux gastritis. Am. J. Surg. 129, 82 (1975)
18. Borg, I.: Bile admixture in gastric juice in health and in peptic ulcer before and after operation according to Billroth II and Billroth I. Acta Chir. Scand. (Supplement) 251, 97 (1959)
19. Gadacz, Th.R., Zuidema, G.D.: Bile acid composition in patients with and without symptoms of postoperative reflux gastritis. Am. J. Surg. 135, 48 (1978)
20. Kilby, J.O.: Duodenogastric reflux and pyloric surgery. Gastroenterology 58, 594 (1970)
21. Keighley, M.R.B., Asquith, P., Alexander-Williams, J.: Duodenogastric reflux: a cause of gastric mucosal hyperemia and symptoms after operations for peptic ulceration. Gut 16, 28 (1975)

22. Hoare, A.M., Keighley, M.R.B., Storkey, B., Alexander-Williams, J.: Measurement of bile acids in fasting gastric aspirates: an objective test for bile reflux after gastric surgery. Gut 19, 166 (1978).

23. Byers, F.M., Jordan, P.H.: Effect of bile upon gastric mucosa. Proc. Exp. Biol. Med. 110, 864 (1962)

24. Wickbom, G., Bushkin, F.L., Linares, C. et al.. On the corrosive properties of bile and pancreatic juice on living tissue in dogs. Arch. Surg. 108, 680 (1974)

25. Belowski, H.: Does the duodenal content exert a harmful effect on the gastric mucosa? Gastroenterologia 98, 233 (1962)

26. Sander, S., Myren, J., Helsingen, N.: The effect of bile reflux on the gastric mucosa. Gastroenterologia 101, 3 (1964)

27. Lawson, H.H.: Effect of duodenal contents on the gastric mucosa under experimental conditions. Lancet I, 469 (1964)

28. Lawson, H.H.: The reversibility of postgastrectomy alkaline gastritis by a Roux-en-Y-loop. Brit. J. Surg. 59, 13 (1972)

29. Menguy, R., Max, M.H.: Influence of bile on the canine gastric antral mucosa. Am. J. Surg. 125, 29 (1973)

30. Delaney, J.P., Butler, B.A., Cheng, J.W.B., et al.: Gastritis induced by intestinal juices. Bull. Soc. Int. Chir. 3, 176 (1972)

31. Kirk, R.M.: Experimental gastric ulcers in the rat; the separate and combined effects of vagotomy and bile duct implantation into the stomach. Brit. J. Surg. 57, 521 (1970)

32. Dragstedt, L.R., Woodward, E.R., Seito, T., et al.: The question of bile regurgitation as a cause of gastric ulcer. Ann. Surg. 174, 548 (1971)

33. Hollander, F.: The mucosa barrier in the stomach in peptic ulcer. W.B. Saunders, Philadelphia, 65 (1951)

34. Grant, R., Grossman, M.I., Wang, K.J., Ivy, A.C.: The cytolytic action of some gastro-intestinal secretions and enzymes on the epithelial cells of the gastric and duodenal mucosa. J. Cell. Comp. Physiol. 37, 137–161 (1951)

35 van Geertruyden, J.: Altérations de la physiologie gastrique sous l'influence de la bile. Leur importance pour la pathogénie de l'ulcère peptique récidivant après gastrectomie. Bull. de l'Academie Roy. Médicine de la Belgique 1, 53 (1961)

36. Black, R.B., Hole, D., Rhodes, J.: Bile damage to the gastric mucosal barrier: the effect of pH and bile acid concentration. Gastroenterology 61, 178 (1971)

37. Eastwood, G.L.: Effect of pH on bile salt injury to mouse gastric mucosa. Gastroenterology 68, 1456–1465 (1975)

38. Ritchie, W.R., Shearburn, E.W.: Acute gastric mucosal ulcerogenesis is dependent on the concentration of bile salts. Surgery 80, 98 (1976)

39. Ritchie, W.P., Shearburn, E.W.: Influence of isoproterenol and cholestyramine on acute gastric mucosal ulcerogenesis. Gastroenterology 73, 62 (1977)

40. Rees, W., Rhodes, J.: Bile reflux in gastrooesophageal disease. In: Clinics in Gastroenterology. p. 179. London: W.B. Saunders 1977

41. Davenport, H.W.: Absorption of taurocholate 24 ^{14}C through the canine gastric mucosa. Proc. Soc. Exp. Biol. Med. 125, 670 (1967)

42. Ivey, K.J., DenBesten, L., Bell, S.: Absorption of bile salts from human gastric mucosa. J. Appl. Physiol. 29, 806 (1976)

43. Johnson, A.R., Moran, N.C.: Release of histamine from rat mast cells: a comparison of the effects of 48/80 and two antigen-antibody systems. Fed. Proc. 28, 1716 (1969)

44. Gottfried, E.L., Rapport, M.M.: The biochemistry of plasmalogens: 2. haemolytic activity of some plasmalogen derivatives. J. Lipid. Res. 4, 57 (1963)

45. Davenport, H.W.. Effect of lysolecithin, digitonin and phospholipase A upon dog's gastric mucosal barrier. Gastroenterology 59, 505 (1970)

46. Johnson, A.G., McDermott, S.J.: Lysolecithin: a factor in the pathogenesis of gastric ulceration. Gut 15, 710–713 (1974)

47. Clemençon, G., Bürgi, W., Kaufmann, H.: Lysolecithin im Mageninhalt. Z. Gastroent. 13, 1 (1975)

48. Schumpelick, V., Begemann, F., Bandomer, G., Großner, D., Doehn, M.: Intragastrale Gallensauren und Lysolecithin bei klinischer Streßulkus-Gefährdung. Dtsch. med. Wschr. 103, 735 (1978)

49. Scudamore, H.H., Eckstam, E.E., Fencil, W.J., Jaramillo, C.A.: Bile reflux gastritis. Am. J. Gastroent. 60, 9 (1973)

50. Meshkinpour, H , Elashoff, H., Stewart, H., Sturdevant, R A.L.: Effect of cholestyramine on the symptoms of reflux gastritis. A randomized double blind crossover study Gastroenterology *73*, 441–443 (1977)

51a. Caspary, W.F., Graf, S . Bindung von Gallensauren an Antacida. Dtsch. Med. Woschr. *103*, 825 (1978)

51. Eastwood, G.L.: Failure of cholestyramine to prevent bile salt injury to mouse gastric mucosa. Gastroenterology *68*, 1466 (1975)

52. Anderson, D.L., Boyce, A W. Use of parenteral hyperalimentation in the diagnosis and treatment of alkaline reflux gastritis. Gastrointestinal Endoscopy *20*, 15 (1973)

53. Herrington Jr., J L , Sawyers, J.L., Whitehead, W.A : Surgical management of reflux gastritis. Ann. Surg. *180*, 526 (1974)

54. Drapanas, T., Bethea, M · Reflux gastritis following gastric surgery. Ann. Surg. *179*, 618–627 (1974)

55. Joseph, W.L., Rivera, R A , O'Kieffe, D.A., et al.· Management of postoperative alkaline reflux gastritis. Ann. Surg. *177*, 655 (1973)

56. Bushkin, F.L., Woodward, E.R.. Alkaline reflux gastritis. In Postgastrectomy syndromes. Bushkin, F.L., Woodward, E.R. (eds), p 49 Philadelphia. W.B. Saunders 1976

57. Coppinger, W R., Job, H , De Lauro, J.E , et al.. Surgical treatment of reflux gastritis and esophagitis. Arch. Surg. *106*, 463 (1973)

14 Postoperative Reflux Oesophagitis

14.1 Incidence

The postoperative syndrome of reflux oesophagitis is now being more frequently recognised in patients after gastric surgery, owing to the development of modern gastro-intestinal endoscopy. Scott and Longmire [1] recognised in 1949 that heartburn and dysphagia were frequent after total gastrectomy. They attributed these symptoms to regurgitation of bile and pancreatic juice into the oesophagus. It was later reported by Longmire and Beal [2] and by Helsingen [3] that reconstruction of a Braun entero-anastomosis between the afferent and efferent limbs of the oesophagojejunostomy resulted in reduced incidence of oesophageal reflux symptoms. Helsingen [3] reported in 1959, in a follow-up examination of nine patients who had undergone total gastrectomy 5 years previously, the presence of mild to moderate oesophagitis in eight of the nine patients. The frequency with which oesophageal stenosis occurs after oesophagogastric operations had already been pointed out by Barrett and Franklin [4] and Ripley et al. [5]. The occurrence of oesophageal strictures after uncomplicated partial gastrectomy had been reported by Douglas [6] and McKeown [7] and oesophageal strictures after partial gastrectomy with complications had been reported by Benedict and Daland [8] and Craighead [9]. Oesophageal strictures after gastrojejunostomy had been reported by several other authors [10–15].

Postoperative reflux oesophagitis was also seen after total gastrectomy with loop oesophagojejunostomy [3, 5, 16, 17]. Paulson [18], using endoscopic methods, observed that oesophagitis began early after total gastrectomy, and Nissen described strictures occurring within a few months after total gastrectomy.

Postoperative reflux oesophagitis after lesser gastric procedures was first described by McKeown in 1958 [7]. He reported two patients with oesophageal stricture after Polya partial gastrectomy. Conversion to gastroduodenostomy and bougienage of the stricture were effective in both cases. Reflux of alkaline duodenal material was considered to have been the cause. Cox [19] reported later three cases with oesophageal stricture after partial gastrectomy. He also suggested that oesophageal strictures were caused by regurgitation of alkaline-tryptic jejunal content into the oesophagus [19].

That postoperative reflux oesophagitis was not a rare condition as later pointed out by Windsor [20], who studied 61 unselected patients undergoing distal partial gastrectomy and reported that 50% of Billroth I patients and 27% of Billroth II patients had radiological evidence of reflux. Thirty per cent of the Billroth I group and 20% of the Billroth II group complained of heartburn. Only very few patients had a demonstrable hiatal hernia. Himal and MacLean [21] and Coppinger et al. [22] reported in 1973 that these patients could be successfully treated by Roux-en-Y diversion of duodenal contents.

14.2 Pathogenesis

The pathogenesis of the destructive mucosal changes seen in postoperative reflux oesophagitis remains unclear and controversial. Experimental results in animals have produced conflicting and variable results. Cross and Wangensteen [23] demonstrated in cats and dogs that either bile or pancreatic juice or mixture of the two caused erosions of the oesophagus. They suggested that a Roux-en-Y reconstruction should be used in total gastrectomy to avoid reflux of duodenal contents. Bleeding from erosions resulted in anaemia. Moffat et al. [24] demonstrated in dogs that whole bile and extracted bile salts were able to produce severe erosive oesophagitis, independently of the pH and in the absence of pancreatic juice.

Redo and Barnes [25] showed in the dog that bile did not produce oesophagitis, but that gastric juice induced deep penetrating ulcers. Gastric juice mixed with duodenal contents or duodenal contents alone produced only superficial linear oesophagitis. Dragstedt et al. [26] drained duodenal secretions into the oesophagus using a jejunal conduit and found no significant oesophagitis in 2–7 months. Helsingen [27] found the rat to be a better model animal. After total gastrectomy, typical oesophagitis developed in all animals in which oesophago-intestinal reconstruction permitted regurgitation of duodenal secretions into the oesophagus. Severe oesophagitis was found in oesophagoduodenostomy, oesophagojejunostomy, oesophagojejunostomy and Braun entero-anastomosis. The performance of a Roux-en-Y type of reconstruction or interposition of a large jejunal segment between oesophagus and duodenum could prevent oesophagitis in long-term follow-up studies in rats. Lambert [28] observed in rats that pancreatic juice, more than bile, produced severe oesophagitis, but pure acid had no damaging effect.

Gillison [29] compared the effects of bile-free and bile-contaminated unaltered gastric juice on oesophageal mucosa in Rhesus monkeys after performing an operation promoting reflux to the oesophagus (oesophagogastrostomy, after resecting 1 cm of proximal stomach and 2 cm of distal oesophagus). Oesophagitis was rare when pure gastric juice refluxed, but all degrees of oesophagitis were produced when bile-contaminated gastric juice was allowed to reflux up the oesophagus. Oesophagitis occurring after gastric surgery most likely results from reflux of duodenal contents. Regurgitation of duodenal contents or bilious vomiting is fairly common. In the Leeds/York trial, bilious vomiting occurred in about 10% to 15% of patients who had undergone subtotal gastrectomy or vagotomy with drainage or antrectomy [30, 31]. Unfortunately there are few oesophageal manometric studies in patients undergoing gastric operations.

Weakening of the lower oesophageal sphincter has been reported to occur after partial gastrectomy [32], but the effects of truncal vagotomy on the sphincter are controversial [33–35]. There is evidence that vagotomy per se does not increase the tendency for gastro-oesophageal reflux [34, 35]. It seems likely that regurgitation or vomiting of duodenal contents results in a decrease of the lower oesophageal sphincter pressure, since experimental induction of oesophagitis lowers the sphincter pressure [36].

14.3 History and Clinical Symptoms

The clinical history of patients with postoperative reflux oesophagitis is similar to that of patients with peptic reflux oesophagitis. The patients complain primarily of heartburn, substernal burning sensations occurring most dramatically postprandially and aggravated by reclining positions. The history differs, however, in some respects from peptic reflux oesophagitis: the patient has had gastric surgery for ulcer and has no hiatal hernia, the pain often persists between meals and is merely aggravated be meals, and pain may be experienced on swallowing. Since the patient avoids meals, malnutrition may be a consequence. Antacid therapy as used in peptic oesophagitis is not effective, and even cholestyramine, known to bind bile acids potently, at least at neutral pH, is not effective in most cases.

An interesting study was recently published by Pellegrini et al. [37]. In 100 patients with symptoms of gastro-oesophageal reflux, they monitored the pH of the lower oesophagus over 24 h. On the basis of this 24-h monitoring, they divided the patients into four groups: acid refluxers (51), acid-alkaline refluxers (25), alkaline refluxers (6), and non-refluxers (18). Alkaline refluxers had a lesser incidence of heartburn, but a greater incidence of regurgitation. Similar incidences of oesophagitis were seen in all refluxer groups. The mean lower oesophageal sphincter pressure was significantly lower in refluxers than in asymptomatic patients. Among the 100 patients studied, vagotomy and drainage procedure had been previously performed in 6 of the 25 (24%) acid-alkaline refluxers, 1 of the 6 alkaline refluxers (17%) and 1 of the 51 acid refluxers (2%). It was concluded by the authors that symptomatic gastro-oesophageal reflux is a mixture of both acid and alkaline secretions, with one or both abnormal owing to different degrees of acid production and pyloric regurgitation. Patients with alkaline reflux may develop serious complications of reflux in the absence of typical symptoms of heartburn.

Complications include strictures and haemorrhage, but acute haemorrhage is less common than in peptic reflux oesophagitis; chronic blood loss may result in iron-deficiency anaemia. Endoscopy is the most important diagnostic procedure. Mucosal changes are often severe and diffusely spread over the mucosa, which is dark, necrotic and extremely friable. Endoscopy will not, however, be able to differentiate between alkaline and peptic reflux oesophagitis. History of previous gastric surgery and a gastric analysis will help to establish the diagnosis. Owing to the presence of heavily bile-stained regurgitated duodenal juice, gastric analysis may be difficult to interpret, but the presence of acid after histalog or pentagastrin stimulation casts doubt on the condition's being postoperative alkaline reflux oesophagitis. The diagnosis of alkaline or peptic reflux oesophagitis has to be established with certainty, because any operation performed to prevent reflux, such as the Roux-en-Y anastomosis or the interposition of a jejunal segment, may provoke peptic ulcer.

14.4 Therapy

Cross and Wangensteen [23] suggested that a Roux-en-Y anastomosis should prevent reflux. Animal experiments by Helsingen [27] demonstrated clearly that a Roux-en-Y anastomosis in rats was able to prevent injurious mucosal changes induced by bile acids. The principle proved valid in man. Bushkin and Woodward [38] reported on 18 operative procedures in 15 patients with reflux oesophagitis, performed from 1958 to 1974. Isoperistaltic jejunal interposition or Henley loop procedures resulted in a recurrence of reflux oesophagitis in two of five patients. Ten patients were treated by a Roux-en-Y duodenal diversion, and the operation followed by prompt disappearance of the endoscopically visible gross microscopical changes of the oesophageal mucosa. The authors concluded that the Roux-en-Y anastomosis with its more extensive diversion of duodenal contents was more effective in treating postoperative reflux oesophagitis than the interposition of a jejunal segment. Thus the most effective operation for reflux oesophagitis after gastric surgery is one that effectively diverts duodenal contents from the oesophagus. This is best accomplished by a Roux-en-Y procedure [22, 39]. In order to be effective the distance between the oesophageal anastomosis and the jejunostomy of the Roux-en-Y drainage must be at least 60 cm, in order to ensure prevention of reflux [40].

References

1. Scott, H.W. Jr., Longmire, W.P. Jr.: Total gastrectomy. Surgery 26, 488 (1949)
2. Longmire, W.P. Jr., Beal, J.M.: Construction of a substitute gastric reservoir following total gastrectomy. Ann. Surg. 135, 637 (1952)
3. Helsingen, N. Jr.: Oesophagitis following total gastrectomy: a follow-up study on nine patients five years or more after operation. Acta chirurg. Scand. 118, 190 (1959)
4. Barrett, N.R., Franklin, R.H.: Concerning the unfavourable late results of certain operations performed in the treatment of cardiospasm. Brit. J. Surgery 37, 194 (1949)

5. Ripley, H.R., Olsen, A.M., Kirklin, J.W.: Esophagitis after esophagogastric anastomosis. Surgery *32*, 1 (1952)
6. Douglas, W.K.: Oesophageal strictures associated with gastroduodenal intubation. Brit. J. Surgery *43*, 404 (1956)
7. McKeown, K.C.: Oesophageal stenosis after partial gastrectomy. Brit. Med. J. *2*, 819 (1959)
8. Benedict, E.B., Daland, E.M : Benign stricture of the esophagus complicating duodenal ulcer. New Engl. J. Med. *218*, 599 (1938)
9. Craighead, C.C.: Esophagitis: a review with special reference to effects of subtotal gastrectomy on esophagitis. Amer. J. Surg. *20*, 760 (1954)
10. Klein, L., Hochbaum, W.: Stenosing esophagitis associated with duodenal ulcer. Am. J. Roentgenol. *42*, 724 (1939)
11 Larson, E.M., Layne, J.A., Howard, L.C.: Benign stricture of esophagus: complication of duodenal ulcer. Lancet *62*, 304 (1942)
12. Paul, L.W.: Roentgenologic aspects of acute and chronic esophagitis. Radiology *41*, 421 (1943)
13. Bergquist, B.: Contribution to the question of limited oesophagitis. Acta oto-laryng. *34*, 256 (1949)
14. Allison, P.R.: Peptic ulcer of the oesophagus. Thorax *3*, 20 (1948)
15. Bingham, J.A.W.: Oesophageal strictures after gastric surgery and naso-gastric intubation. Brit. Med. J. *2*, 817 (1958)
16. Kelly, W.D., MacLean, L.D., Perry, J.F., Wangensteen, O.H.: A study of patients following total or near-total gastrectomy. Surgery *35*, 964 (1954)
17. Pontes, J.E., Polak, M., Campos, C.: Total gastrectomy Physiopathology, symptomatology and medical management. Gastroenterologia *85*, 80 (1956)
18. Paulson, M.: Peroral jejunoscopy and duodenoscopy. Endoscopy of the uppermost small intestine Gastroenterology *23*, 593 (1953)
19 Cox, K.R.: Oesophageal stricture after partial gastrectomy. Brit. J Surg. *49*, 307 (1961)
20. Windsor, C.W.O.: Gastro-oesophageal reflux after partial gastrectomy. Brit. Med. J. *2*, 1233 (1964)
21. Himal, H.S., MacLean, L.D.: Bile esophagitis. Can. J. Surg. *16*, 1 (1973)
22. Coppinger, W.R., de Lauro, J.E., Westerbuhr, L.M., McGlone, F B., Phillips, R.G.: Surgical treatment of reflux gastritis and oesophagitis. Arch. Surgery *106*, 463 (1973)
23. Cross, F.S., Wangensteen, O.H.: Role of bile and pancreatic juice in production of esophageal erosions and anemia. Proc. Exp. Biol Med. *77*, 862 (1951)
24. Moffat, R.C., Berkas, E.M.: Bile esophagitis. Arch. Surg. *91*, 963 (1965)
25. Redo, S.F., Barnes, W.A.: Effects of the secretions of the stomach, duodenum, jejunum and the colon on the esophagus of dogs. Surg. Gynecol. Obstet. *106*, 337 (1958)
26. Dragstedt, L.R , Woodward, E.R , Seito, T., et al.· The question of bile regurgitation as a cause of gastric ulcer. Ann Surg *174*, 548 (1971)
27. Helsingen, N , Jr.: Oesophagitis following total gastrectomy; a clinical and experimental study. Acta chirurg. Scand. Suppl. *273*, 1 (1961)
28 Lambert, R.: Relative importance of biliary and pancreatic secretions in the genesis of esophagitis in rats. Am. J Dig. Dis. *7*, 1026 (1962)
29. Gillison, E.W., de Castro, V.A.M., Nyhus, L.M , Kusakari, K., Bombeck, C.T : The significance of bile in reflux esophagitis. Surg. Gynecol Obstet *134*, 419–424 (1972)
30 Goligher, J.C., Pulvertaft, C.N., DeDombal, F T., et al : Five-to-eight year results of Leeds/York controlled trial of elective surgery for duodenal ulcer. Brit. Med. J. *2*, 781 (1968)
31. Goligher, J.C., Pulvertaft, C.N., Irvin, T.T., et al.· Five-to-eight year of truncal vagotomy and pyloroplasty for duodenal ulcer. Brit. Med. J. *1*, 7 (1972)
32. Earlam, R.J., Thomas, P A.: The gastroesophageal junction in duodenal ulcer after operations. Gastroenterology *62*, 746 (1972)
33. Williams, J.A., Woodward, D.A.K.: The effect of subdiaphragmatic vagotomy on the junction of the gastroesophageal sphincter. Surg. Clin. North Amer. *47*, 1341 (1967)
34. Mann, C V., Greenwood, R.K., Ellis, F.H.· The esophagogastric junction. Surg Gynec Obstet *118*, 853 (1969)
35. Balison, J.R., Woodward, E.R.: Effect of hiatus hernia repair and truncal vagotomy on human lower esophageal sphincter pressure. Ann. Surg. *177*, 554 (1973)
36. Eastwood, G.L., Castell, D O , Higgs, R H.: Experimental esophagitis in cats impairs esophageal sphincter pressure. Gastroenterology *69*, 146 (1975)

37. Pellegrini, C.A., DeMeester, T.R., Wernly, J.A., Johnson, L.F., Skinner, D.B.: Alkaline gastro-esophageal reflux. Am. J. Surg. *135*, 177 (1978)
38. Bushkin, F.L., Woodward, E.R.: Alkaline reflux esophagitis. In: Postgastrectomy syndromes, Bushkin, F.L., Woodward, E.R., eds. W. B. Saunders, 64 (1976)
39. Herrington, J.L., Mody, B.: Total duodenal diversion for treatment of reflux esophagitis uncontrolled by repeated antireflux procedures. Ann. Surg. *183*, 636 (1976)
40. Wells, C., Johnston, J.H.: Revision of the Roux-en-Y anastomosis for postgastrectomy syndromes. Lancet *II*, 479 (1956)

15 Gastro-Ileostomy

An anastomosis between the stomach and the ileum instead of a proximal jejunal loop is a rare but well-known complication of gastric surgery (Fig. 50). The error in choosing a wrong small-bowel loop may be caused by a fixation of the terminal ileal loop to the retroperitoneal fixed caecum, thus imitating the first jejunal loop and the ligament of Treitz [1].

The clinical picture is characterised by considerable weight loss immediately after operation, despite a good appetite, the loss of large volumes of fluid and electrolytes, and voluminous stools, which very often contain undigested food particles [2–4]. At the same time, peripheral neuropathia, oedema and ascites – signs of hypoalbuminaemia – are observed. The anaemia may be more or less pronounced, and both microcytic and macrocytic types have been described, indicating malabsorption of vitamin B_{12}, folate or iron [5, 6].

If the last ileal loop has been anastomosed to the stomach as a simple gastro-enterostomy and the pylorus is patent. ileus symptoms will occur, since the food will partly pass through the pylorus, but will be hindered in its passage by the anastomosis and reflux into the stomach [2, 6]. If the pylorus remains closed, or if a Billroth II resection has been performed, diarrhoea will be the principal symptom, often accompanied by subileus symptoms. In most patients diarrhoea occurs a few days after operation, as soon as the patients start eating solid food [4, 5]. Nearly half the patients show severe vomiting and often a type of faeculent vomiting.

In most patients anastomotic ulcerations will occur in the region of the gastro-ileostomy, especially after simple gastro-ileostomy without resection [2].

A gastro-ileostomy always has to be differentiated from a gastrojejunocolic fistula [4]. An important differential diagnostic sign is the time of occurrence of symptoms after operation. While in most patients with gastrojejunocolic fistula there is a long interval between operation and onset of symptoms, in most cases accompanied by ulcer symptoms, with gastro-ileostomy the symptoms will occur immediately after operation. The diagnosis of gastro-ileostomy will be verified by X-ray examination. If the pylorus is intact and large amounts of contrast medium pass through the pylorus, the gastric anastomosis may be overlooked [2, 5]. However, an important radiological sign is the fast passage of barium into the

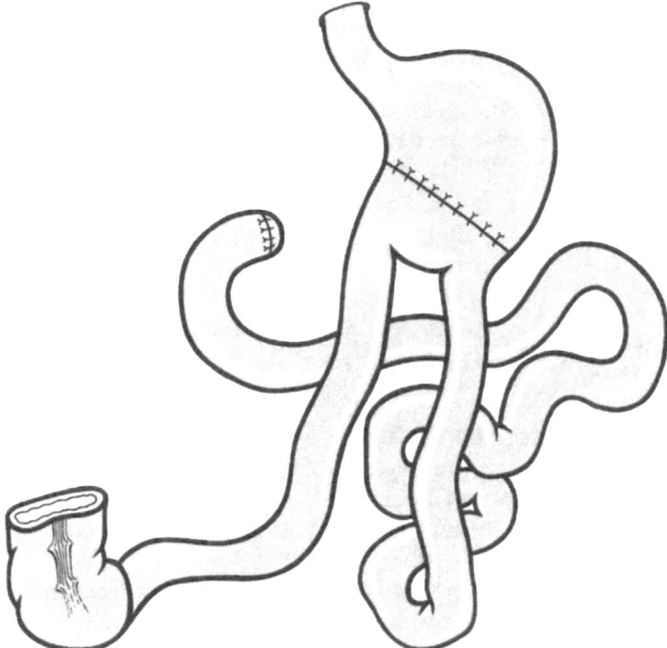

Fig. 50. Erroneous anastomosing of the stomach to the ileum after Billroth II resection

ascending colon. For differentiation from a gastrojejunocolic fistula, a barium enema has to be performed. An early positive ^{14}C-glycocholic acid breath test and a very marked decrease in intestinal transit time, measured after lactulose ingestion by hydrogen breath exhalation, will help to confirm the presence of a gastro-intestinal shunt. When the diagnosis is verified, the treatment of choice is surgical correction of the anastomotic error. After removal of the anastomosis, the appropriate therapy for the primary disease has to be carried out.

References

1. Nissen, R.: Eingriffe an Magen und Duodenum. In: Brandt, G., Kunz, H., Nissen, R.: Intra- und postoperative Zwischenfalle. Stuttgart: Thieme-Verlag 1970
2. Fromm, D.: Complications of gastric surgery. Clin. Gastroent. Monograph Series. New York: Wiley Sons 1977
3. Castleton, K.B., Bailey, F.B.: Syndrome following gastroileostomy. Amer. J. Surg. *79*, 736 (1950)
4. Landry, R.M.: Gastroileostomy and gastrocolostomy. Surgery *30*, 528 (1951)
5. Gross, J.B., Waugh, J.M.: The clinical manifestations of gastroileal anastomosis. Arch. Int. Med. *102*, 722 (1958)
6. Palumbo, P.J., Sardamore, H.H., Gross, J.B., Ferris, D.O.: Inadvertent gastroileostomy. Gastroenterology *45*, 505 (1963)

16 Recurrent Peptic Ulceration

A very serious organic complication after definitive surgery for peptic ulcer disease is a recurrent ulcer. It is characterised by a high mortality rate and presents considerable therapeutic problems. The ulcer may develop in the stomach or duodenum or in the region of the anastomosis. In most cases the ulceration is located in the intestinal mucosa distal to the anastomosis.

In the majority, an inadequate initial surgical treatment is responsible for the recurrence, besides endocrine disorders which cause hypersecretion in the stomach. In a large number, the cause of the recurrence remains uncertain.

Clear principles for the surgical therapy of recurrent ulceration have not yet been defined, though the syndrome was first described by Braun in 1899. This chapter deals with recurrent ulcerations after simple gastrojejunostomy or the various types of resection; recurrences after vagotomy are described in Chapt. 26.

16.1 Incidence

Recurrences after the different types of gastric resection (Billroth I, Billroth II) can be expected in 1%–5% of patients [2–5]. However, the absolute incidence can be determined, if in prospective studies regular endoscopic controls are performed postoperatively. The frequency of recurrent ulcers is five to ten times higher in men than women [6, 7]. More than 95% of recurrences develop in patients whose first operative procedure was because of a duodenal ulcer, in 2%–4% it was a case of gastric ulcer, and in 2% combined ulcer (duodenal plus gastric).

Although the majority of recurrent ulcers occurs within a few years after operation, comparison of results after 10 years with results at 5 years suggests a further increase during the second 5 years. Wychulis and co-workers [8] observed a mean time interval of 1–2 years between gastric resection or vagotomy and the development of recurrences; on the other hand the mean time interval after simple gastro-enterostomy was 7.4 years. Cleator et al. [11] reported a mean interval between original and subsequent operation of 3.4 years after Billroth II resection, 5.4 years after Billroth I resection, 3.6 years after vagotomy and gastro-enterostomy, and 2.8 years after vagotomy plus antrectomy, but 17.3 years after simple gastro-enterostomy. Several other studies were also able to demonstrate that recurrences after gastro-enterostomy occur much later than after gastric resection [6, 8].

Stomal ulcerations are usually located in the intestinal mucosa, seldom traversing the gastro-intestinal suture line [11, 12]. To what extent local factors may be responsible for the development of recurrent ulcers is not known, but stomal ulcers are often found close to non-resorbable sutures.

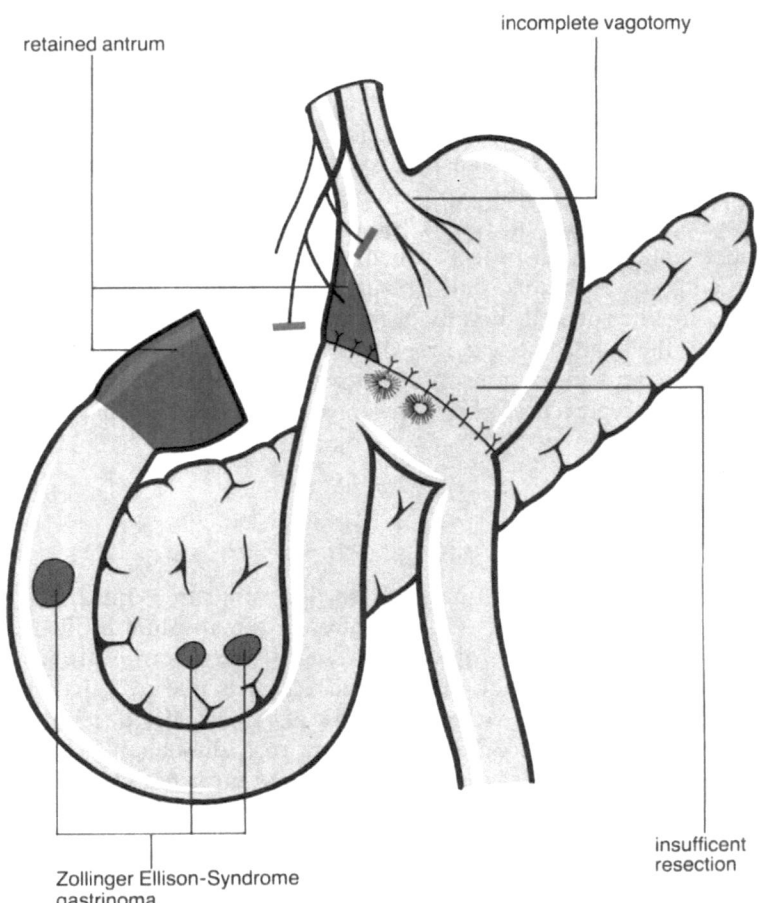

Fig. 51. Pathogenetic factors in recurrent peptic ulceration after Billroth II resection

16.2 Aetiology

Several pathogenetic factors may be involved in the development of recurrent ulcerations (Fig. 51, Table 33). In most instances, however, recurrences are caused by inadequate primary surgical therapy. By comparison, conditions are rare which cause gastric acid hypersecretion. Furthermore, ulcerogenic drugs have to be taken into consideration, since their consumption has increased tremendously over the last few years.

16.2.1 Inadequate Surgery

Simple gastro-enterostomy was widely used in the early years of surgical treatment of peptic ulcer disease, but it was accompanied by a high recurrence

Table 34. Aetiologic factors for recurrent peptic ulcer

  I. *Inadequate surgical procedure*
     Simple gastro-enterostomy
     Incomplete vagotomy
     Inadequate gastric resection
     Long afferent jejunal loop after B II
     Insufficient antral drainage
     Non-absorbable mucosal suture

 II. *Gastric hypersecretion*
     Retained gastric antrum
     Zollinger-Ellison syndrome
     Hypercalcaemia
     Other endocrine disorders

III. *Ulcerogenic drugs*
     Salicylates
     Phenylbutazone
     Indomethacin
     Reserpine
     Corticosteroids?
     Alcohol

---

rate of 34% [13]. The high recurrence rate was due to the non-reduction of gastric acid secretion. Although the method is no longer used nowadays, occasionally patients are observed who received a gastro-enterostomy several decades ago and are now developing stomal ulceration.

Incomplete vagotomy plays a major role in the development of recurrences after vagotomy; this problem will be discussed in Chap. 26. However, in Billroth I resection with resection of a major part of the lesser curvature, an extensive vagal denervation of the stomach is performed, so that the therapeutic effect of the operation comprises both gastric resection and vagotomy. Likewise, if in a Billroth I resection the lesser curvature is preserved, vagal denervation will be much less, which results in a higher recurrence rate.

Inadequate gastric resection is the main factor favouring recurrent ulceration. It can be clearly demonstrated that the recurrence rate in duodenal ulcer patients is directly correlated to the amount of the stomach resected [14, 15]. Incomplete antrectomy is not of major importance in Billroth I gastroduodenostomy. In patients with Billroth II gastrojejunostomy, however, a retained antrum at the duodenal stump leads to a picture similar to the Zollinger-Ellison syndrome, since the lack of acid inhibition of antral gastrin release results in hyper-gastrinaemia, with subsequent gastric hypersecretion. This pathogenetic principle is responsible for the high recurrence rate in patients with the antrum exclusion procedure of von Eiselsberg. Only reduction of the amount of antral mucosa or its resection (the modifications of Finsterer, Plenk, Bancroft) have resulted in a decrease of recurrences to an acceptable level.

A long afferent loop after Billroth II resection and an erroneously performed gastro-ileostomy are also considered to be causes of a high recurrence rate [6, 19], since the neutralisation of acid in the anastomotic region is inadequate.

16.2.2 Hypersecretion of Acid

The problems associated with a retained antrum at the duodenal stump were mentioned above. Most patients show hypergastrinaemia and hypersecretion, as in Zollinger-Ellison syndrome. In cases of hypergastrinaemia, the differentiation may be done by the secretin test [20]: while patients with the Zollinger-Ellison syndrome show an increase in serum gastrin levels after intravenous injection of secretin, in patients with a retained antrum gastrin levels will fall or be unchanged. The incidence of retained antrum in patients with recurrent ulcer after partial gastrectomy amounts to about 9% [6].

Zollinger-Ellison syndrome. The most fulminant type of peptic ulcer disease is found in the Zollinger-Ellison syndrome (ZES), which is caused by a gastrin-producing tumour in the pancreas or duodenum. Since most patients produce large quantities of gastric acid, diarrhoea is a common clinical symptom. About 1.8% of all recurrent ulcers after gastric surgery suggest ZES [6]. More frequent use of serum gastrin determination and better knowledge of the syndrome will possibly contribute to an increase in the number of verified cases of ZES.

Hypercalcaemia. On the basis of several single observations, a direct correlation between hypercalcaemia and peptic ulcer disease has been suggested. Barreras [21] supposed that patients with hyperparathyroidism have a ten times higher incidence of peptic ulcer disease than a normal population. Furthermore, hyperparathyroidism is ten times more frequent in ulcer patients than in non-ulcer patients. Also, the combination of gastrinomas and hyperparathyroidism within the scope of multiple endocrine adenomatosis has to be considered.

Other Endocrine Disorders. Pituitary adenomas have been thought responsible for recurrent ulcerations, mainly in connection with multiglandular endocrine adenomatosis. Recurrent ulcers have also been observed in patients with tumours of the adrenal cortex and Cushing's syndrome [6].

16.2.3 Ulcerogenic Agents

Cleator et al. [11] observed that in their series, patients with recurrent ulcers regularly took salicylates: 11% used aspirin more than once a week; 30% of the patients drank alcohol, and in 14% an alcohol-dependency of varying degrees was observed.

16.3 Diagnosis

The use of non-absorbable suture material for the mucosa involves the hazard of suture granulomas, which sustain chronic ulcerations. Probably less than 2% of recurrent ulcerations are due to suture material.

16.3.1 Clinical Symptoms

Recurrent ulcer is not difficult to diagnose, because of the typical ulcer symptoms. The patients complain of pain in the epigastrium, which is similar to their previous ulcer symptoms. There are also complications that very often lead to therapeutic efforts. In 56% of their patients, Bushkin and Woodward [23] observed bleeding, not massive in most cases; in 4% perforation occurred, and 9% had an obstruction.

Postoperative ulceration tends to penetrate into the neighbouring organs. Depending on the type of anastomosis, the penetration may be into the pancreas or colon or under the surface of the liver. In rare cases the ulcer may penetrate into the abdominal wall, with subsequent fistula.

After penetration of the ulcer into the colon, a gastrojejunocolic fistula will develop; this is thought to occur in about 6% of patients with simple gastro-enterostomy [23]. Up till about 1950, gastrojejunocolic fistulas were observed quite frequently, but today this complication is rare: it is mainly a complication of simple gastro-enterostomy, which is no longer used in the surgical treatment of peptic ulcer disease. This complication tends to occur more frequently in male patients. The main symptoms are rapid weight loss and voluminous stools with undigested material, occasionally accompanied by diarrhoea. Often copremesis occurs and patients complain of foul breath. The continuing malabsorption results in progressive anaemia, osteoporosis, dehydration and cachexia. Subjective complaints include upper abdominal pain of changing intensity, faeculent breath, weight loss and diarrhoea. Diagnosis is in most cases confirmed by a barium enema with retrograde visualisation of small bowel or stomach.

16.3.2 Radiological Examination

In patients with recurrent ulcerations after gastric surgery the evidence of X-ray examination is limited: recurrent ulcerations can be demonstrated definitely in only 50%–65% [8, 11]. A specific ulcer niche is the most important radiological sign, but there may be problems in interpretation, especially due to bulging in the anastomotic area.

16.3.3 Gastroscopy

In the interpretation of pathological findings after gastric surgery, gastroscopy is superior to X-ray examination. By direct view, a recurrent ulcer can be verified in about 90%. Furthermore, by taking biopsy specimens several other pathological conditions, such as the various forms of gastritis, which may result in similar symptoms, can be differentiated.

16.3.4 Gastric Analysis

A gastric analysis is indicated in all patients with recurrent ulceration after gastric surgery, since the amount of acid secreted by the stomach may influence the choice of operative procedure. Both basal acid output (BAO) and maximal acid output (MAO) after pentagastrin stimulation are significantly higher in patients with recurrent ulcer than in control patients without recurrences. MAO over 15 mval/h and BAO over 6 mval/h can be found in most patients with recurrent ulcerations. The results of the insulin test are discussed in the Chap. 2.3.2 [3.3.5.3].

In all patients, determination of serum gastrin levels is mandatory, in order to be able to exclude Zollinger-Ellisson syndrome. However, almost all patients show elevated serum gastrin levels after the various types of vagotomy. A discrimination between the different forms of hypergastrinaemia and the Zollinger-Ellison syndrome may be achieved by several endocrine provocation tests (calcium, secretin, glucagon; see Chap. 2.4).

Chaundhuri and co-workers [25] reported that technetium is enriched in the retained antrum, which can be demonstrated by radio-isotopic scanning. However, the evidence of this test requires further evaluation.

16.4 Conservative Treatment

In patients with recurrent ulceration after gastric surgery and without complications, conservative treatment is indicated. Since the discovery of histamine H_2-receptor antagonist (Cimetidine) a potent agent is available, which can be successfully used. However, definite demonstration of the effectiveness of cimetidine in treating recurrent ulceration is still lacking: a first controlled randomized study showed no influence of cimetidine on healing rate, but a relatively low dosage was used [25a]. For the healing of recurrent ulcerations it is of great importance to avoid ulcerogenic drugs and to restrict alcohol, coffee and smoking. Furthermore, antacids, anticholinergics and sedatives may additionally be given.

The results of conservative treatment of recurrent ulcers were not promising before the development of the H_2-receptor antagonist. In a review Stabile and Passaro [6] reported in 297 patients an ulcer specific mortality of 10.8% and a recurrence or persistence rate of 42.1%; in only 31.6% of all patients recurrent ulcerations healed permanently.

16.5 Surgical Therapy

Surgical therapy is the most effective treatment of recurrent ulceration after operations. The approach depends on the previous procedure.

Recurrence after simple gastro-enterostomy can be treated surgically in four ways, indicated in Fig. 52. The best results are obtained after subtotal gastrectomy or vagotomy plus gastrectomy; the resection procedures have the highest mortality, while vagotomy gives a high recurrence rate (Table 35).

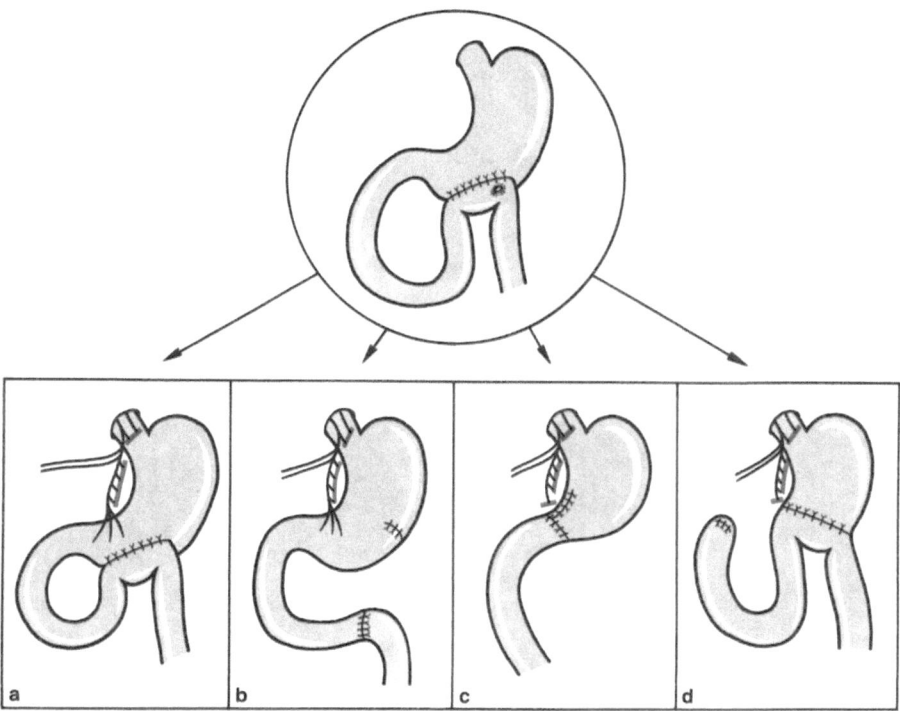

Fig. 52 a–d. Treatment of recurrent ulceration after simple gastro-enterostomy

Table 35. Results of treatment of recurrent ulcers after simple gastroenterostomy [6]

Procedure	Number of patients	Operative mortality (%)	Recurrence (%)	Good results
Vagotomy	180	1.7	23.9	57.8
Resection	826	2.7	11.3	70.8
Vagotomy + resection	67	9.0	7 5	64.2
Vagotomy + pyloroplasty	5	0	60.0	20.2

For *recurrence after gastric resection*, the operative tactics depend on the type of previous anastomosis (Billroth I or Billroth II); the possibilities are shown in Figs. 53 and 54. Vagotomy alone results in a much lower mortality than reresection; the recurrence rate is similar after vagotomy and after resection plus vagotomy, but reresection alone has a high mortality and recurrence rate (Table 36). Naturally, these guidelines are only valid if during operation an adequate primary resection (70% or more) can be verified. If the primary resection was too limited, vagotomy plus reresection has to be performed.

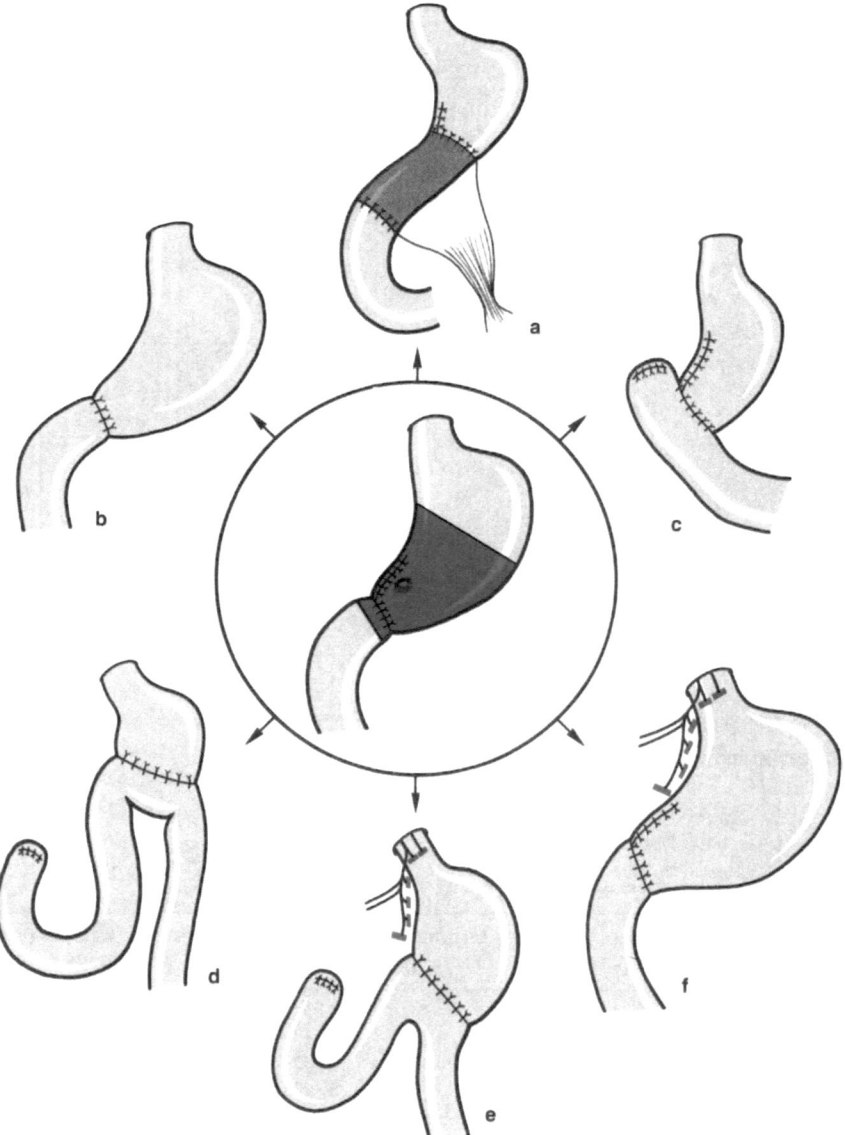

Fig. 53. Treatment of recurrent ulceration after Billroth I resection

16.6 Therapy of Gastrojejunocolic Fistula

The operative procedure of choice in patients with gastrojejunocolic fistula depends on the general condition of the patient and on local findings, mainly with regard to the defect of the colon wall. In primary definitive surgery, one performs reresection, vagotomy and sewing over the small colonic defect. In patients in poor general condition, gastric resection can be done in two steps.

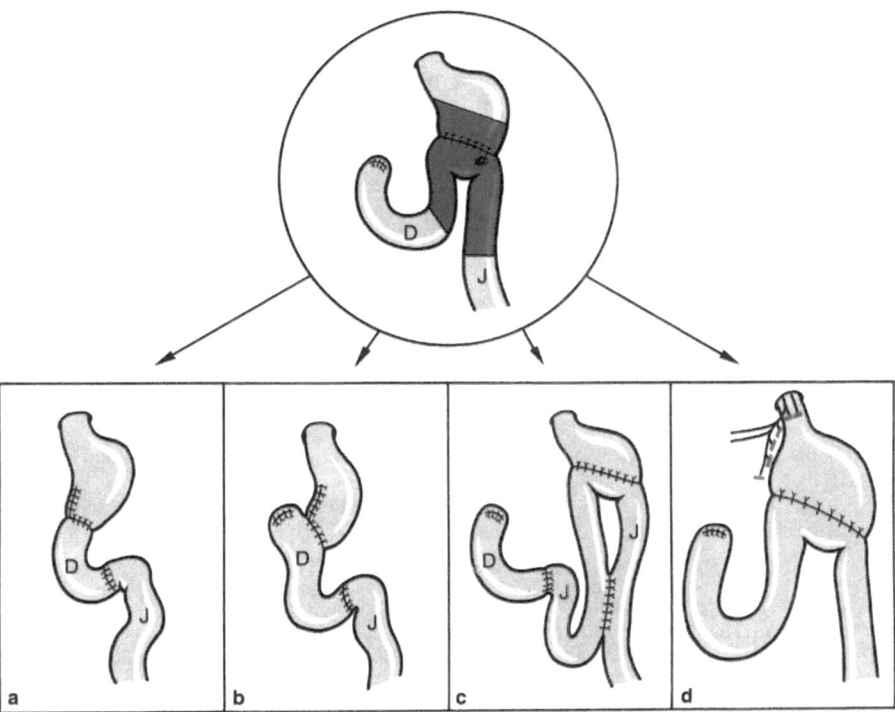

Fig. 54. Treatment of recurrent ulceration after Billroth-II resection. *D*, duodenum; *J*, jejunum

Table 36. Results of treatment of recurrent ulcers after gastric resection

Procedure	Number of patients	Operative mortality (%)	Recurrence (%)	Good results (%)
Vagotomy	624	1.0	12.0	66.2
Reresection	366	6.8	20.2	58.2
Reresection + vagotomy	225	5.3	8.0	67.1

In the first operation, a new antecolic gastro-enterostomy with a wide entero-anastomosis is established above the old anastomosis. In the second operation, resection of the anastomosis together with the spontaneously shrinking gastro-jejunocolic fistula is performed. If the colon defect is large, a resection of the colon with end-to-end anastomosis has to be added. If the colon defect cannot be closed by direct suture, but resection is indispensable and the patient in bad condition, then resection is done, the distal (aboral) colonic stump is closed and the proximal (oral) colonic part brought to the abdominal wall as an artificial anus. Reconstruction of the continuity can be accomplished, according to Nissen [26], with an interposed small-bowel loop.

The mortality and recurrence rate used to be extremely high for the one-step procedure; choosing the two-step procedure or modern therapeutic efforts to improve the patients' general condition have brought the mortality down to 0–3% [10, 27]. The recurrence rate using the procedures proposed here is about 4% [27].

References

1. Braun, H.: Demonstration eines Praeparates einer 11 Monate nach Ausfuhrung der GE entstandenen Perforation des Jejunums Verh dtsch. Ges Chir. *28*, 95 (1899)
2. Goligher, J.C., Pulvertaft, C.N., Ironi, T T , Jonston, D., Walker, B., Hall, R.A., Willson-Pepper, J., Matheson, T.S : Five to eight – year results of truncal vagotomy and pyloroplasty for duodenal ulcer. Brit. med. J. 7 (1972)
3. Hoffmann, V.: Das Anastomosengeschwur nach Magenoperation. Munch. med. Wschr. *106*, 592 (1964)
4. Zenker, R., Reichel, K., Rueff, F.: Indikation zur klassischen Resektion und Vagotomie beim peptischen Ulcus. Langenbeck's Arch. Klin Chir. *320*, 223 (1968)
5. Postlethwait, R.W.: Five year follow up results of operations for duodenal ulcer. Surg Gynec. Obstet. *137*, 387 (197)
6 Stabile, B E., Passaro, E.: Recurrent peptic ulcer. Gastroenterology *70*, 124 (1976)
7. Kronberger, L.: Korrekturoperationen beim operierten Ulcusmagen Stuttgart: Enke-Verlag 1970
8. Wychulis, A.R., Priestly, J.T., Foulk, W T.: A study of 360 patients with gastrojejunal ulceration. Surg. Gynec. Obstet. *122*, 89 (1966)
9. Walters, W., Chance, D P., Berkson, J A.: A comparison of vagotomy and gastric resection for gastrojejunal ulceration· a follow up study of 301 cases. Surg. Gynec. Obstet. *100*, 1 (1955)
10. Fromm, D.: Complications of gastric surgery. Clin. Gastroent. Monogr. Series. New York: Wiley Publication 1977
11. Cleator, I.G.M., Hollubitsky, I.B , Harrison, R.C.: Anastomotic ulceration. Ann Surg. *179*, 339 (1974)
12. Small, W.P.. The recurrence of ulceration after surgery for duodenal ulcer. J. R. Coll. Surg. Edinb. *9*, 255 (1974)
13. Lewisohn, R.: Frequency of gastrojejunal ulcer Surg Gynecol. Obstet. *40*, 70 (1925)
14. Holle, F : Spezielle Magenchirurgie. Heidelberg: Springer-Verlag 1968
15. Gobbel, W.G , Shoulders, H H., Jr.. Gastric resection In: Postlethwait, R.W.: Results of surgery for peptic ulcer Philadelphia Saunders 1963
16 von Eiselsberg, A.· Zur Behandlung des Ulcus ventriculi et duodeni Arch. Klin Chir. *114*, 539 (1920)
17. Krause, U.: Long term results of medical and surgical treatment of peptic ulcer Acta chir. Scand. Suppl. 310 (1963)
18. Kunz, H., Schenka, G.. Spätergebnisse der praepylorischen Resektion zur Ausschaltung nach Finsterer. Wien klin. Wschr 76, 739 (1964)
19 Kirulik, L.B., Merendino, K.A.. An elucidation of the intestinal sensitivity factor and the distance factors in the incidence of stomach ulcer in the Billroth II type of gastrectomy. Surgery 35, 538 (1954)
20 Korman, M.G., Scott, D.F., Hansky, J.: Hypergastrinemia due to an excluded gastric antrum. a proposed method for differentiation from Zollinger-Ellison syndrome. Aust. N Z.J. Med. 2, 266 (1972)
21. Barreras, R.F : Calcium and gastric secretion. Gastroenterology *64*, 1168 (1973)
22. Black, B.M.· Primary hyperparathyroidism and peptic ulcer. Surg. Clin. N. Amer. *51*, 955 (1971)
23 Bushkin, F.L , Woodward, E.R Postgastrectomy syndromes. Major problems in clinical surgery. Vol. XX. Philadelphia. Saunders 1976
24 Scobie, B.A., Rovelstad, R A.: Anastomotic ulcer: Significance of the augmented histamine test. Gastroenterology *48*, 318 (1965)

25. Chaudhuri, T.K., Shirazi, S.S., Condon, R.E.: Radioisotopic scan – a possible aid in differentiating retained gastric antrum from Zollinger-Ellison syndrome in patients with recurrent peptic ulcer. Gastroenterology *65*, 697 (1973)

25a Kennedy, T., Spencer, A.: Cimetidine for recurrent ulcer after vagotomy or gastrectomy: a randomized controlled trial. Brit. med. J. *1*, 1242 (1978)

26. Brandt, G., Kunz, H., Nissen, R.: Intra- und postoperative Zwischenfälle. Band II. Stuttgart: Thieme-Verlag 1970

27 Localio, S.A., Stone, P, Hinton, J.W.: Gastrojejunocolic fistula. Surg. Gynecol. Obstet. *96*, 455 (1953)

17 Gastric Remnant Carcinoma

Surgical treatment of gastroduodenal ulcer disease by resection or simple gastro-enterostomy was popular at the beginning of this century. The first carcinoma in the gastric remnant after resection for benign ulcer disease was described in 1922 by Balfour. Up to the 1950s this complication of gastric surgery was rare [1–3]. Thus, K.H. Bauer [4] was able to give a survey of 27 cases in 1951. In the last few decades, however, the number of cases reported in the literature has increased steadily, so that at the moment about 300 cases of carcinoma in the gastric remnant have been described [5–10].

17.1 Definition

Primary gastric stump cancer has been defined as follows [11, 12]:
1) Primary gastric surgery has been performed because of a histologically verified benign disease (gastroduodenal ulcer, gastritis, polyps, trauma of the stomach or duodenum).
2) The interval between primary surgery and appearance of the tumour has to be at least 5 years. Only after this interval primary malignant disease can be excluded.

17.2 Incidence, Risk and Interval after Operation

Although the number of observed gastric stump cancer has increased significantly, the incidence rate after the various operative procedures (Billroth I or II resection, simple gastro-enterostomy, vagotomy plus drainage) is unknown. Also, the influence of the primary disease on the occurrence of postoperative gastric remnant cancer is not clear. A definite answer can only be achieved by controlled prospective studies, which must involve a follow-up period of 15–30 years, since the mean free interval between the primary gastric procedure and the appearance of malignant tumour is about 20 years [7, 11].

In several clinical publications the number of observed gastric stump cancers has been correlated to the number of primary gastric cancers treated during the same period [14–17] or related to the number of gastric resections for peptic ulcer disease during a certain period [15, 17, 18]; on the basis of these studies, relatively low gastric stump cancer rates of 0.8%–2% have been reported [19].

Evaluation of large series of autopsies by Kühlmayer and Rokitansky [20] and by Hilke and co-workers [21] demonstrated a tendency for the resected stomach to develop cancer of 8.9%–10.7%; this frequency is double that of the gastric cancer lethality of their controls. Current statistics based on autopsies should demonstrate even higher cancer rates, since more patients with gastric resection survive an interval of 25 years and more and may therefore be included in the figures.

To evaluate the exact incidence in retrospective long-term follow-up studies it is necessary to keep a check on all patients who had gastric surgery 5–40 years before, to detect any tumour in the gastric stump. Helsingen and Hillestad [22] followed 303 patients with Billroth II resection: 38 patients died during the follow-up period, with a 3.3% rate of gastric stump cancer. Krause [23], who studied 361 patients with gastric resection for 20–50 years after operation, found a cancer rate of 7.7%. Grieser and Schmidt [7] observed a gastric stump cancer rate of 13.3% in patients who had undergone Billroth II resection for gastric ulcer.

The incidence of malignant tumours in the gastric remnant varies widely between 1.3% and 28.9%, depending on the follow-up period and the number of patients who die [8, 12]. Furthermore, the gastric stump cancer rate is influenced by the primary disease which leads to gastric surgery. Retrospective long-term follow-up studies after gastric resection for gastric ulcer show a cancer rate between 13.2% and 16% [7, 11]. On the other hand, it is known that about 10% of patients with conservatively treated gastric ulcer will develop gastric cancer after a long enough follow-up period [7, 27], and in chronic atrophic gastritis after a follow-up of 10–15 years 10% will develop gastric cancer [24–26]. These findings are important, since in most studies the incidence of gastric stump cancer has been compared with the gastric cancer incidence in the normal population and not with the already elevated cancer risk of gastric ulcer patients.

If gastric resection was performed because of duodenal ulcer, the gastric cancer rate is significantly lower. Of patients who die 5 years or more after gastric resection for duodenal ulcer, death is caused by a gastric stump cancer in 7%–9% [7]. However, a control group of conservatively treated duodenal ulcer patients with a follow-up period of 5–30 years is not available for comparison.

A direct correlation between cancer rate and length of follow-up can be demonstrated. Between the 5th and 25th year after gastric resection, a gastric stump cancer will be found in 1.9%–7.9% of patients; during this period patients mainly die because of suicide or bronchial carcinoma. After the 20th year of follow-up, the cancer disposition of the gastric stump increases and reaches a peak of 22% after the 25th year [11]. A comparison of gastric cancer risk after resection for gastric ulcer and in patients with chronic atrophic gastritis demonstrates that gastric resection protects against cancer during the first

5–8 years after operation, since it is well documented that in the intact stomach cancer will develop mainly in the antrum, which in gastric surgery is resected [9].

Very few reports deal with gastric cancer after Billroth I resection. Only Griesser and Schmidt [7], in a retrospective study of 104 patients with Billroth I resection for gastric ulcer disease, found a cancer rate of 8.3%; this is significantly lower than in Billroth II patients and slightly lower than in conservatively treated ulcer patients. Similar results have been reported in patients with simple gastro-enterostomy, but there are no prospective studies and retrospective results are rare. Griesser and Schmidt [7] reported a 20% incidence of gastric cancer in 124 patients with primary gastric ulcer in whom a simple gastro-enterostomy had been performed.

17.3 Pathogenetic Factors

As pointed out earlier, there is strong evidence that the gastric stump cancer risk is higher in gastric ulcer patients than in patients with duodenal ulcer disease. This is in good correlation with the higher primary cancer rate in gastric ulcer patients. Furthermore, malignant gastric remnant tumours have been observed mainly in central Europe, but not in the USA. In Japan, primary gastric cancer is six times more frequent than in the USA and about four times more frequent than in Europe, but gastric remnant tumours are a rare finding [8]. Men develop this complication four to seven times more frequently than women [12, 18], whereas the sex ratio in primary gastric cancer is 1.5:1.

Causal factors for the increased incidence of malignant tumours after partial resection of the stomach may include damage to the mucosal barrier by the increased reflux of duodenal contents, with subsequent chronic atrophic stump gastritis, or chronic irritation in the transient zone between the gastric and jejunal or gastric and duodenal mucosa. The chronic damage to gastric mucosa by duodenal contents causes the development of chronic atrophic gastritis, which is found in all patients about 10 years after Billroth II resection. Especially the hyperplastic – hypertrophic types of gastritis with intestinal metaplasia and cystic dilatation of the glands may represent a facultative precancerous disease [28]. In about 10% of gastroscopically controlled patients with previous gastric resection, polypous lesions are found, which histologically represent degenerative or inflammatory polyps and which are caused by chronic gastritis.

The precancerous lesions are mainly found in the anastomotic area; it is also mainly in this region that the polyps are localised. Furthermore, about two-thirds of manifest cancers develop in this area [8, 12, 17, 18]. Hammar [29] observed precancerous lesions and infiltrating tumours mainly at the posterior wall, close to the efferent loop.

According to Lauren [30], a diffuse type of gastric cancer may be separated from a so-called intestinal type, which has a significantly better prognosis [31]. In gastric remnant carcinoma Hammar [29] observed the intestinal type in almost all precancerous lesions, but in infiltrating tumours mainly the diffuse type was found. Furthermore, the shift to the intestinal type in elderly people that is found in primary gastric cancer does not exist in gastric stump cancer [33].

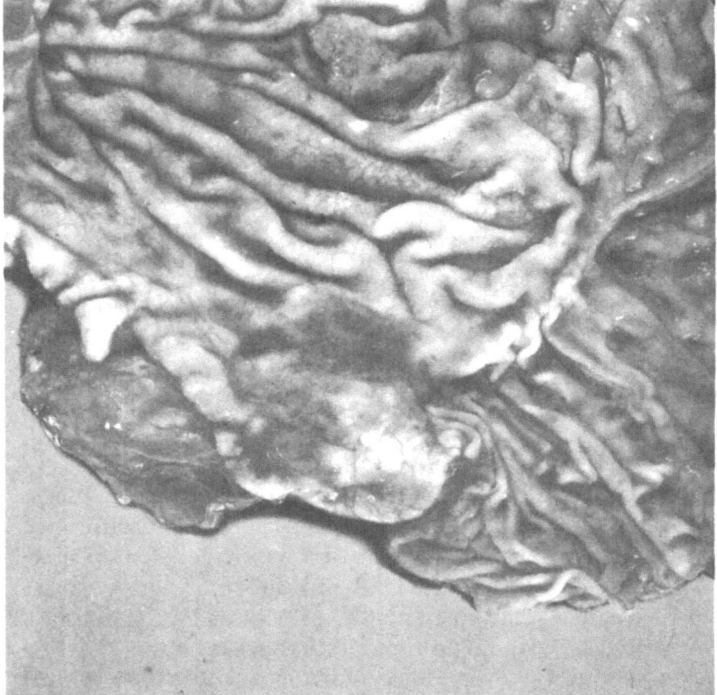

Fig. 55. Small gastric remnant carcinoma in the anastomic region

17.4 Symptoms

The symptoms in gastric remnant tumours are not characteristic; mainly epigastric fullness, vomiting, dysphagia, weight loss, minor gastro-intestinal bleeding, weakness, obstruction and diarrhoea are reported. In most cases complaints are so unspecific that there is a significant delay in diagnosis [33].

It may be difficult to differentiate between a stump tumour and a peptic jejunal ulcer; however, ulcus pepticum jejuni occurs mainly during the first 10 years after operation, whereas gastric remnant tumours will develop mainly after the 20th postoperative year.

17.5 Diagnostic Procedures

With the introduction of flexible glass-fibre instruments and their technical improvement, endoscopy represents the main diagnostic procedure after gastric surgery. The radiological examinations often present problems in the exact interpretation of the mucosal relief of the gastric stump, anastomotic region and adjacent small bowel (Fig. 55). Therefore the accuracy of X-ray examination of operated stomachs is not much higher than 50% [19, 33, 34].

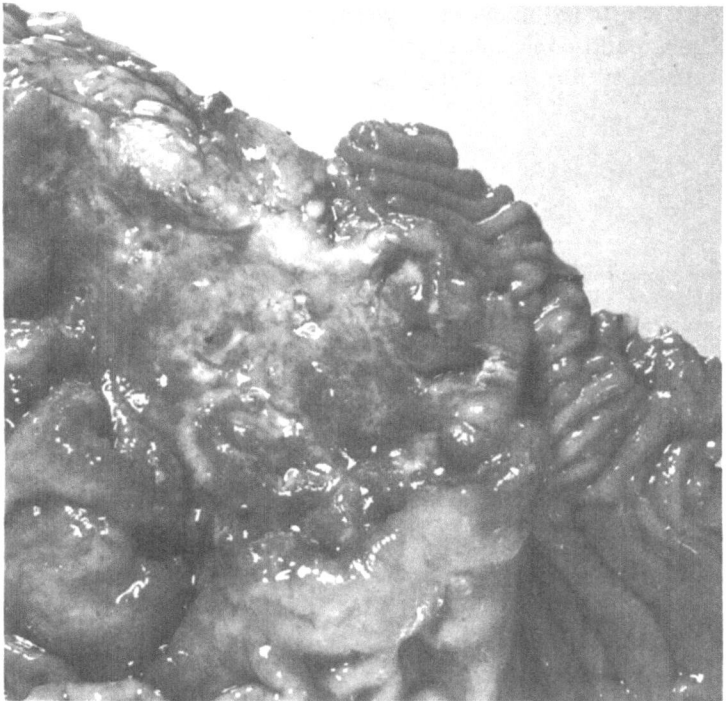

Fig. 56. Diffus infiltrating tumour of the gastric remnant

The great advantage of endoscopic examination is in the detection of precancerous lesions in the operated stomach, since only at this stage of the disease prognosis is good. Furthermore, gastric cancer may develop multifocally, this finding being of special interest, since the surgical procedure depends on the origin and extent of the tumour.

17.6 Therapy, Prognosis

The only successful therapy in patients with gastric stump cancer is surgical excision of the tumour (Fig. 56). Since in most cases the tumour will be widespread at the time of operation, the surgeon will be forced to do a total gastrectomy, as a simple by-pass procedure may be technically unsatisfactory. Saegesser and Jämes [9] were able to demonstrate that the duration of symptoms did not influence the resection rate of gastric stump cancer. Furthermore, they showed that palliative resection produced the best subjective results. However, the overall prognosis of gastric stump cancer is depressing; only very few patients will survive for 5 years [9, 13]. In most series the longest survival time is 1–2 years [12, 35]. A better prognosis can be reached by early recognition of precancerous and cancerous lesions of the operated stomach. Therefore it seems necessary for patients who have undergone gastric resection for gastric ulcer disease to receive regular endoscopic check-ups after the 10th postoperative year. That is the only possibility for improving the prognosis in gastric remnant cancer.

References

1. Balfour, D.C.: Factors influencing the life expectancy of patients operated on for gastric ulcers. Ann. Surg. 76, 405 (1922)
2. Beatson, G.T.: Carcinoma of the stomach after gastrojejunostomy. Brit. med. J. 1, 15 (1926)
3. Schwarz, H.: Operationsbefunde an Gastroenterostomierten. Aussprache. Zbl. Chir. 53, 3000 (1926)
4. Bauer, K.H.: Das Krebsproblem. Berlin, Heidelberg: Springer Verlag 1963
5. Clemencon, G., Baumgartner, R., Leuthold, E., Miller, G., Neiger, A.: Das Karzinom des operierten Magens. Dtsch. med. Wschr 101, 1015 (1976)
6. Domellof, L., Eriksson, S., Janunger, K.G.: Late precancerous changes and carcinoma of the gastric stump after Billroth I resection. Amer. J. Surg. 132, 26 (1976)
7. Griesser, G., Schmidt, H.: Statistische Erhebungen uber die Haufigkeit des Karzinoms nach Magenoperation wegen eines Geschwürleidens. Med. Welt 35, 1836 (1964)
8. Dahm, K., Rehner, M.: Das Karzinom im operierten Magen. Stuttgart: Thieme-Verlag 1975
9. Saegesser, F., James, D.: Cancer of the gastric stump after partial gastrectomy (Billroth II principle) for ulcer. Cancer 29, 1150 (1972)
10. Stalsberg, H., Taksdal, S.: Stomach cancer following gastric surgery for benign conditions. Lancet 2, 1175 (1971)
11. Peitsch, W., Becker. H.D · Frequency and prognosis of primary gastric stump carcinomas. Front. Gastroint Res 5, 170 (1979)
12. Morgenstern, L., Yamabawa, T., Selker, D.: Carcinoma of the gastric stump. Amer. J. Surg. 125, 29 (1973)
13. Terjesen, T., Ericksen, H.G.: Carcinoma of the gastric stump after operation for benign gastroduodenal ulcer. Acta chir. scand. 142, 256 (1976)
14. Laroczi, G, Metzl, J.: Über das sog. Magenstumpfkarzinom. Bruns Beitr. klin. Chir. 198, 401 (1959)
15. Becker, Th., Freund, E.: Magenkarzinom und Ulkuschirurgie. Zbl Chir. 89, 455 (1964)
16. Schreiber, H.W., Bernhard, B., Kuss, B.. Über das Karzinom im Magenstumpf. Zbl. Chir 89, 577 (1964)
17. Kootz, F.: Das Stumpfkarzinom nach Operation wegen eines benignen Magenleidens. Bruns Beitr. klin. Chir. 215, 275 (1967)
18. Kronberger, L., Hafner, H.: Über das primäre Stumpfcarcinom nach Ulkusresektion. Chirurg 39, 118 (1968)
19. Pack, G.T., Banner, R.L : The late development of gastric cancer after gastroenterostomy and gastrectomy for peptic ulcer and benign pyloric stenosis. Surgery 44, 1024 (1958)
20. Kühlmayer, R., Robitansky, O.: Das Magenstumpfkarzinom als Spatproblem der Ulkuschirurgie. Langenb. Arch. klin. Chir. 278, 361 (1954)
21. Hilbe, G., Salzer, G.M., Hussel, H., Kutschera, H.: Die Carcinomgefahrdung des Resektionsmagens. Langenb. Arch. klin. Chir. 323, 142 (1968)
22. Helsingen, N., Hillestad, L.: Cancer development in the gastric stump after partial gastrectomy for ulcer Ann. Surg. 143, 173 (1956)
23. Krause, U.: Late prognosis after the partial gastrectomy for ulcer Acta chir. scand. 114, 341 (1957)
24. Siurala, M., Varis, K., Wiljasolo, M.: Studies of patients with atrophic gastritis: a 10–15 year follow-up. Scand. J. Gastroent. 1, 40 (1966)
25. Siurala, M., Salmi, H.J.: Long term follow-up subjects with superficial gastritis or a normal gastri mucosa. Scand. J. Gastroent. 6, 559 (1971)
26. Walker, J.R., Strickland, R.G., Ungar, B., Mackay, J.R.: Simple atrophic gastritis and gastric carcinoma. Gut 12, 906 (1971)

27. Peitsch, W., Becker, H.D.: Was ist gesichert in der Pathogenese und Häufigkeit des primaren Karzinoms im operierten Magen. Chirurg 50, 33 (1979)
28. Domelhöf, L., Eriksson, S, Janunger, K G . Carcinoma and possible precancerous changes of the gastric stumps after Billroth II resection. Gastroenterology 73, 462 (1977)
29. Hammar, E.: The localisation of precancerous changes and carcinoma after previous gastric operation for benign conditions. Acta path. microbiol. scand 84, 495 (1976)
30. Lauren, P.: The two main histological types of gastric carcinoma. Diffuse and so-called intestinal type carcinoma – an attempt at a histo-clinical classification. Acta path. microbiol. scand 64, 31 (1965)
31. Inberg, M.V., Lauren, P., Vuori, J., Viibari, S.J.: Prognosis in intestinal-type and diffuse gastric carcinoma with special reference to the effect of stromal reaction. Acta chir. scand 139, 273 (1973)
32. Taksdal, S., Stalsberg, H.: Histology of gastric carcinoma occurring after gastric surgery for benign conditions. Cancer 32, 162 (1973)
33. Berkowitz, D., Cooney, P., Bralow, S.P.: Carcinoma of the stomach appearing after previous gastric surgery for benign ulcer disease. Gastroenterology 36, 691 (1959)
34. Boeckl, O., Lill, H.: Über das Magenstumpfcarcinom. Münch. med. Wschr. 105, 615 (1963)
35. Nicholls, J.C.: Carcinoma of the stomach following partial gastrectomy for benign gastro duodenal lesion. Brit. J. Surg. 61, 244 (1974)

18 Postgastrectomy Malabsorption

18.1 Incidence of Weight Loss and Steatorrhoea

Although the majority of patients do relatively well following gastric surgery, some develop severe malabsorption and present difficult problems of nutritional management. Partial gastric resection was the procedure most frequently performed for peptic ulcer disease up to a decade ago and is still performed today. These patients, particularly those with Billroth II gastric resection, present potentially serious malabsorption problems. Weight loss commonly occurs after gastrectomy, the incidence being variously reported between 30% and 84% (1–13). The most common cause of postgastrectomy weight loss, although it may be multifactorial, is not malabsorption but inadequate food intake, due to poor appetite early sensations or fear of postcibal symptoms [7, 12]. Weight changes are found mostly in the first year after operation, but thereafter small changes are observed. Johnston et al. [12] observed that those patients who had lost weight prior to subtotal gastrectomy tended to gain afterwards, but those who had maintained a steady weight or had had an increase in weight before the operation tended to lose afterwards (Fig. 57). After truncal vagotomy, Wastell [13] found that the method of drainage (pyloroplasty or gastro-enterostomy) did not influence the loss of weight, and about half or more of the patients lost weight after vagotomy and drainage. Wheldon et al. [5] found a weight more than 4 kg below standard in 47% of men and in 64% of women after truncal vagotomy with gastro-enterostomy.

Preliminary results with proximal gastric vagotomy suggest that the incidence and degree of weight loss are less than those observed after other procedures.

In a prospective study, Jordan observed that 67% of patients with a parietal cell vagotomy equalled or exceeded their preoperative weight, whereas this was

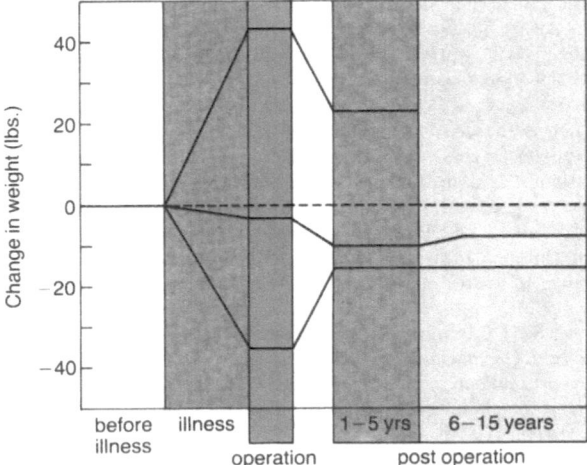

Fig. 57. Effect of subtotal gastrectomy on body weight. Patients who had lost weight prior to subtotal gastrectomy tended to gain afterwards, but those who had maintained a steady weight or had an increased weight before the operation tended to lose afterwards. After Johnston et al., 1958

found in only 25% of patients who had undergone selective vagotomy combined with a Billroth I partial gastrectomy [13a].

Malabsorption of fat (faecal fat excretion >6 g/day), however, is common in postgastrectomy patients, the incidence varying between 60% and 70% [14–17]. The vast majority, however, have only mild steatorrhoea and the condition is chemical rather than clinical and cannot account for the weight loss observed in these patients. The incidence is higher after large resections [14], after operations producing duodenal by-pass [14, 18] and in Polya resection with long afferent loops [14, 19, 20], and it increases as the postoperative interval lengthens. A small minority of patients [7, 14] have severe malabsorption and may present problems in postoperative management.

Thus patients on a provocative 200 g fat diet have been found to have a 41% increase in faecal fat excretion after Billroth I reconstruction, versus a 129% increase after Billroth II resection [21].

Using a ^{131}I-triolein test meal, blood values of radioactivity were significantly lower and faecal radioactivity higher in a group of postgastrectomy patients (Billroth II) than in corresponding healthy controls [22], thus exhibiting malabsorption of fat. Eleven of the abnormal results occurred in the patients who were below ideal weight.

Malabsorption of fat in postgastrectomy malabsorption is much more important than that of protein or carbohydrates [7]. There are no common accurate methods to measure protein malabsorption besides determination of faecal nitrogen. Gastrectomy per se does not affect protein absorption [14, 16]. Severe protein malnutrition has been described, but it is usually due to additional complications such as bacterial overgrowth of the small bowel or pancreatic disease [23–26]. Fat malabsorption is relatively easy to detect and is often associated with loss of important fat-soluble vitamins (vitamins A, D, E, K).

In order to elucidate the mechanism which might be responsible for post-gastrectomy malabsorption, especially fat malabsorption, knowledge of the physiology of fat absorption is necessary.

18.2 Physiology of Fat Digestion and Absorption (Fig. 58)

Dietary fat, ingested as long-chain triglycerides, is converted to an emulsion in passing from the stomach to the duodenum. This process is supposed to increase the total surface area of the fat particles by a factor of 8×10^{12}. Gastric lipase does not seem to play an important role in fat digestion. Pancreatic lipase, which is inhibited by an acid pH, hydrolyses triglycerides to monoglycerides and free fatty acids. In order to make these products water-soluble, micelle formation by bile acids has to take place. Optimal micelle formation by bile acids occurs with monoglycerides and free fatty acids, but not with unhydrolysed triglycerides. By the formation of micelles, the surface area of the fat particle is further increased, by an additional factor of 2×10^6. Thus by emulsification, lipolysis and micelle formation, the surface area of a fat droplet is increased by a factor of up to 17×10^{18}. More important than bile acids seems to be pancreatic lipase, the action of which is a prerequisite for subsequent micelle formation and absorption of fat. Steatorrhoea after total pancreatectomy is more severe than after complete biliary obstruction. After entering the mucosal epithelial cells, monoglycerides and fatty acids are resynthesised to triglycerides, which are subsequently discharged as chylomicrons and transported via the lymphatics to the systemic circulation.

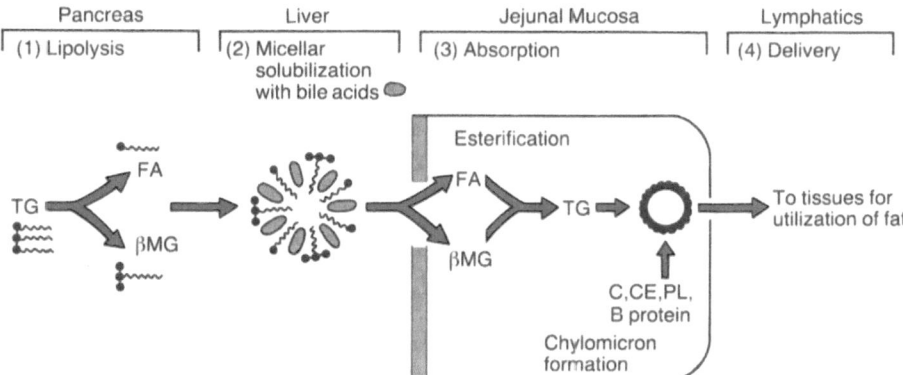

Fig. 58. Diagrammatic representation of the major steps in the digestion and absorption of dietary fat. Depicted is the lipolysis of dietary triglyceride (TG) by pancreatic lipase, operating under optimal conditions by protection of bicarbonate (1). The second step (2) requires micellar solubilization of the resulting long-chain fatty acids (FA) and β-monoglyceride (βMG) by bile acids secreted into the intestinal lumen by the liver. This step is followed by absorption (3) of the fatty acids and β-monoglyceride into the mucosal cell, subsequent re-esterification, and formation of chylomicrons, which finally move out from the mucosal cell into the intestinal lymphatic system (4). During the process of chylomicron formation small amounts of cholesterol (C), cholesterol esters (CE) and phospholipids (PL) as well as triglycerides are incorporated into this specific lipoprotein section. After Wilson and Dietschy, Gastroenterology, *61*, 911–931 (1971)

Table 37. Physiology of absorption of medium-chain triglycerides (MCTs) and therapeutic consequences

---

MCTs can be hydrolysed by gastric lipase; absorption may already start in the stomach
Indication: small-bowel resection

MCTs are hydrolysed by pancreatic lipase faster than long-chain triglycerides (LCTs)
Indications: exocrine pancreatic insufficiency, resection

Lipolysis is not a prerequisite for MCT absorption
Indication: exocrine pancreatic insufficiency

Micelle formation with bile acids is not necessary
Indications: deficiency of intraluminal bile acids, as in extrahepatic biliary obstruction, cholestasis, decompensated enteral loss of bile acids (ileal resection), fatty acid diarrhoea

MCTs will be absorbed faster than LCTs by mucosal cells
Indications: small-bowel resection, coeliac disease

No resynthesis of fatty acids or 2-monoglycerides to triglycerides within the enterocyte as prerequisite for discharge
Indications: Abetalipoproteinaemia, coeliac disease

MCTs are cleared via the portal venous system
LCTs are cleared via the lymphatic system
Indications: Whipple's disease, lymphangiectasia, other causes of lymphatic obstruction

---

The absorptive mechanism for medium-chain triglycerides (C_6–C_{10}) is different. They can be absorbed more effectively than long-chain triglycerides, they do not necessarily require pancreatic lipolysis and micellar solubilisation, and they are cleared from the mucosal cells via the portal venous system instead of the lymphatic system (Table 37).

These differences in the physiological absorptive mechanisms are the basis for the treatment of severe fat malabsorption with medium-chain triglycerides.

18.3 Pathophysiology of Postgastrectomy Steatorrhoea (Fig. 60)

18.3.1 Gastric Mechanism

The stomach begins the digestive process, primarily as a reservoir for food until gastric secretion has normalised the tonicity of the meal, and gradually empties a more isotonic stream of food into the duodenum. Antral contraction achieves a more thorough mixing and emulsification of the food with gastric juice. In addition, protein digestion is initiated by pepsin in the presence of hydrochloric acid.

After gastrectomy the gastric remnant empties rapidly [14, 9, 28]. Emptying is even more rapid when the duodenum is by-passed.

Presumably duodenogastric reflexes which normally seem to control the rate of gastric emptying are lost [28]. Thus, less time is allowed for gastric predigestion, which is already less efficient owing to the reduced or absent secretion of acid and pepsin. Food is passed directly into the upper part of the small intestine; the effect of the duodenum in making the gastric contents iso-osmolar has been well documented.

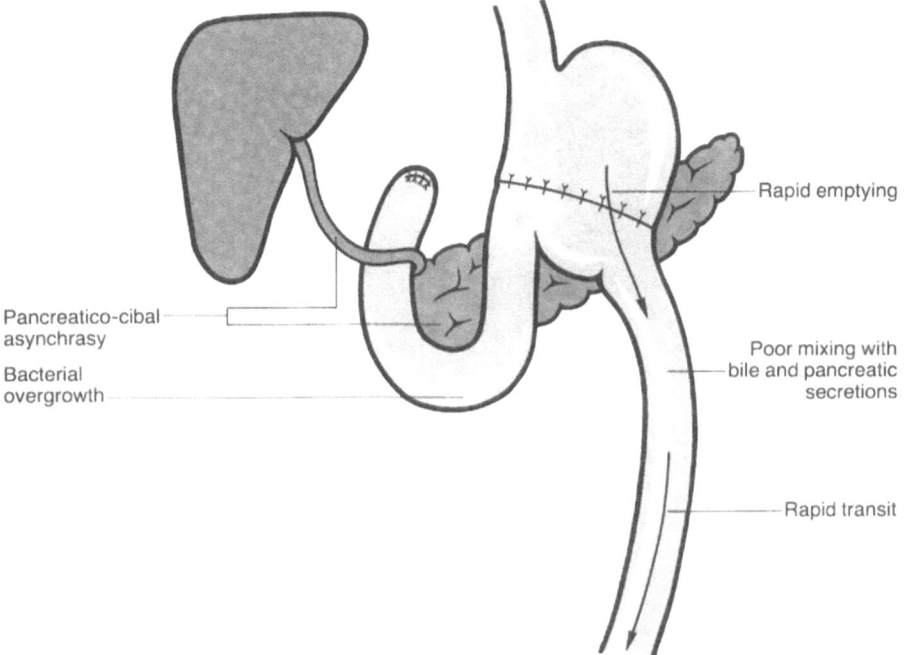

Rapid emptying

Pancreatico-cibal
asynchrasy

Poor mixing with
bile and pancreatic
secretions

Bacterial
overgrowth

Rapid transit

Fig. 59. Pathogenetic factors responsible for postgastrectomy steatorrhoea

A variety of postulates have been formulated to explain postoperative malabsorption:
1) Loss of peptic digestion in the resected stomach [17]
2) Stasis and/or bacterial overgrowth in the afferent loop resulting in deconjugation of bile salts or destruction of pancreatic enzymes [29, 30]
3) Primary pancreatic insufficiency [10, 31]
4) Loss of absorbing surface or of surface that releases pancreatic stimulating hormones, when the afferent loop is by-passed [9]
5) Rapid intestinal transit of chyme resulting in poor mixing of digestive pancreatic secretion with food [32, 33]
6) Diminished CCK-pancreozymin release from the vagally denervated small intestine [34, 35]

One of the most thorough older studies is that of Lundh [9] who studied intraluminal digestive events in patients with subtotal gastrectomy (STG) and found abnormally low concentrations of bile (bile pigment) and pancreatic enzymes (trypsin) in the proximal gut lumen in patients with STG during the first hour after a liquid meal. These defects were later confirmed by others [31, 36]. Fields and Duthie [37] described low postcibal concentrations of bile salts and lipase after liquid test meals following vagotomy and pyloroplasty. These low concentrations were associated with subnormal fat solubilisation.

These studies clearly indicated that intraluminal digestive events are abnormal in patients with STG and vagotomy with pyloroplasty (V + P), but they could not

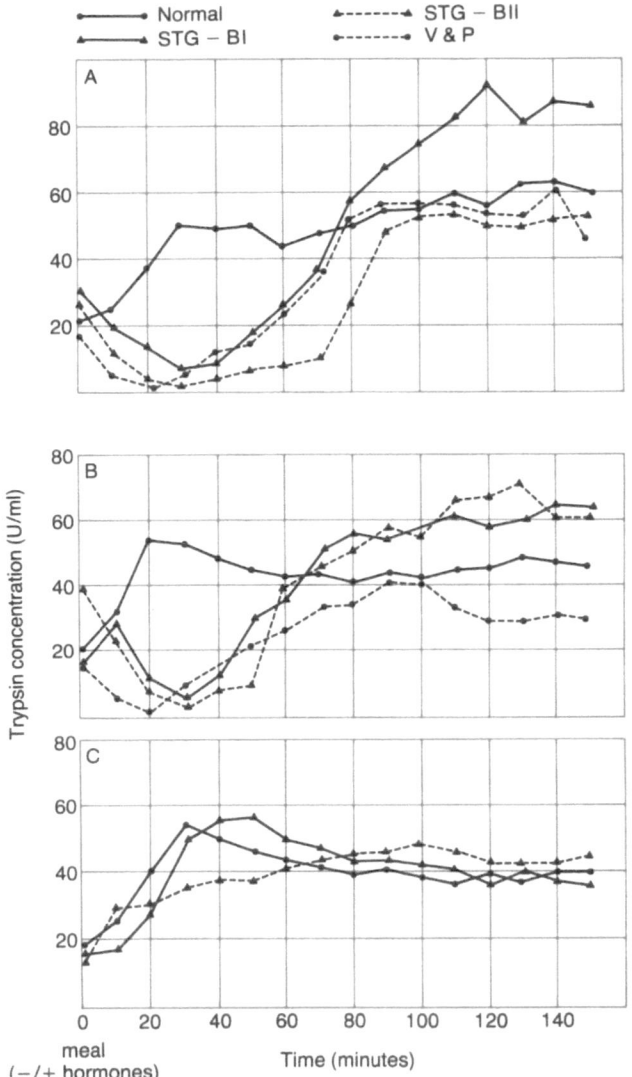

Fig. 60 A–C. Mean trypsin concentration at proximal jejunal sampling site after liquid test meal (LTM) alone **A**; LTM + hormones (CCK) **B**; and CCK alone **C**. Meals were taken and intravenous hormone infusion started at zero time. Trypsin concentration was significantly lower than normal ($P < 0.05$): subtotal gastrectomy with gastroduodenostomy (STG-BI), **A** 30 min, **B** 20 and 30 min; subtotal gastrectomy with gastrojejunostomy (STG-BII), **A** 20, 30, 60, and 70 min, **B** 20, 30, 40, and 50 min; truncal vagotomy and pyloroplasty (V + P), **A** 20 and 30 min, **B** 20 min. Following hormone infusion no significant differences were seen between the four groups. After MacGregor et al., 1977

give information on the underlying cause of the decreased intraluminal concentration of bile acids and exocrine pancreatic enzymes. Does a primary pancreatic insufficiency exist, or a decreased release of CCK, or were secretory outputs normal, but only diluted owing to rapid entry of fluid into the proximal small intestine?

18.3.2 Pancreaticocibal Asynchrasy

In a very complex and careful study MacGregor et al. [35] examined by intestinal perfusion technique the biliary and pancreatic secretory responses of patients with STG and V + P. Since their methods measured not only bile acid and pancreatic enzyme concentrations, but also the rates of entry of a liquid meal from the stomach into the intestine, they were able to provide information on the extent by which rapid gastric emptying diluted biliary and secretory outputs. Their studies were performed in controls and in patients with STG-BI, STG-BII, and V + P. In all subjects operated upon, the jejunal flow rates were markedly increased compared to normals in the first 40–50 min after a meal. Addition of hormones (CCK-PZ) changed flow patterns only a little. As expected from the high flow rates, gastric emptying was markedly increased in the operated patients. The half-time (in normals 75.3 min) was markedly decreased in STG-BI (43.1 min), STG-BII (44.3 min) and V + P (34.2 min).

The intraluminal concentration of trypsin rose postcibally in normals after 20–30 min from 21 to 50 U/ml and remained constant over more than 2 h (Fig. 60), while at the same time concentration of trypsin decreased below fasting values in all operated patients and began slowly to rise after 50 min, reaching supranormal values in STG-BI patients. Exactly the same pattern was observed after additional administration of CCK, but the pattern was nearly equal for all groups of patients after hormonal stimulation alone. Thus, rapid gastric emptying diluted intraluminal contents, with subsequent initially low concentrations of trypsin and bile salts, a pattern which was not corrected by intravenous addition of hormones to the meal stimulus.

Trypsin output in V + P subjects after a test meal was significantly depressed to 40% of normals', but was normal in the STG groups (Fig. 61). The delay of trypsin and bile salt concentrations in reaching normal values was more marked in STG-BII patients, owing to sequestration of secretions in the afferent loop. The low luminal concentration of digestive secretions was therefore attributable to rapid gastric emptying in all operated groups; in V + P patients additionally a depressed response of pancreatic enzymes was observed. In STG-BII patients, afferent-loop sequestration exaggerated the delay in attaining normal intraluminal concentrations of bile acids and pancreatic enzymes. The combined disturbance in STG-BII produced greater malabsorption than that seen in STG-BI patients. The study thus indicated that in patients with vagotomy and pyloroplasty maximal pancreatic secretory capacity is markedly reduced.

A reduced concentration of bile acids following a liquid test meal was also found by MacGregor et al. [35], especially in patients with V + P (Fig. 62). The consequence of the pancreaticocibal asyncrasy consisting in a relative pancreatic

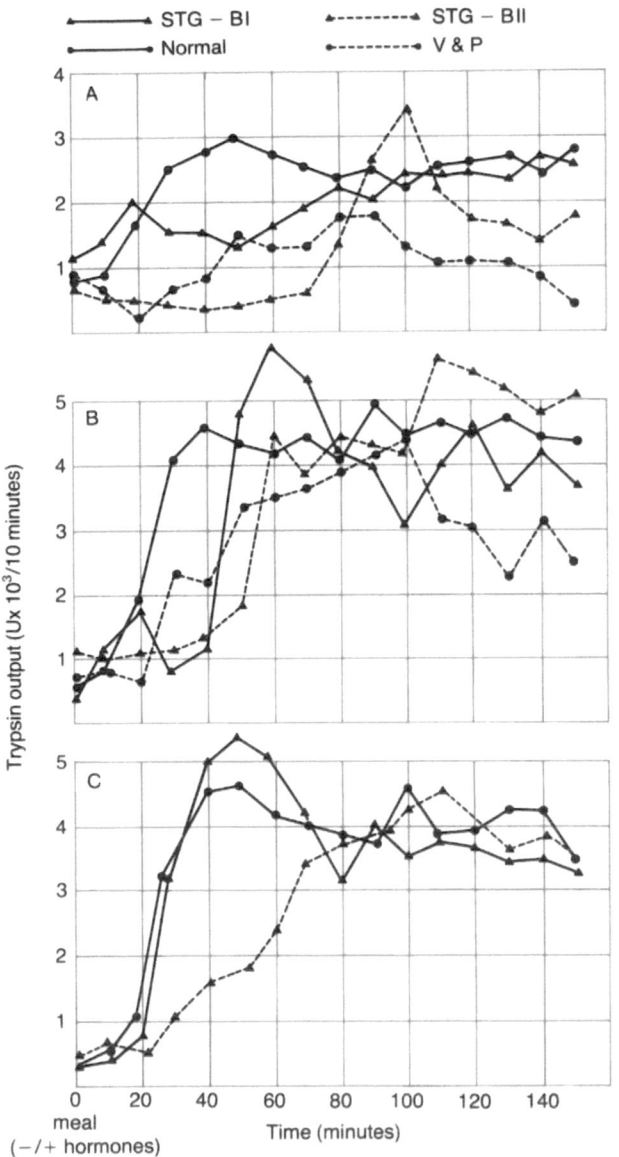

Fig. 61 A–C. Mean trypsin passage past proximal jejunal sampling site after liquid test meal (LTM) alone **A**, LTM + CCK **B**, and CCK alone **C**. Meals were taken and intravenous hormone infusion started at zero time. Trypsin output was significantly below normal ($P < 0.05$), as indicated by an asterisk (**A**, STG-BII 30–60 min). After MacGregor et al., 1977

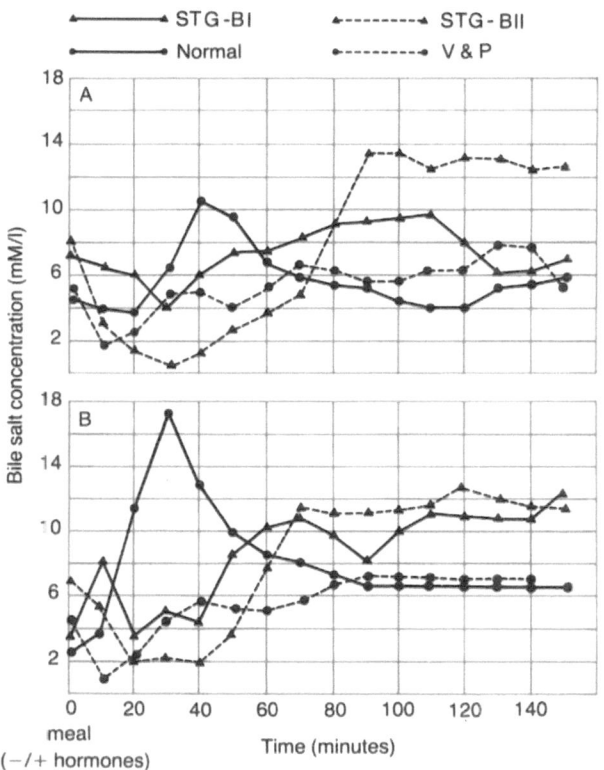

Fig. 62 A, B. Mean bile salt concentrations at proximal jejunal sampling site after liquid test meal (LTM) alone **A** and LTM + CCK **B**. Meals were taken and intravenous hormone infusion began at zero time. Bile salt concentration was significantly below normal ($P < 0.05$). **A**: subtotal gastrectomy with gastrojejunostomy (STG-BII), 30 and 40 min. **B**: subtotal gastrectomy with gastroduodenostomy (STG-BI), 20 min; subtotal gastrectomy with gastrojejunostomy (STG-BII), 20, 30, and 40 min; truncal vagotomy and pyloroplasty (V + P), 10, 20, 30, and 40 min. After MacGregor et al., 1977

insufficiency and a decreased concentration of bile acids is a reduced capacity for fat absorption and possibly in addition for absorption of carbohydrates and proteins. This has for example been shown for digestion of gelatin infused into the jejunum, which was impaired in patients with BII gastrectomy [38] compared to normal controls who had gelatin infused into the duodenum. An indirect evidence of the existence of relative exocrine pancreatic insufficiency emerges from the results of Hillman [10], who showed that exocrine pancreatic insufficiency after gastrectomy can be sufficiently treated by pancreatic enzyme replacement, resulting in reduced faecal fat excretion (Fig. 63).

18.3.3 Small-intestinal Factors

It is generally agreed, on the basis of light and electron microscopy, that gastrectomy does not affect the structure of the small-bowel mucosal cells [16, 39, 40]. Postgastrectomy malabsorption seems to be due to a luminal rather than a

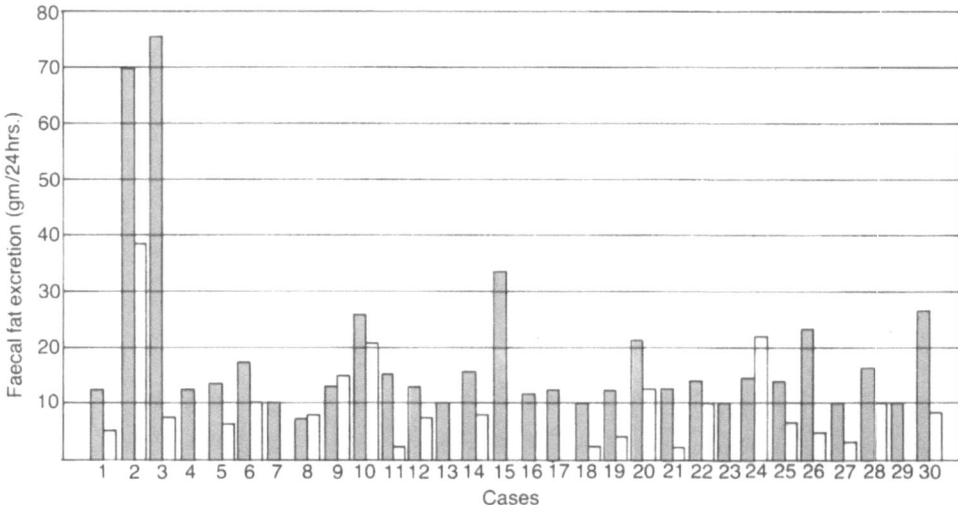

Fig. 63. Influence of pancreatic enzyme replacement therapy on faecal excretion of fat (before treatment, red columns, during treatment, white columns). The mean percentage decrease in excretion during treatment was 49.7, SE 7.7; $P < 0.001$ (22). After H.S. Hillman, 1968

cellular defect. However, for unknown reasons some of the most severe cases have been due to unmasking of latent coeliac disease [41]. A previously latent malabsorption becomes manifest when both maldigestion in the proximal gastrointestinal tract and more rapid transit allow less time for the absorptive process. Lactose intolerance thus may become manifest, since the enzyme lactase is already in any case a weak element in terminal carbohydrate digestion in normals. In addition, lactase deficiency seems to be more frequent in postgastrectomy patients [42], and the condition may symptomatically be aggravated owing to the by-passing of digestive duodenal surface in Billroth II resected patients and rapid intestinal transit. The loss of the reservoir function of the stomach, the by-passing of the duodenum and the shorter intestinal transit time may even result in malabsorption of glucose from the upper small bowel [43]. The reduced small-intestinal transit time in some patients with gastrectomy will allow D-glucose, which is so avidly absorbed from the upper small bowel, to reach the colon, where it is fermented by the colonic flora to H_2 and other products. Levitt and Bond [43] have demonstrated an increased H_2 production in these patients following glucose ingestion and have shown that glucose malabsorption increased with decreasing small-intestinal transit time (Fig. 64).

18.3.4 Bacterial Overgrowth

Bacterial proliferation of the small bowel can also produce malabsorption. There is a tendency for the number of bacteria present in the small intestine to be increased after gastrectomy [44–46, 29]. The postgastrectomy state attributable to proximal intestinal bacterial overgrowth has been termed, in addition to blind-loop syndrome, stagnant-loop or stasis syndrome.

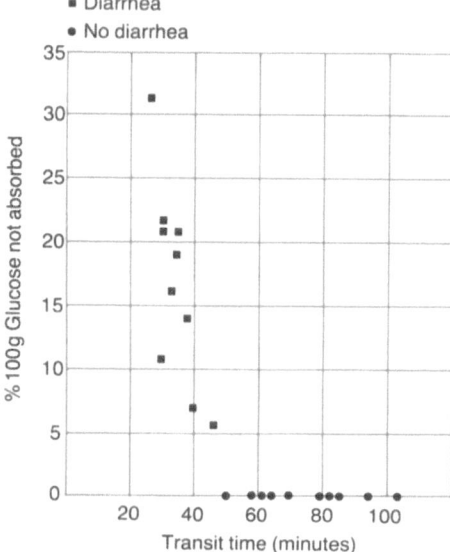

Fig. 64. Correlation of small-bowel transit time with glucose absorption in postgastrectomy patients with diarrhoea (■) and without diarrhoea (●). Rapid transit in gastrectomised patients with diarrhoea resulted in malabsorption of glucose. Thus malabsorption of glucose can be considered to be the cause of diarrhoea. After Bond and Levitt, 1977

In a study involving 70 dogs, Greenlee et al. [47] performed various degrees of vagal denervation and gastric resection and obtained postoperative cultures of the stomach and small bowel via laparotomy at intervals up to 1 year. Quantitative aerobic and anaerobic bacterial studies demonstrated a persistent and marked increase in the number of micro-organisms comparing the flora of the upper small bowel after each of these operations, with the exception of parietal cell vagotomy [47] (Figs. 65–67). Normal jejunal bacterial flora contains 10^4 or fewer aerobes and anaerobes per millilitre [48]. During bacterial overgrowth as many as 10^8 or 10^9 organisms, aerobes or anaerobes, are found per millilitre [49].

In addition to the quantitative difference in bacterial counts, there is the qualitative difference between normal aspirates – mostly showing only two or three species (mostly Gram-positive, coccal, facultatively anaerobic lactobacilli, with non-anaerobic bacteroides) – and the colon-like flora harbouring many species of aerobes and anaerobes that is seen in the stasis syndrome. Normal motility and gastric acid output seem to be the main factors maintaining normal levels of small-intestinal flora, whereby decreased acid output possibly might alter intestinal motility. It has recently been shown that absence of the so-called inter-digestive motor complex, which serves a 'housekeeping' function for the intestine in the absence of food, was associated with intestinal bacterial over-growth, demonstrated by a positive ^{14}C-glycocholate breath test [50]. Alterations of intestinal motility, as in truncal vagotomy or as occur with anatomical stagnation, e.g. in the afferent-loop syndrome of a Billroth II anastomosis, present a common setting for small-intestinal bacterial overgrowth. The incidence of

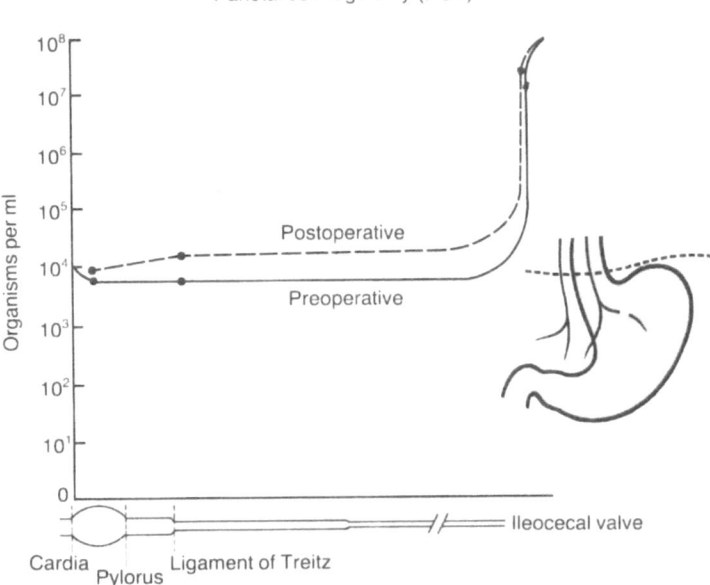

Fig. 65. No significant changes in stomach and jejunal flora were found after parietal cell vagotomy compared to controls. After Greenlee et al , 1977

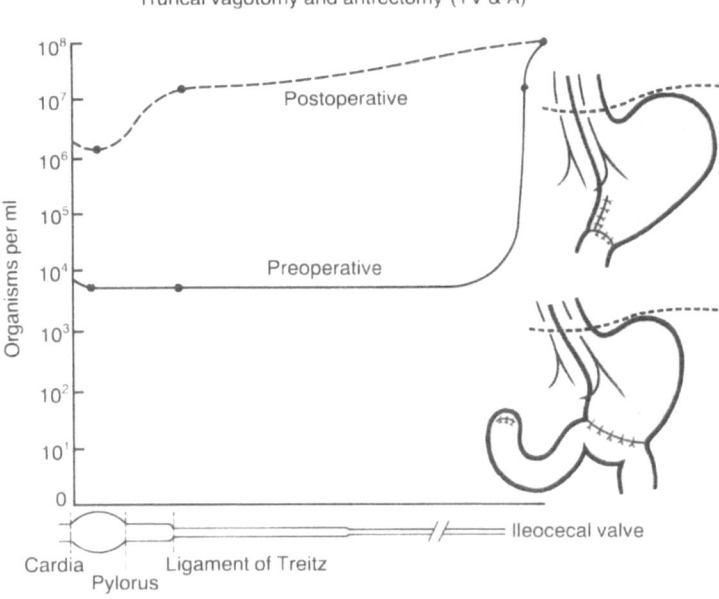

Fig. 66. Significant bacterial overgrowth was found in both the stomach and jejunum after truncal vagotomy and antrectomy. After Greenlee et al., 1977

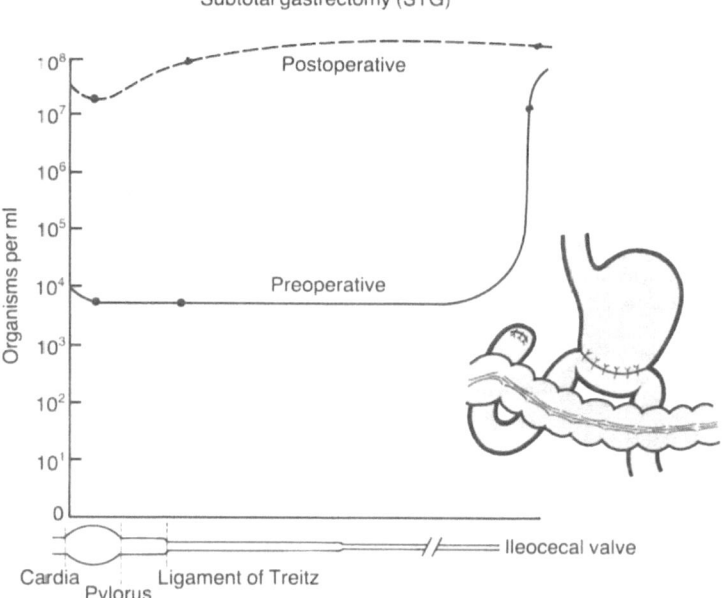

Fig. 67. Massive bacterial overgrowth was found in the stomach and jejunum following subtotal gastrectomy. After Greenlee et al., 1977

significant bacterial overgrowth in Billroth II patients has been estimated at 30%–50% [49, 51]. Malabsorption due to the blind-loop syndrome may be severe in postgastrectomy patients. Highest bacterial counts in the upper intestine are due to a gastrojejunocolic fistula, allowing colonic bacteria direct access to the stomach or jejunum. Bacteria themselves seem not to be toxic to the intestinal epithelial cells, as judged by light microscopy, since jejunal biopsy specimens in patients with small-intestinal bacterial overgrowth appear normal [44]. This does not, however, mean that morphological or functional changes resulting from the intraluminal dysfunction induced by bacterial overgrowth are not present at all. Paulley [52] observed microscopic changes of the mucosal epithelium. Since several laboratories have shown functional mucosal changes in addition to morphological changes, the concept of gut damage as an important etiological factor in the malabsorption due to bacterial overgrowth seems to be established. Gracey et al. [53] observed a defect of active monosaccharide transport in experimental animals with bacterial overgrowth. Similar changes [54, 55], consisting in microscopical changes, functional alterations of glucose and leucine transport, and depression of vitamin B_{12}, with only partial correction by antibiotics, have been demonstrated. A defect in intracellular fat transport and a patchy morphological abnormality ranging from mild broadening of villi to complete villous atrophy were shown by Ament et al. [56] in three patients with the stasis syndrome, changes only partially corrected by antibiotic treatment.

An intraluminal effect induced by bacterial overgrowth seems to be operative.

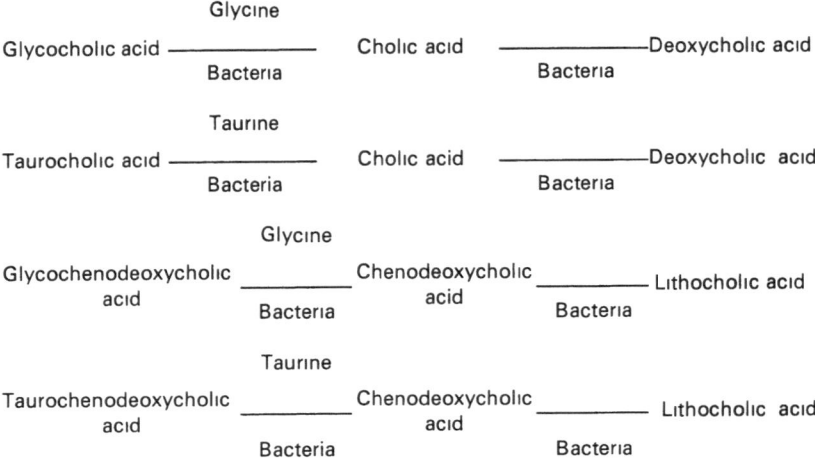

Fig. 68

18.3.5 Bacteria and Bile Acid Metabolism (Fig. 68)

Bacteria in the upper small intestine (bacteroides, clostridia, other anaerobes and enterococci) deconjugate and dehydroxylate conjugated bile acids, thus converting taurine and glycin conjugates to free bile acids. In addition, bacteria may convert primary bile acids to secondary bile acids (cholic acid→deoxycholic acid, chenodeoxycholic acid→lithocholic acid). This may lead to malabsorption of fat in three ways [44, 57, 58]:
1) Free bile acids, unlike conjugated bile acids, owing to their pK values are largely absorbed in the non-ionic form at the pH of the intestinal contents in the upper intestine. They do not therefore participate optimally in micelle formation.
2) Free bile acids are therefore absorbed predominantly by non-ionic diffusion from the upper small intestine, whereas the most important mechanism for conjugated bile acids is the active ileal transport system. Thus they may have left the upper small intestine without participating in micelle formation.
3) Free bile acids are relatively insoluble at the pH of the intestinal contents, tend to precipitate and may be excreted in the faeces, resulting in impaired micelle formation.

The increased deconjugation of bile acids can now be easily detected by a simple $^{14}CO_2$ breath test [59–61] (see Chap. 2.7.3.2).

In the presence of bacterial overgrowth and bile acid deconjugating bacteria, ^{14}C-glycocholate will be deconjugated, the ^{14}C-glycine moiety will be absorbed like any other amino acid, metabolized and finally exhaled as $^{14}CO_2$ in the breath. Bacteria may even be able to metabolize glycine, thus $^{14}CO_2$ diffusing through the intestinal membrane may be detected directly in breath. This test has become popular owing to its non-invasive nature and to its giving information on one of the functional consequences of bacterial overgrowth. The test is not, however, specific for the detection of bacterial overgrowth of the small intestine,

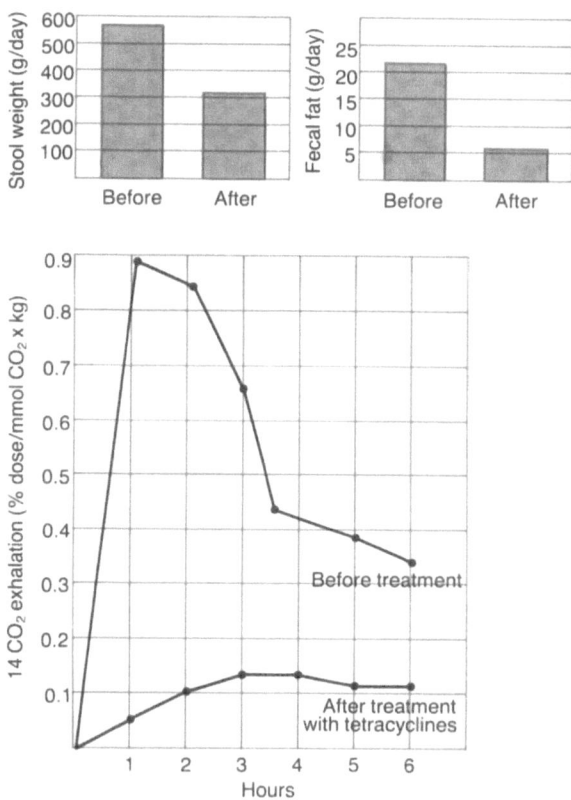

Fig. 69. ^{14}C-glycocholate breath test, faecal fat excretion and stool weights in a patient with bacterial overgrowth after a Billroth II subtotal gastrectomy: 5 days after treatment with tetracyclines the increased deconjugation of glycocholate and the steatorrhoea were normalised, the stool weight reduced

since it may also be positive in ileal resection, when owing to malabsorption of bile acids deconjugation of bile acids takes place in the colon. Simultaneous measurement of ^{14}C in faeces will enable to differentiate between increased deconjugation of glycocholic acid due to malabsorption and bacterial overgrowth of the small intestine. Since micelle formation is necessary for absorption of fat-soluble vitamins, absorption of these vitamins may be decreased, too, in the bacterial overgrowth syndrome often following gastrectomy. A typical phenomenon is the response of fat malabsorption caused by bacterial overgrowth to antibiotic treatment (Fig. 69). An increased deconjugation of glycocholic acid may be present, too, in cases of entero-enteric fistula after gastric surgery (Fig. 70). Vitamin B_{12} malabsorption not responding to administration of intrinsic factor but responding to antibiotic treatment is a typical finding in the bacterial overgrowth syndrome. The mechanism underlying vitamin B_{12} malabsorption is uptake of the vitamin B_{12} by numerous bacteria proliferating in the intestinal lumen. Certain bacteria have as great an avidity for vitamin B_{12} as does gastric intrinsic factor [62]. These bacteria can incorporate vitamin B_{12} and keep

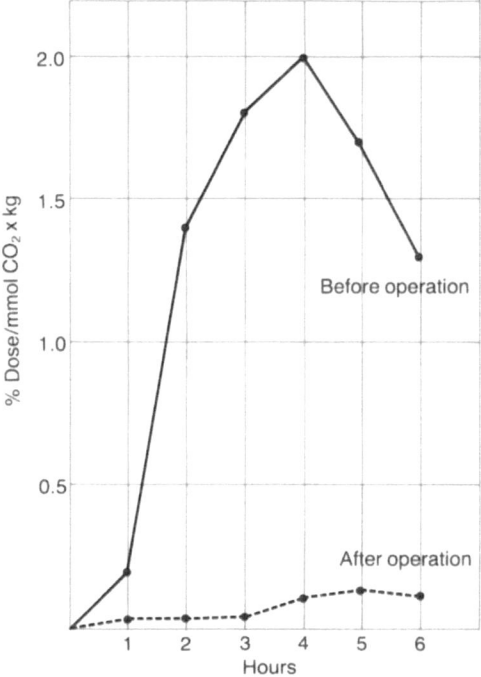

Fig. 70. ^{14}C-glycocholate breath test in a patient with a choledochoduodenocholic fistula before and after operation for removal of the fistula. The preoperatively markedly increased deconjugation of the bile acid glycocholic acid suggested massive bacterial overgrowth of the upper small intestine, which was completely normalised 4 weeks after he operation

it from the human host. Although vitamin B_{12} bound to gastric intrinsic factor is not taken up as freely by bacteria as vitamin B_{12} alone, both in animal experiments [63] and in patients [64] uptake of gastric intrinsic factor – vitamin B_{12} complex by intestinal bacteria has been demonstrated.

Thus it can be stated that vitamin B_{12} malabsorption associated with bacterial overgrowth results from bacterial ingestion of dietary vitamin B_{12}.

In contrast to vitamin B_{12} and fat absorption, the absorption of carbohydrates, protein, salt and water in the blind-loop syndrome has received less attention. Decreased urinary D-xylose excretion, depressed serum protein and diarrhoea have been frequently observed in patients and experimental animals with this syndrome [30].

Goldstein et al. [65] suggested that the low urinary D-xylose values in patients with bacterial overgrowth might be secondary to bacterial utilization of this carbohydrate. This assumption was based on a perfusion study with D-xylose in the intestine of a single patient with the blind-loop syndrome. By the use of $^{14}CO_2$-xylose breath test Spivey et al. [66] and Gianella et al. [54] showed that as much as 40% of D-xylose may be metabolized by intraluminal bacteria. Metz et al. [67] have shown that oral administration of glucose to patients with bacterial overgrowth may result in increased breath H_2 due to the bacterial action on D-glucose. A pathological D-xylose test with normalization after a week's course of antibiotic treatment may be taken as an indirect proof of bacterial overgrowth of the small intestine. The diarrhoea observed in bacterial overgrowth may be due to various factors [68].

1) Morphological changes of the mucosa induced by secondary free bile acids, which may alter secretory function or the motility pattern of the intestine.

2) Owing to fat malabsorption, hydroxy fatty acids will exert a cathartic effect on the colon, as do bile acids.

18.4 Diagnosis

Patients with postgastrectomy steatorrhoea should be fully investigated to exclude specific causes such as unmasked coeliac disease, pancreatic insufficiency, afferent-loop stasis, gastrojejunocolic fistula, inadvertent gastro-ileostomy. The routine haematological and metabolic investigations should be extended to include: small-bowel biopsy, secretin-pancreozymin test, radiological studies such as upper gastro-intestinal series, a barium enema when fistula is assumed, ^{14}C-glycocholate breath test, D-xylose test, Schilling test, and intestinal transit time (H_2 measurement after 10 or 15 g of lactulose).

18.5 Treatment

When investigation reveals a specific cause of postgastrectomy steatorrhoea the appropriate therapy should be started. This will be gluten-free diet in coeliac disease, substitution of pancreatic enzymes in absolute or relative pancreatic insufficiency and antibiotics in small-intestinal bacterial overgrowth. Tetracyclines (500 mg four times a day) are the drugs of first choice followed by ampicillin. Neomycin is not appropriate, since the drug may itself induce malabsorption due to precipitation of bile acids and to its possible toxic effects on the mucosa. Most easily correctable is vitamin B_{12} malabsorption (by antibiotics), probably because the total number of organisms present seems to be related to the vitamin B_{12} malabsorption [69]. Treatment is continued for 2 weeks, and improvement in the D-xylose and Schilling tests as well as normalisation of the ^{14}C-glycocholate breath test can be used as objective measures for the success of treatment. If unsuccessful, a course with ampicillin may improve symptoms and objective tests. If relapse occurs after discontinuation of treatment, we advise patients to take the antibiotic 10 days a month and have had good results.

Long-standing malabsorption of fat induced by alterations of bile acid metabolism in the blind-loop syndrome will result in malabsorption of fat-soluble vitamins, which should be replaced (vitamins A, D, E, K). Indeed, decreased levels of 25-hydroxycholecalciferol (25-OHCC) have been found in gastrectomised patients not receiving vitamin D supplements. Gertner et al. [70] reported decreased 25-OHCC levels in six postgastrectomy patients. Schoen et al. [71] studied 29 patients following gastrectomy; 10 were taking supplemental vitamins

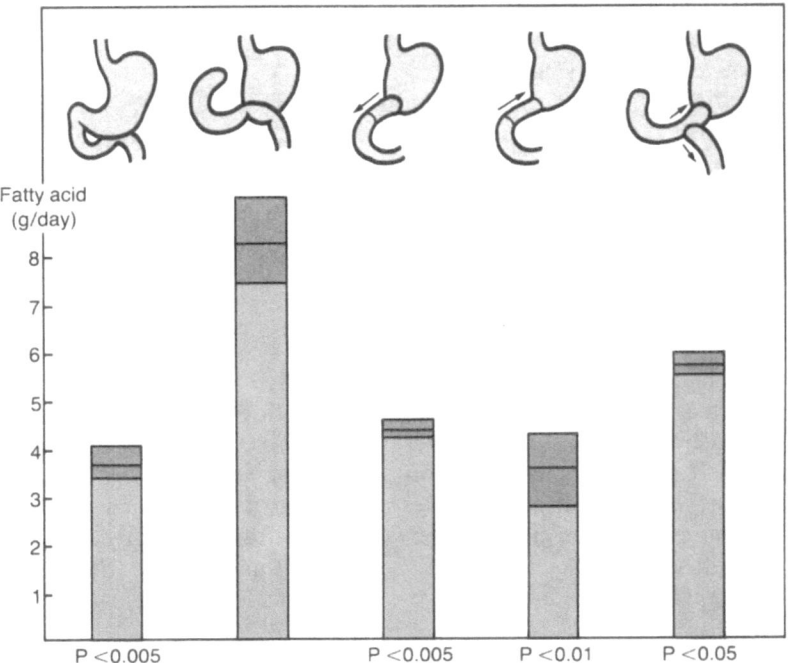

Fig. 71. Faecal fat excretion in dogs after gastrectomy and reoperation with different kinds of jejunal interposition. After C. MacKay, 1970

and had normal 25-OHCC levels, whereas over 40% of the remaining 19 patients, without supplemental vitamins, had low 25-OHCC levels.

When despite thorough investigation no specific cause is revealed, the non-specific medical treatment is indicated. This is frequent small meals, which have the effect of compensating for the lost reservoir function of the resected stomach. Pancreatic enzymes and antibiotics are less effective when used empirically than when used specifically. Surgical treatment is indicated when investigation reveals a surgically remediable cause such as gastrocolic fistula, gastro-ileostomy or obstructed afferent loop syndrome. Operation may also be indicated when no specific cause can be demonstrated and medical treatment has failed. Clear-cut correction of fat loss and vitamin B_{12} malabsorption and of bacterial overgrowth by revison of BII gastrojejunostomy to BI gastroduodenostomy has been documented.

Conversion to BI gastrectomy is the most common kind of operation for the treatment of postgastrectomy malabsorption. Good results by this kind of operation have been reported [14, 72], but it is not invariably successful [73, 74]. Other remedial operations have been developed; they have been reviewed by Rutledge [75]. The most popular has been the interposition of an iso- or aniso-peristaltic segment of jejunum between the gastric remnant and the duodenum [76–81]. Restoration of the duodenal passage certainly will be beneficial, but there has been some disagreement regarding the effect of the operation on gastric emptying. Herrington [82, 83] found that an isoperitaltic segment

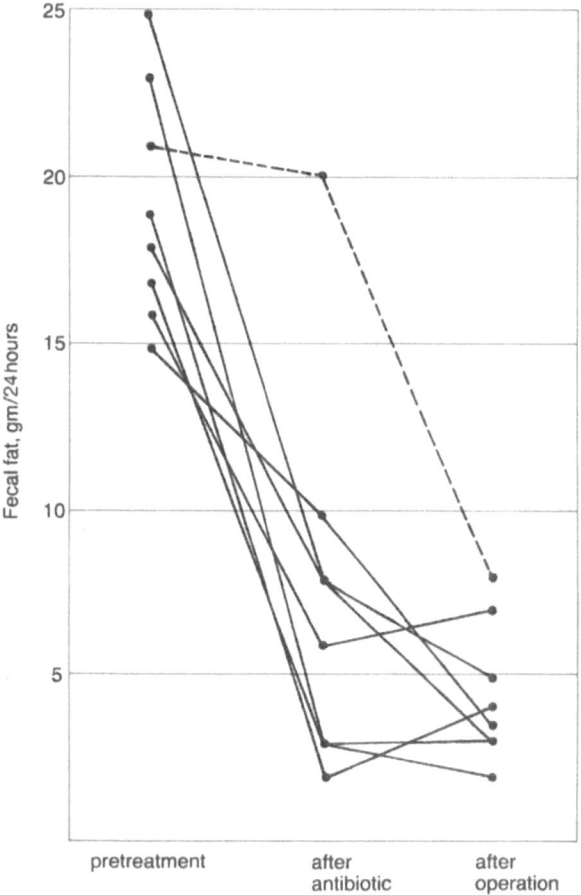

Fig. 72. Faecal fat excretion in patients with partial gastrectomy before and after antibiotic and subsequent surgical treatment (isoperistaltic jejunal loop interposition between the stomach and the duodenum) The dashed line represents patients who did not have impressive response to antibiotics but did respond to isoperistaltic loop interposition. After Fineberg et al., 1973

produced no delay in gastric emptying, whereas Hedenstedt found the opposite [84]. In a very elegant study MacKay [85] examined the effect of jejunal interposition on the gastric emptying in partially gastrectomised dogs. Dogs were subjected to a 80% gastrectomy and a gastrojejunostomy. Three months later they were reoperated: one group received no jejunal interposition, a second group an interposition of an isoperistaltic jejunal segment between the stomach and the duodenum, a third group an anisoperistaltic jejunal segment, and a fourth group an anisoperistaltic jejunal segment between the gastric remnant and jejunum just distal to the duodenojejunal flexure. Each of the groups had lost weight 3 months after gastrectomy. Jejunal interposition resulted in weight gain in all groups, but most markedly in the groups with interposition of an isoperistaltic segment. Faecal fat excretion was significantly lower in all groups with jejunal interposition than in that with gastrectomy alone (Fig. 71). The mean rate of gastric emptying was increased by the gastrectomy, but jejunal interposition delayed the rate of gastric emptying. Gastroduodenal interposition more effectively reduced the rate of gastric emptying than gastrojejunal interposition.

Fineberg et al. [86] measured faecal fat excretion after antibiotic treatment and found a marked reduction of steatorrhoea in most of the patients. Isoperistaltic jejunal loop interposition between the stomach and duodenum in patients with previous Billroth II gastrectomy caused a striking improvement in fat absorption (Fig. 72).

References

1 Wall, A.J., Ungar, B., Baird, C.W., Langford, I.M., MacKay, I.R.: Malnutrition after partial gastrectomy. Am. J. Dig Dis. *12*, 1077 (1967)
2. Magnuson, F.K., Judd, E.S., Dearing, W.H.: Comparison of postgastrectomy complications in gastric and duodenal ulcer patients. Ann. Surg. *32*, 375 (1966)
3. Cox, A.G.· The outcome of truncal vagotomy and a drainage procedure. Chapt. 5. In: Vagotomy on Trial, A.G. Cox, I.A. Williams, eds. Heinemann Medical Books 67 (1973)
4. Goligher, J.C., Pulvertaft, C.N., Watkinson, G.: Controlled trial of vagotomy and gastroenterostomy in elective treatment of duodenal ulcer: Interim report. Brit. med. J. *1*, 455 (1969)
5. Wheldon, E.J., Venables, C.W., Johnston, I.D.A.: Late metabolic sequelae of vagotomy and gastroenterostomy. Lancet *I*, 437 (1970)
6. Williams, J.A.: Partial gastrectomy. The late nutritional and metabolic effects. Am J. Proctol. *17*, 288 (1966)
7. Williams, J.A.: Postgastrectomy problems II. Brit. Med. J. *4*, 467 (1967)
8. Mac Lean, L.D., Perry, J.F., Kelly, W.D., et al.: Nutrition following subtotal gastrectomy of four types (Billroth I and II, segmental and tubular resections). Surgery *35*, 705 (1954)
9. Lundh, G.: Intestinal digestion and absorption after gastrectomy. Acta Chir. Scand. Suppl. *231*, 1 (1958)
10 Hillman, H.S.: Postgastrectomy malnutrition. Gut *9*, 576 (1968)
11. Pryor, J.P., O'Shea, M.J., Brooks, P.L., Datar, G.K.: The long-term metabolic consequences of partial gastrectomy Am J Med *51*, 5 (1971)
12. Johnston, I.D.A ,Welbourne, R , Acheson, K.: Gastrectomy and loss of weight. Lancet *1*, 1242 (1968)
13 Wastell, C.: Long-term clinical and metabolic effects of vagotomy with either gastrojejunostomy or pyloroplasty. Ann. Roy. Coll. Surg. Engl. *44*, 193 (1969)
13a. Jordan, P.H., Jr.: A prospective study of parietal cell vagotomy and selective vagotomy-antrectomy for treatment of duodenal ulcer. Ann. Surg. *183*, 183 (1976)
14. Welbourne, R.B.: Nutritional aspects of gastric surgery. Rev. Surg. *24*, 233 (1967)
15. Butler, T.J.: A study of the pancreatic response to food after gastrectomy in man. Gut *1*, 55 (1960)
16. Corsini, G., Gandolfi, E., Bonecki, I., Cerri, B.: Post-gastrectomy malabsorption. Gastro-enterology *50*, 358 (1966)
17. MacKay, C.: Postgastrectomy steatorrhea. Am. J. Surg. *120*, 324 (1970)
18 Capper, W M., Welbourne, R.B.: Early post-cibal symptoms following gastrectomy. Brit. J. Surg. *43*, 24 (1955)
19. Orr, J.: Physiological considerations in the surgery of peptic ulcer. Ann. Roy. Coll. Surg. Engl. *34*, 314 (1964)
20 Herrmann, G., Axtell, H.K., Starzl, T.E.: Fat absorption and the afferent loop. Surgery *57*, 291 (1965)
21. Wollaeger, E.E., Waugh, J.M., Power, M.H.: Fat assimilation capacity of the GI tract after partial gastrectomy and gastroduodenostomy. Gastroenterology *44*, 25 (1963)
22. Shingleton, W.W., Isley, J.K., Floyd, R D., et al.: Studies on postgastrectomy steatorrhea using radioactive triolein. Surgery *42*, 12 (1957)
23. Krikler, D.M., Schrire, V.: Kwashiorkor in an adult due to an intestinal blind loop. Lancet *I*, 510 (1958)

24. Neale, G., Antcliff, A.C., Welbourne, R.B., et al.: Protein malnutrition after partial gastrectomy. Quarterl. J. Med. *36*, 469 (1967)
25. Booth, C.C., Brain, M.C., Jeejeebhoy, K.N.: Late postgastrectomy syndromes. Hypoproteinemia after partial gastrectomy. Proc. Roy. Soc. Med. *57*, 582 (1964)
26. Brain, M.C., Unstall, H.B., Jeejeebhoy, K.N.: Postgastrectomy hypoproteinemia. Am. J. Med. *39*, 674 (1965)
28. Buckler, K.G.: Effects of gastric surgery upon gastric emptying in cases of peptic ulceration. Gut *8*, 484 (1965)
29. Wirts, L.W., Goldstein, F.: Studies on the mechanism of postgastrectomy steatorrhea. Ann. Internal Med. *58*, 25 (1963)
30. Tabaqchali, S.: The pathophysiological role of small intestinal flora. Scand. J. Gastroenterol. (Suppl. 6) *5*, 139 (1970)
31. Worning, H., Mulleritz, S., Hess Thaysen, E., et al.: pH and concentration of pancreatic enzymes in aspirates from the human duodenum during digestion of a standard meal in patients with duodenal ulcer and in patients subjected to different operatons Scand. J. Gastroenterol. *2*, 23 (1967)
32. Glazebrook, A.J., Welbourne, R.B.: Some observations on the function of the small intestine after gastrectomy. Br. J. Surg. *40*, 111 (1952)
33. Annis, D., Hallenbeck, G.A.: The effects of partial gastrectomy on canine external pancreatic secretion. Surgery *31*, 517 (1952)
34. Malagelada, J.R., Go, V.L.W., Summerskill, W.J.H.: Altered pancreatic and biliary function after vagotomy and pyloroplasty. Gastroenterology *66*, 22 (1974)
35. MacGregor, I.L., Parent, J., Meyer, J.H.: Gastric emptying of liquid meals and pancreatic and biliary secretion after subtotal gastrectomy or truncal vagotomy and pyloroplasty in man. Gastroenterology *72*, 195 (1977)
36. Lagerlof, H.O., Rudewald, M B., Perman, G.: The neutralization process in duodenum and its influence on the gastric emptying in man. Acta med. Scand *168*, 269 (1960)
37. Fields, M., Duthie, H.L.: Effect of vagotomy on intraluminal digestion of fat in man. Gut *6*, 301 (1965)
38. Toskes, P.P., Cerda, J.J.: The value of the gelatine infusion test in the diagnosis of pancreatic exocrine insufficiency in patients with Billroth II anastomosis. Am. J Dig. Dis. *18*, 147 (1973)
39. Scott, G.B., Williams, M.J., Clark, C.G.: Comparison of jejunal mucosa in postgastrectomy states, idiopathic steatorrhoea and controls using the dissecting microscope and conventional histologic methods. Gut *5*, 553 (1964)
40. Rubin, C.E., Dobbins, W.O.: Peroral biopsy of the small intestine. A review of its diagnostic usefulness. Gastroenterology *49*, 676 (1965)
41. Hedberg, C.A., Melnyk, C.S., Johnson, C.F.: Gluten enteropathy appearing after gastric surgery. Gastroenterology *50*, 796 (1966)
42. Gryboski, J.D., Thayer, W R., Gryboski, W.N., et al.: A defect in disacharide metabolism after gastrojejunostomy. N. Engl. J. Med. *268*, 78 (1963)
43. Bond, J.H., Levitt, M.D.: Use of breath hydrogen (H_2) to quantitate small bowel transit time following partial gastrectomy. J. Lab Clin. Med. *90*, 30 (1977)
44. Donaldson, R.M.: Small bowel bacterial overgrowth. Adv. Intern. Med. *16*, 191 (1970)
45. Ballinger, W.F., Lida, J., Padula, R.T., et al.: Bacterial inflammation and denervation atrophy of the small intestine. Surgery *57*, 535 (1965)
46. Bishop, R.F.: Bacterial flora of stomach and small intestine after gastric surgery. Ernahrungsforschung *10*, 417 (1965)
47. Greenlee, H.B., Gelbart, S.M., De Orio, A.J., et al.: The influence of gastric surgery on the intestinal flora Am. J. Clin. Nutr. *30*, 1826 (1977)
48. Gorbach, S.L., Plant, A.G., Nahas, L., et al.: Studies of intestinal microflora I. Microorganisms of the small intestine and their relations to oral and rectal flora. Gastroenterology *53*, 856 (1967)
49. Draser, B.S., Shiner, M.: Studies on the intestinal flora. Part II: Bacterial flora of the small intestine in patients with gastrointestinal disorders. Gut *10*, 812 (1969)
50. Vantrappen, G., Janssens, J., Hellemans, J., et al.: The interdigestive motor complex of normal subjects and patients with bacterial overgrowth of the small intestine. J. Clin. Invest. *59*, 1158 (1977)
51. Browing, G.G., Buchan, K A., Mackay, C.: The effect of vagotomy and drainage on the small bowel flora. Gut *15*, 139 (1974)

52. Paulley, J.W.: The jejunal mucosa in malabsorptive states with high bacterial counts. In: Girwood, R.H., Smith, A.N., eds. Malabsorption. p 171 Edinburgh: University of Edinburgh Press 1969

53. Gracey, M., Burke, V., Oshin, A., et al.: Bacteria, bile salts and intestinal monosaccharide absorption. Gut *12*, 683 (1971)

54. Gianella, R.A., Rout, W.R., Toskes, P.P.: Jejunal brush border injury and impaired sugar and amino acid uptake in the blind loop syndrome. Gastroenterology *67*, 965 (1974)

55. Toskes, P.P., Gianella, R.A., Jervis, H.R., et al.: Small intestinal mucosal injury in the experimental blind loop syndrome: light- and electron-microscopic and histochemical studies. Gastroenterology *68*, 1193 (1975)

56. Ament, M.E., Shimoda, S.S., Saunders, D.R., et al : Pathogenesis of steatorrhea in three cases of small intestinal stasis syndrome. Gastroenterology *63*, 728 (1972)

57. Donaldson, R.M.: Studies on the pathogenesis of steatorrhea in the blind loop syndrome. J. Clin. Invest. *44*, 1815 (1965)

58. Kim, Y.S., Spritz, N., Blum, M., et al.: The role of altered bile acid metabolism in the steatorrhoea of experimental blind loop. J. Clin. Invest. *45*, 956 (1966)

59. Fromm, H., Hofmann, A.F.: Breath test for altered bile acid metabolism. Lancet *II*, 621 (1971)

60. Caspary, W.F., Reimold, W.V.: Klinische Bedeutung des ^{14}C-Glykocholat-Atemtestes in der gastroenterologischen Diagnostik bei Erkrankungen mit gesteigerter Dekonjugation von Gallensäuren. Dtsch. med. Wschr. *101*, 353 (1976)

61. Caspary, W.F.. Breath tests. In: Clinics in Gastroenterology Vol. 7, 351 (1978)

62. Gianella, R.A., Broitman, S A , Zamcheck, N.: Vitamin B_{12}-uptake by intestinal microorganisms: mechanism and relevance to syndromes of intestinal bacterial overgrowth. J. Clin. Invest. *50*, 110 (1971)

63. Donaldson, R.M.: Malabsorption of Co^{60}-labeled cyanocobalamin in rats with intestinal diverticula. I. Evaluation of possible mechanisms. Gastroenterology *43*, 271 (1962)

64. Schjonsky, H.: The absorption of vitamin B_{12} in the blind loop syndrome. Scand. J. Gastroenterology (Suppl.) *29*, 65 (1974)

65. Goldstein, F., Karacadag, S., Wirts, C.W., et al.: Intraluminal small intestinal utilization of D-xylose by bacteria. Gastroenterology *59*, 380 (1970)

66. Spivey, J., Lorenz, E., Manderli, W., et al.: Evaluation of carbohydrate metabolism in patients with the blind loop syndrome. Gastroenterology *68*, 1001 (1975)

67. Metz, G., Gassull, A.M , Drasar, B.S., et al.: Breath hydrogen test for small intestinal bacterial colonization. Lancet *I*, 668 (1976)

68. King, C.E , Toskes, P.D.· Small intestine bacterial overgrowth Gastroenterology *76*, 1035 (1979)

69. Campbell, C B , Cowen, A E., Harper, J.: Duodenal bacterial flora and bile salt patterns in patients with gastrointestinal disease. Austral. N.Z. J. Med. *3*, 339 (1973)

70. Gertner, J.M., Lilburn, M., Domnech: 25-hydroxycholecalciferol absorption in steatorrhea and postgastrectomy osteomalacia. Brit. Med. J. *1*, 1310 (1977)

71 Schoen, M.S., Lindenbaum, J., Rogiusky, M.S , et al.: Significance of serum levels of 25-hydroxycholecalciferol in gastrointestinal disease. Am. J. Dig. Dis. *23*, 137 (1978)

72. Engstrom, J., Hellstrom, K., Lundh, G., et al.: Microflora of small intestine, incidence of steatorrhea and indicanuria before and after conversion of Billroth II to Billroth I type of gastric resection. Acta chir. Scand. *139*, 546 (1973)

73. Buchan, R., Clark, C G., Downie, R.W.M.: Conversion to Billroth I anastomosis or enteroanastomosis for postgastrectomy states. Brit. J. Surg. *52*, 651 (1965)

74. Borg, I., Borgstrom, S.G., Haeger, K.: The value of the BII-BI conversion operation in the treatment of the postgastrectomy syndrome. Acta chir. Scand. *134*, 655 (1968)

75. Rutledge, R.H : Jejunal segments for the postgastrectomy syndromes. Ann. Surgery *169*, 810 (1969)

76. Wirts, C.W , Templeton, J.Y , Fineberg, C., et al : The correction of postgastrectomy malabsorption following a jejunal interposition operation. Gastroenterology *49*, 141 (1965)

77. Henley, F.A.: Gastrectomy with replacement. a preliminary communication. Brit. J. Surg. *40*, 118 (1952)

78. Hedenstedt, S., Lundqvist, G.: Antiperistaltic jejunal segment in gastric surgery. Acta chir. Scand. *133*, 545 (1967)

79. Hedenstedt, S., Lundqvist, G.: Antrectomy plus jejunal transposition plus selective vagotomy. Acta chir. Scand. *134*, 373 (1968)

80. Herrington, J.L.: Jejunal interposition for certain postgastrectomy syndromes. Surg. Clin. North Am. *46*, 441 (1966)
81. Kay, A.W., Cox, A.G.: Jejunal transposition for the postgastrectomy patient. Brit. J. Surg. *51*, 763 (1964)
82. Herrington, J.L : Remedial operations for severe postgastrectomy symptoms. Ann. Surg *162*, 789 (1965)
83. Herrington, J.L.: Utilization of small bowel segments as a gastric reservoir for control of the dumping syndrome. Am. J. Surg. *111*, 89 (1969)
84. Hedenstedt, S.: Gastrectomy with jejunal replacement. Acta Chir. Scand *117*, 295 (1959)
85. Fineberg, C., Templeton, J.Y. III, Wirts, C.W., et al.: The correction of postgastrectomy malabsorption by jejunal interposition. Surg. Clin. N. Amer. *53*, 581 (1973)

19 Postgastrectomy Anaemia

19.1 Incidence

Alterations in haematological parameters often resulting in anaemia are among the major clinical complications encountered in patients who have had gastric surgery. The reported incidence of anaemia following partial gastrectomy has ranged from 3% to 63% [1]. Examination of the peripheral blood smear of anaemia patients after gastric surgery may be confusing, because iron-deficiency anaemia and vitamin-deficiency anaemia may coexist [2]. The reported incidence of anaemia depends on how carefully it is looked for. Although not anaemic, many more patients have low serum iron or vitamin B_{12} levels [3]. The incidence of anaemia increases with time. In one study, anaemia was found to be present in 9% of patients (iron-deficiency anaemia) during the first year after gastrectomy, but later 30% of the patients were found to have anaemia [4].

Johnston noted that 20 years after truncal vagotomy, 30% of men and 52% of women were anaemic [5]. The incidence of anaemia was about the same after vagotomy with gastro-enterostomy as after partial gastrectomy.

The pathogenesis of postgastrectomy anaemia is complex, depending on the inter-relationship between iron, vitamin B_{12} and folic acid. Iron deficiency has been the most frequent and often the only haematologic abnormality detected in patients after gastric surgery [4, 6–8]. More recent reports, however, have stressed the importance of vitamin B_{12} deficiency in the pathogenesis of postgastrectomy anaemia. Mahmud et al. [9, 10], in a recent series of 107 patients, emphasised the equal importance of iron deficiency and vitamin B_{12} deficiency. Hines et al. [11] did not find a relationship between the location of the preoperative ulcer and the type of surgery performed in the development of postoperative anaemia, but others have stressed that all types of anaemia were more common after surgery for gastric ulcer [12]. It was also found that patients with a Billroth II anastomosis are more likely to develop anaemia than patients with a Billroth I operation [1, 10, 12]. In a study including 292 patients with partial gastrectomy, Hines et al. [11] found that 30% of the patients with gastric ulcer developed vitamin B_{12} deficiency, compared to 9% with a duodenal ulcer.

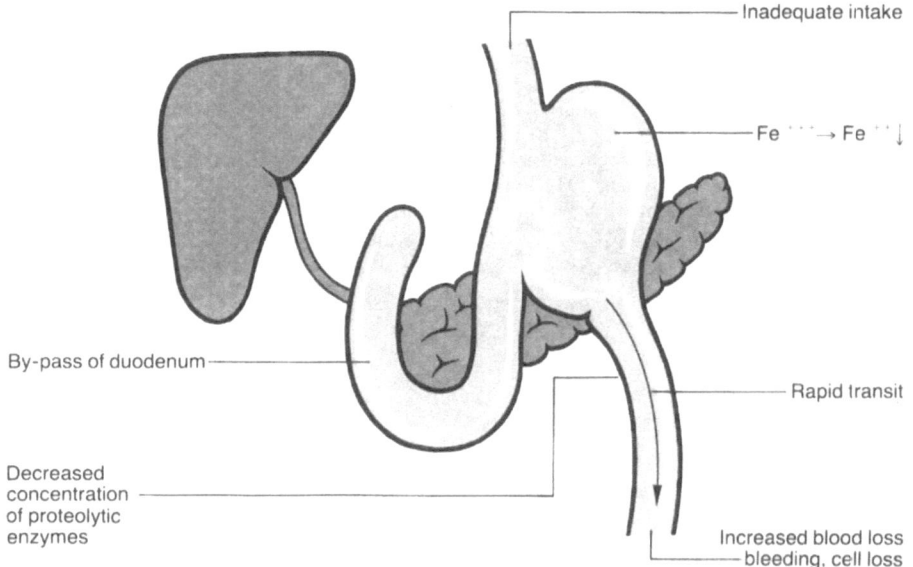

Fig. 73. Pathogenic factors responsible for postgastrectomy iron-deficiency anaemia

19.2 Iron-Deficiency Anaemia

Iron-deficiency anaemia after partial gastrectomy is the most common type of postgastrectomy haematological abnormality. The increased incidence of post-gastrectomy iron-deficiency anaemia can be attributed to several factors (Fig. 73).
1) Inadequate dietary intake of iron
2) Decreased bio-availability of iron
3) Impaired absorption
4) Increased blood loss.

Iron-deficiency anaemia has been found in 33%–50% of patients following partial gastric resection [1, 9–11, 13]. Inadequate iron intake has been assumed to contribute to the development of iron-deficiency anaemia after gastric surgery, but inadequate intake cannot account completely for the cause of anaemia [6]. Another factor which has to be seriously considered as the cause is an increased blood loss from the remnant of the stomach, especially in the presence of postoperative reflux oesophagitis or gastritis.

Results in the literature are controversial, however: Baird et al. [6, 8] did not find significantly increased blood loss in 18 postgastrectomy patients with un-explained anaemia, compared with 13 controls. Aspirin-induced blood losses were identical in postgastrectomy subject and controls. Considerably higher were the blood losses reported by Kimber et al. [14], who reported ^{51}Cr-labelled red blood cell stool losses between 3.2 and 6.5 ml/day, a finding supported by Holt et al. [15, 16], who found blood losses between 150 and 200 ml/month in patients with partial gastrectomy. Thus, increased blood loss after gastric surgery seems to be a contributing factor for the development of iron-deficiency anaemia, when the adaptive process in the intestine may not compensate effectively enough for loss of iron due to the increased blood loss. Effectiveness of intestinal absorption of iron is normally increased following an increased blood loss. In patients with damage to the stomach or intestine (i.e. adult coeliac disease) there may be loss of iron due to an increased cell turnover, an increase of sloughing-off of cells, or an iron-losing enteropathy. Since absorption of iron is facilitated by hydrochloric acid, reduced acid secretion may be responsible for the decreased bio-availability of ferrous iron. An important factor contributing to iron-deficiency anaemia is by-pass of the duodenum, the major site for iron absorption in Billroth-II operations. Since organic iron in food seems to be absorbed differently from inorganic iron, digestive processes responsible for liberation of food iron might become rate-limiting. A decreased contact time of digestion of food, due to rapid intestinal transit, and pancreaticocibal asyncrasy, leading to a relative pancreatic insufficiency, are contributing factors for decreased bio-availability of food iron after gastrectomy. The relative pancreatic insufficiency results from a lack of food-stimulated release of intestinal hormones eliciting pancreatic secretion. In the case of vagotomy, a decrease of maximal pancreatic enzyme secretion has in addition been reported [17]. Thus resected patients whose most important source of iron is meat may not be able to increase absorption appropriately in times of need. They may, however, respond well to administration of inorganic iron salts [6, 7, 11].

19.3 Vitamin B_{12} Deficiency

Vitamin B_{12} malabsorption after partial gastrectomy is well known, though megaloblastic anaemia from this cause is rare. Only 18 patients with megaloblastic anaemia were detected in a combined series of 2,180 patients after gastrectomy examined by four groups of workers [1, 18–20]. Hines et al. [11] reported a 2%–4% incidence of defective peripheral blood maturation. However, as subacute degeneration of the spinal cord complicating neglected vitamin B_{12} deficiency after gastrectomy is well recognized [21], the importance of vitamin B_{12} deficiency lies in an early diagnosis and treatment. The principal cause of vitamin B_{12} deficiency has long been considered to be shortage or absence of intrinsic factor. Large body stores of vitamin B_{12} and the progressive atrophy of the mucosa of the gastric remnant delay the onset of this deficiency. Based on five studies in 1284 patients, Table 38 shows the percentages of patients with a subnormal vitamin B_{12} level below 140 pg/ml.

The study of Mahmud et al. [10] stressed the importance of vitamin B_{12} deficiency after gastric surgery. They found vitamin B_{12} deficiency to be the most common haematological abnormality, occuring in 68% of 107 patients with partial gastrectomy. Their parameter was the red cell vitamin B_{12} level. Whether red cell vitamin B_{12} levels are a specific indicator for vitamin B_{12} deficiency has, however, been seriously questioned [22]. Nevertheless Rygvold et al. [23] found that in a series of 351 patients with Billroth II anastomosis, 20% had B_{12} levels below 150 pg/ml and 16% had levels between 150 and 200 pg/ml. Thus 36% of

Table 38. Subnormal levels of serum vitamin B_{12} after partial gastrectomy (lower limit of normal $= 140$ pg/ml)

Authors	No. of patients	% Subnormal
Deller and Wilts, 1962	265	14
Weir et al., 1963	315	11.5
Mollin and Hines, 1964	212	13
Hoffbrand, 1967	292	20
Lee and Clark, 1970	200	12
Total	1,284	14%

of these patients were considered to have vitamin B_{12} deficiency. Hines et al. [11] found decreased vitamin B_{12} absorption in 58 of their 59 patients. Repeated Schilling tests with intrinsic factor in 40 patients resulted in normalization of vitamin B_{12} absorption in 35%, suggesting that a decrease of intrinsic factor was the most likely cause of the vitamin B_{12} malabsorption observed in these patients.

This finding is not, however, shared by other workers. Rygvold et al. [23] observed a lack of intrinsic factor in only one-third of their patients with decreased vitamin B_{12} levels. By examination of vitamin B_{12} absorptive capacity before and soon after partial gastric resection, a reduced absorption of vitamin B_{12} could not be demonstrated [24]. The time elapsed after gastric resection, however, may have been too short to take into account the decreased intrinsic factor production following postoperative atrophic gastritis.

In contrast to normal vitamin B_{12} absorption, in two-thirds of their patients with low vitamin B_{12} levels assessed by the Schilling test, Mahmud et al. [10] found that absorption of vitamin B_{12} was lower when it was incorporated into eggs. Thus these workers stress that two-thirds of the patients after partial gastfectomy were able to absorb vitamin B_{12} in the crystalline form, but unable to absorb it in a normal manner from food. Thus there seems to be a parallel to iron absorption, where absorption of food iron seems to be more seriously impaired than absorption of inorganic iron (Fig. 74).

When abnormally low vitamin B_{12} levels occur together with a normal vitamin B_{12} absorption test after gastric surgery, this means that there is impaired release of food-bound vitamin B_{12}. Doscherholmen and Swaim have shown that ^{57}Co-labelled vitamin B_{12} incorporated into scrambled eggs may be poorly absorbed after partial gastrectomy [25].

A recent report [26] showed that malabsorption of vitamin B_{12} bound to chicken serum occured in patients who had just undergone vagotomy and a drainage procedure, but these patients absorbed crystalline vitamin B_{12} in a normal fashion. They demonstrated a correlation between the amount of bound vitamin B_{12} absorbed and the amount of gastric acid produced. Patients with a positive Hollander test 5 years after vagotomy and drainage absorbed more bound vitamin B_{12}, whereas patients with a negative Hollander test exhibited markedly reduced absorption of bound vitamin B_{12}. Since a decrease of pancreatic exocrine function does occur after vagotomy and pancreatic exocrine insufficiency

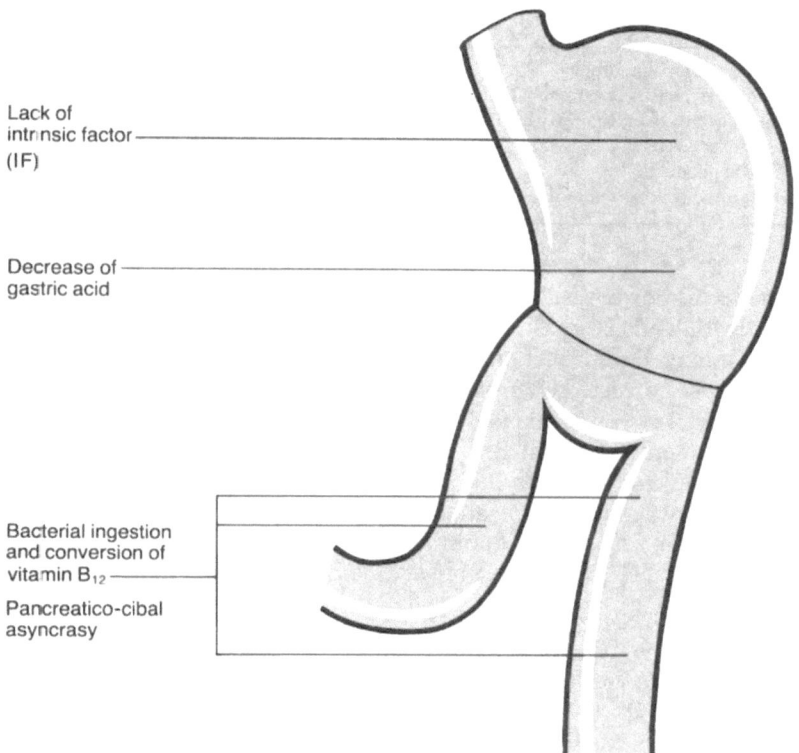

Lack of
intrinsic factor
(IF)

Decrease of
gastric acid

Bacterial ingestion
and conversion of
vitamin B$_{12}$

Pancreatico-cibal
asyncrasy

Fig. 74. Pathogenesis of vitamin B$_{12}$ deficiency after gastric resection

[17] favours vitamin B$_{12}$ malabsorption, a decrease of exocrine pancreatic function may be another explanation for the findings of this group.

An implication of the results of Doscherholmen [25] and Streeter [26] is that it may be unnecessary to give vitamin B$_{12}$ parenterally to all patients with low vitamin B$_{12}$ levels. If the Schilling test is normal, administration of crystalline vitamin B$_{12}$ between meals should be adequate. Parenteral Vitamin B$_{12}$ administration will be required if a lack of intrinsic factor exists.

Forty per cent of patients with exocrine pancreatic deficiency develop vitamin B$_{12}$ malabsorption, which can be corrected by administration of pancreatic extracts or intestinal secretions obtained from normal subjects [27]. Vitamin B$_{12}$ malabsorption may also occur following vagotomy without gastric reresection [28] and after gastro-enterostomy without vagotomy [26]. Another important factor contributing to vitamin B$_{12}$ deficiency is the bacterial overgrowth syndrome often developing after gastric resection. Vitamin B$_{12}$ deficiency in the bacterial over-growth syndrome is due to binding or even ingestion of the vitamin by bacteria, so that it becomes unavailable for absorption. Thus bacteria decrease the bio-availability of vitamin B$_{12}$. Bacteria take up vitamin B$_{12}$ bound to intrinsic factor as well as the free vitamin.

Table 39. Role of bacteria in vitamin B_{12} malabsorption

1) Uptake and use of cyanocobalamine
2) Uptake of the intrinsic factor – cyanocobalamine complex
3) Release of intrinsic factor from the intrinsic factor – cyanocobalamine complex
4) Alteration of intrinsic factor
5) Production of toxic products
6) Conversion of ingested cyanocobalamine to inactive analogues

Stasis of the small bowel resulting in small-intestinal bacterial overgrowth is more common in Billroth II anastomoses than is generally appreciated. Some of these patients may develop vitamin B_{12} malabsorption and vitamin B_{12} deficiency that may be corrected by broad-spectrum antibiotics. Vitamin B_{12} malabsorption in bacterial overgrowth results from competition by bacteria with the human host for the dietary vitamin B_{12}. It has been recently shown that intra-luminal bacteria can take up vitamin B_{12} attached to gastric intrinsic factor [29]. There is evidence that vitamin B_{12} analogues (cobamides) are produced by intestinal bacteria from ingested vitamin B_{12}, thus making the vitamin B_{12} unavailable for absorption [30]. The role of bacteria in vitamin B_{12} malabsorption is detailed in Table 39.

19.4 Folate Deficiency

Although the major cause of megaloblastic anaemia after gastric surgery is vitamin B_{12} deficiency, folic acid deficiency may also contribute [31]. Although Hines et al. [11] found 41% of their patients to have subnormal folate levels, Pryor et al. [12] found no evidence of folate deficiency. Mahmud et al. observed a folate deficiency in about 33% of patients followed for a mean of $8^1/_2$ years after subtotal gastrectomy [10]. There may also exist a combined deficiency of folate and vitamin B_{12} [31], since it is generally believed that the major cause for folate deficiency after gastric surgery is inadequate dietary intake [31, 32]. It remains undecided whether decreased serum folate levels are due to folic acid malabsorption or possibly, like vitamin B_{12}, to a decrease of digestion of folate conjugates which are major sources of folate in food.

References

1. Deller, D.J., Wilts, L.J.: Changes in the blood after partial gastrectomy with special reference to vitamin B_{12}. I Serum vitamin B_{12}, hemoglobin, serum iron and bone marrow Quart. J. Med. *31*, 71 (1962)
2. Lous, P., Schwartz, M.: The absorption of vitamin B_{12} following partial gastrectomy. Acta Med. Scand. *164*, 407 (1959)
3. Mollin, D.L., Hines, J.D.: Observations on the nature and pathogenesis of anaemia following partial gastrectomy. Proc. Royal Soc. Med. *57*, 575 (1964)
4. Lyngar, E.: Blood changes after partial gastrectomy for ulcer. Acta Med. Scand. (Suppl.) *1*, 247 (1950)

5. Johnston, I.D.A.: The management of side-effects of surgery for peptic ulceration. Brit. J. Surg. *57*, 787 (1970)
6. Baird, I.McL., Blackburn, E.K., Wilson, G.M.: The pathogenesis of anemia after partial gastrectomy: 1) Development of anemia in relation to time after partial gastrectomy: operation, blood loss, and diet. Quart. J. Med. *28*, 21 (1959)
7. Baird, I.McL., Wilson, G.M.: The pathogenesis of anemia after partial gastrectomy. 2. Iron absorption after partial gastrectomy. Quart. J. Med. *28*, 35 (1959)
8. Baird, I.McL., St. John, D.J.B., Nasser, S.S.: Role of occult blood loss in anemia after partial gastrectomy. Gut *11*, 55 (1970)
9. Mahmud, K., Ripley, D., Doscherholmen, A.: Vitamin B_{12} absorption tests, their unreliability in postgastrectomy states. J.A.M.A. *216*, 1167 (1971)
10. Mahmud, K., Ripley, D., Swaim, W.R., Doscherholmen, A.: Hematologic complications of partial gastrectomy. Ann. Surg. *177*, 432 (1973)
11. Hines, J.D., Hoffbrand, A.V., Mollin, D.L.: The haematological complications of a partial gastrectomy. Am. J. Med. *43*, 555 (1967)
12. Pryor, J.P., O'Shea, M.J., Brooks, P.L., Datar, G.K.: The long-term metabolic consequences of partial gastrectomy. Am. J. Med. *51*, 5 (1971)
13. Hobbs, J.R.: Iron deficiency anemia after partial gastrectomy. Gut *2*, 141 (1961)
14. Kimber, C., Patterson, J.F., Weintraub, C.R.: The pathogenesis of iron deficiency anemia following partial gastrectomy. J. Am. med. Assoc. *202*, 935 (1967)
15. Holt, J.M., Mayet, F.G.H., Warner, G.T. et al.: Iron absorption and blood loss in patients with hiatus hernia. Brit. Med. J. *3*, 22 (1968)
16. Holt, J.M., Gear, M.W.L., Warner, G.T.: The role of chronic blood loss in the pathogenesis of post-gastrectomy iron-deficiency anemia. Gut *11*, 847 (1970)
17. MacGregor, I.L., Parent, J., Meyer, J.H.: Gastric emptying of liquid meals and pancreatic and biliary secretions after subtotal gastrectomy or truncal vagotomy and pyloroplasty in man. Gastroenterology *72*, 195 (1977)
18. MacLean, L.D.: Incidence of megaloblastic anemia after subtotal gastrectomy. New Engl. J. Med. *257*, 262 (1957)
19. Jones, C.T., Williams, J.A., Cox, F.V. et al.: Peptic ulceration. Some hematological and metabolic consequences of gastric surgery. Lancet *II*, 425 (1962)
20. Weir, D.G., Gatenby, P.B.B.: Anaemia following gastric operations for peptic ulceration in Dublin. Brit. J. Med. Science *447*, 105 (1963)
21. Weir, D.G., Gatenby, P.B.B.: Subacute combined degeneration of the cord after partial gastrectomy. Brit. Med. J. *2*, 1175 (1963)
22. Hall, C.A.: Importance of red cell B_{12} and folate levels after partial gastrectomy. Am. J. Clin. Nutr. *27*, 899 (1974)
23. Rygvold, O.: Hypovitaminosis B_{12} following partial gastrectomy by the Billroth II method. Scand. J. Gastroent. (Suppl. 9) *29*, 57 (1974)
24. Loewenstein, F.: Absorption of cobalt (Co) labeled vitamin B_{12} after subtotal gastrectomy. Blood *13*, 339 (1958)
25. Doscherholmen, A., Swaim, W.R.: Impaired assimilation of CO^{57} vitamin B_{12} in patients with hypochlorhydria and achlorhydria after gastric resection Gastroenterology *64*, 913 (1973)
26. Streeter, A.M., Balasubramaniam, D., Boyle, R., et al.: Malabsorption of vitamin B_{12} after vagotomy. Am. J. Surgery *128*, 340 (1974)
27. Toskes, P.P., Deren, J.J.: Vitamin B_{12} absorption and malabsorption. Gastroenterology *65*, 662 (1973)
28. Wheldon, E.J., Venables, C.W., Johnston, I.D.A.: Late metabolic sequela of vagotomy and gastroenterostomy. Lancet *I*, 437 (1970)
29. Schjonsky, H.: The absorption of vitamin B_{12} in the blind loop syndrome. Scand. J. Gastroenterol. *29*, 65 (1974)
30. Brandt, L.J., Bernstein, L.H., Wagle, A.: Production of vitamin B_{12} analogues in patients with small-bowel bacterial overgrowth. Ann. int. Med. *87*, 546 (1977)
31. Deller, D.J., Ibbotson, R.N., Crompton, B.: Metabolic effects of partial gastrectomy with special reference to calcium and folic acid: Part II. The contribution of folic acid deficiency to the anemia. Gut *5*, 225 (1964)
32. Wastell, C.: Malabsorptive states after gastrointestinal surgery. Brit. Med. J. *3*, 661 (1968)

20 Postgastrectomy Bone Disease

20.1 Incidence

Bone disease as a complication of gastrectomy was predicted on the basis on their calcium balance studies by Nicolaysen and Ragard [1], who concluded that the negative balance demonstrated in their patients must inevitably have later metabolic consequences.

The magnitude of metabolic bone disease as a complication of gastrectomy was not recognised until about 1960. The incidence of metabolic bone disease after gastric surgery reported later ranged from 1%–42% in the many reports from all over the world [2–11]. It is now appreciated that frank osteomalacia is a rare complication of gastric surgery, but several authors have argued that there must be a large group of patients with subclinical disease. Three groups of workers set out to investigate this systematically in patients after gastrectomy, and they reported incidences of subclinical osteomalacia in 15%–22% of patients [5, 6, 10, 12].

In 1964 it was reported that peptic ulcer treated by gastrectomy was the most common concomitant condition in cases of fracture of the upper end of the femur [13].

Nilsson [14] observed that men with fractures of the upper end of the femur had been gastrectomised significantly more frequently than randomly selected controls.

Deller and Begley [5] and Deller et al. [6] observed decreased bone mass and osteoporosis in both the peripheral and the axial skeleton after gastrectomy. Louyot et al. [15], Harvald et al. [9], and Thompson et al. [8] found osteomalacia as a frequent complication of gastrectomy. Nilsson and Westlin [16] reported a high incidence of fractures in men 20 years and more after a Billroth II gastrectomy. There was a three fold and highly significant increase in fractures attributable to reduction in quality of the bone – the "fragility fracture" – in gastrectomy patients compared with matched controls. There was also a significantly increased incidence of all other types of fracture compared with the controls. The authors attributed these findings to a gradual loss of quality in bone after gastrectomy (Table 40).

20.2 Osteomalacia and Osteoporosis

No clear-cut differentiation between osteomalacia and osteoporosis is given. Osteomalacia occurs when there is a loss of calcium from bone due to vitamin D deficiency or metabolic changes in the formation of vitamin D hormones (25-hydroxycholecalciferol and 1,25-hydroxycholecalciferol). Osteomalacia usually responds well to physiological doses of vitamin D. Since malabsorption of fat is often accompanied by malabsorption of fat-soluble vitamins such as vitamin D, malabsorbed fat will form calcium soaps with calcium in the lumen of the intestine, and malabsorption of vitamin D and calcium are therefore likely to occur in postgastrectomy malabsorption (Fig. 75).

Table 40. Number of fractures observed in about 20 years in gastrectomised men and random controls. (After Nilsson and Westlin [16])

	No. of patients	No. of fractures	Fragility fractures	Other fractures
Controls	1,098	208 (19%)	33 (3%)	175 (16%)
Gastrectomised patients	549	191 (35%)	50 (9%)	135 (25%)

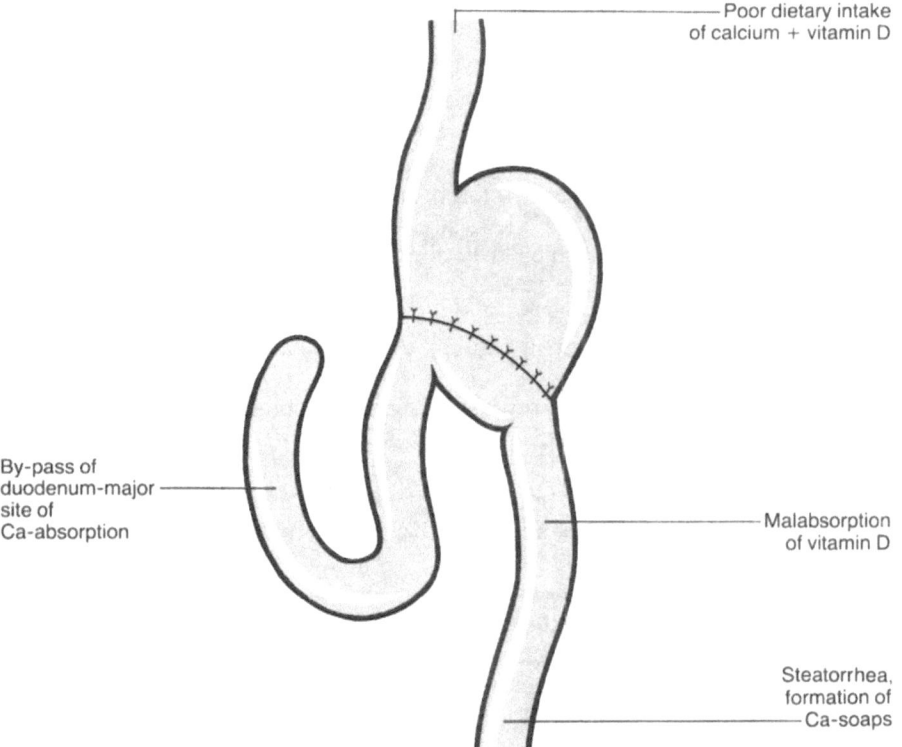

Poor dietary intake of calcium + vitamin D

By-pass of duodenum-major site of Ca-absorption

Malabsorption of vitamin D

Steatorrhea, formation of Ca-soaps

Fig. 75. Pathogenesis of postgastrectomy bone disease

Osteoporosis is usually due to a loss of bone tissue. What remains is normally calcified. Since osteoporosis occurs normally in ageing, the changes in bone due to gastrectomy are superimposed upon, and inseparable from, those due to advancing years. Because of the difficulty of separating osteoporosis from osteomalacia, the term postgastrectomy bone disease has been coined. The assessment of post-gastrectomy bone disease was mostly based on evidence of diminished bone density measured by X-ray and partly on biochemical abnormalities such as a reduction of serum calcium, but the greatest emphasis was placed on the finding of a raised level of serum alkaline phosphatase. Radiological surveys should be viewed with caution, because it takes about a 50% reduction of calcium content in bone before an abnormality can be detected by X-ray. When spinal rarefaction is assessed by subjective methods, Deller et al. [17] found bone disease to be present in 22% of control patients and in 50% of patients after partial gastrectomy. However, using more objective criteria they found that spinal rarefaction was present in only 15% of controls and 35% of patients with partial gastrectomy. Histological evidence of osteomalacia may be found in patients without detectable radiological abnormality [2].

20.3 Metabolic Findings

Morgan and co-workers [3] found a raised level of serum alkaline phosphatase in 18% of patients with gastrectomy over the age of 16. Since they observed a raised serum alkaline phosphatase level in 20% of patients with vagotomy and drainage procedure they considered that a raised serum alkaline phosphatase level after gastrectomy was not a reliable indication of subclinical osteomalacia.

Others have challanged their view, stressing the importance of measuring serum alkaline phosphatase, which they considered indicative of overt or sub-clinical osteomalacia in the absence of Paget's disease or liver dysfunction [8, 18]. The response to vitamin D challenge is another method which demonstrates osteomalacia in patients with a raised serum alkaline phosphatase after gastrectomy [19].

A careful survey by Eddy [20] revealed a significant biostatistical difference in the incidence of metabolic bone disease when 342 patients who had been treated with various types of partial gastrectomy were compared with a series of 180 patients with peptic ulcer of similar age and sex distribution. Thirty per cent of the postgastrectomy patients and only 5% of the non-surgical patients had defects in calcium metabolism.

Statistical correlation between faecal fat excretion and various calcium abnormalities further suggested that malabsorption was the cause.

The most striking biochemical abnormality was a raised serum alkaline phosphatase level in the postgastrectomy group (28%) (Fig. 76). Roentgenograms of the 342 postoperative patients revealed 83 instances (24.4%) of osseous rarefaction (determined by spinal scoring), 2.4% pseudofractures and 5.8% pathological fractures, whereas no fractures or pseudofractures were observed in the peptic ulcer group (Table 41).

Estimates of the incidence vary widely, but postgastrectomy bone disease probably occurs in 5%–15% of patients some 10 years after operation. Some think its incidence to be higher. Until recently no cases of osteomalacia have been reported after vagotomy and drainage procedure, although there have been reports of cases after gastrojejunostomy alone [21, 9]. Long-term studies in England have failed to discover significant osteomalacia or osteoporosis after truncal vagotomy and pyloroplasty or after truncal vagotomy and gastrojejunostomy [22–24]. In a study from Australia [25], however, early bone changes were suspected in a few patients after vagotomy and pyloroplasty. As more patients live longer after vagotomy and gastric drainage, cases of bone disease will probably be seen among them, too.

King Armstrong Units

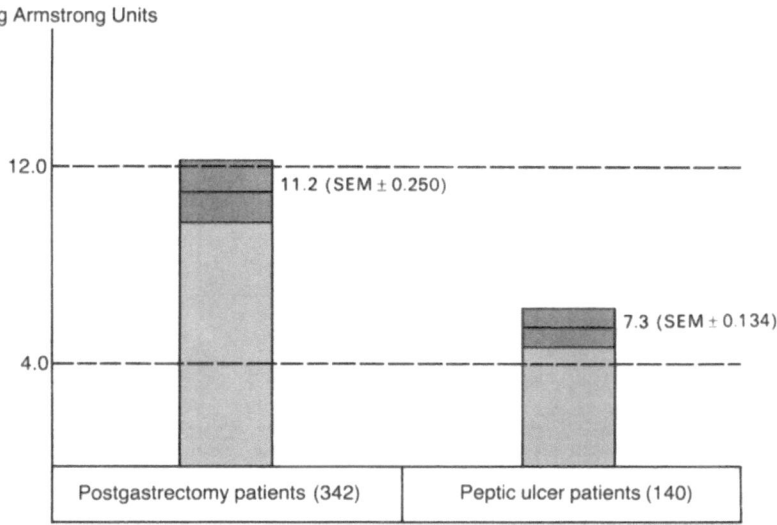

Fig. 76. Serum alkaline phosphatase values in peptic ulcer patients and postgastrectomy patients. The surgical procedures performed in the 342 patients were: Billroth II gastrectomy (212), vagotomy and pyloroplasty (104) and Billroth I gastrectomy (26). The postoperative period ranged from 2–20 years (mean 7.4 years). Normal values: 4.0–12 King-Armstrong units. (After Eddy, 1971 [20])

Table 41. X-ray studies in postgastrectomy patients and patients with peptic ulcer disease. Rarefaction was evaluated by thoracolumbar demineralisation score. (After Eddy, 1971)

X-ray findings	Postgastrectomy patients (342)	Peptic ulcer patients (180)
Osseous rarefaction	83/342 (24.3%)	7/180 (3.9%)
Pseudofractures	7/342 (2.0%)	0/180
Pathological fractures	20/342 (5.8%)	0/180

20.4 Diagnosis and Treatment

Estimation of blood calcium, inorganic phosphate and alkaline phosphatase levels should be the first step in diagnosis, and when there are abnormal arrangements a bone biopsy should be performed. More recently, decreased levels of the first metabolite of vitamin D, 25-hydroxycholecaliferol, have been found in patients after gastric surgery [26–28], as in other gastro-intestinal diseases [29]. There should be a thorough metabolic assessment, but when this is impossible bone disease should be assumed to exist and appropriate treatment started, in order to prevent gross bone disease developing in susceptible patients. Thus those who have had a gastric operation and whose nutrition is poor should be given calcium and vitamin D at intervals or continuously, as appropriate.

Vitamin D administration with or without calcium has been reported to result in biochemical [2, 4, 8, 18], histological [4, 18], radiological [4, 30] and symptomatic

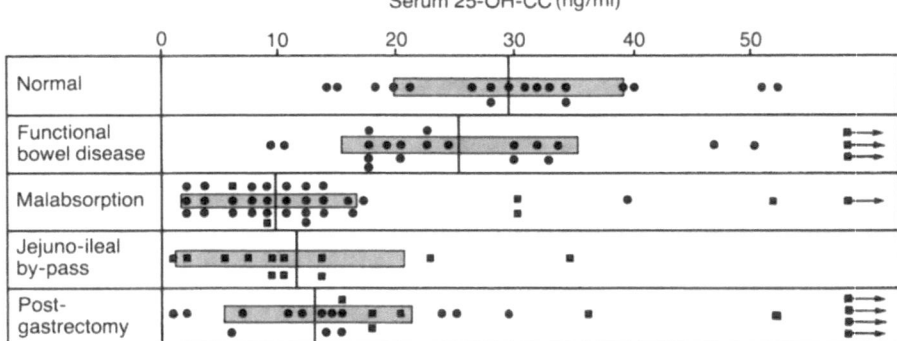

Serum 25-Hydroxycholecalciferol

Fig. 77. Serum 25-hydroxycholecalciferol concentrations in patients with various gastro-intestinal disorders. Groups of normals, patients with functional bowel disease, malabsorption or jejuno-ileal by-pass and 29 postgastrectomy patients, 26 of whom had undergone a Billroth II or Billroth I gastrectomy Studies were performed, with the exception of one postgastrectomy patient, more than 2 years after gastric surgery; ● no supplemental vitamins, ■ taking supplemental vitamins. (After Schoen et al., 1978 [26])

improvement [4, 8]. According to Thompson, a response can usually be observed after 3–6 months [8]. Biochemical improvement may occur, but microscopic changes may not be dramatic after vitamin D treatment [4], or in spite of clinical and biochemical cure the bone may remain histologically abnormal [4].

Alhava et al. [31] observed that treatment with a combination of calcium and vitamin D_2 resulted in increased bone mineral density in men, but not in women. Elevated serum alkaline phosphatase levels also decreased in men but not in women.

Different doses of vitamin D have been recommended for treatment, ranging from 500 to 200,000 U. A dose of 40,000 U given intramuscularly once a month and additional administration of 1–2 g calcium/day seem to be sufficient. Vitamin D should be given parenterally if steatorrhoea exists. The best screening test at the moment seems to be alkaline phosphatase activity. If it is elevated, further diagnostic steps are indicated. Since biochemical abnormalities usually precede overt osteopenic bone disease, proper treatment might prevent postgastrectomy bone disease.

Schoen et al. reported on 25-hydroxycholecalciferol levels in 29 patients following gastrectomy [26]. Ten patients were taking supplemental vitamins and had normal or high 25-hydroxycholecalciferol levels. In the remaining 19 patients the mean serum level was 13.1 ± 7.9 μg/ml (normal: 29.5 ± 9.9 μg/ml), with low determinations in 40% (Fig. 77). There was, however, no correlation between 25-hydroxycholecalciferol values and the length of time following gastric surgery. This was confirmed by Gertner et al. [27], who also found decreased 25-hydroxycholecalciferol levels in patients after gastric surgery, but attributed these findings to poor intake of vitamin D rather than to malabsorption of vitamin D.

References

1. Nicolaysen, R., Ragard, R.: Calcium and phosphorus metabolism in gastrectomized patients. Scand. J. Clin. Labor. Invest. 7, 298 (1955)
2. Williams, J.A.: Effects of upper gastrointestinal surgery on blood formation and bone metabolism. Brit. J Surg. 51, 125 (1964)
3. Morgan, D.B., Patterson, C.R., Pulvertaft et al.: Search for osteomalacia in 1228 patients after gastrectomy and other operations on the stomach. Lancet II, 1085 (1965)
4. Morgan, D.B., Patterson, C.R., Pulvertaft et al.: Osteomalacia after gastrectomy, a response to very small doses of vitamin D. Lancet II, 1089 (1965)
5. Deller, D.J., Begley, M.D.: Calcium metabolism and the bones after partial gastrectomy. I Clinical features and radiology of the bones. Aust. Ann. Med. 12, 282 (1963)
6. Deller, D.J., Edwards, R.G., Addison, M.: Calcium metabolism and the bones after partial gastrectomy. II. Nature and cause of the bone disorder. Aust. Ann. Med. 12, 295 (1963)
7. Higgins, P., Pridie, R.B.: Postgastrectomy osteomalacia: incidence after the no-loop and other types of gastrectomy. Brit. J. Surg. 53, 881 (1966)
8. Thompson, G.R., Watts, J.M., Neale, G., Booth, C.C.: Detection of vitamin D deficiency after partial gastrectomy. Lancet I, 623 (1966)
9. Harvald, B., Krogsgaard, A.R., Lous, P.: Calcium deficiency following partial gastrectomy. Acta Med. Scand. 172, 497 (1962)
10. Clark, C.G.: Disordered calcium metabolism after Polya partial gastrectomy. Lancet I, 734 (1964)
11. Clark, C.G.: Postgastrectomy bone disease. Proc. Royal Soc. Med. 57, 580 (1964)
12. Jones, C.T., Williams, J.A., Cox, E.V. et al.: Peptic ulceration. Some haematologic and metabolic consequences of gastric surgery. Lancet II, 425 (1962)
13. Alffram, P.A.: An epidemiologic study of cervical and trochanteric fractures of the femur in an urbanic population Acta Orthop. Scand. Supp. 65, 1964
14. Nilsson, B.E.R.: Conditions contributing to fracture of the femoral neck. Acta Chir. Scand. 136, 383 (1970)
15. Louyot, P., Mathieu, J., Gascher, A.· L'ostéose raréficante des gastrectomisés. Arch. Mal. Appar. dig. 50, 20 (1961)
16. Nilsson, B.E., Westlin, N.E.: The fracture incidence after gastrectomy. Acta chirurg. Scand. 137, 533 (1971)
17. Deller, D.J., Begley, M.D., Edwards, R.G., et al.: Metabolic effects of partial gastrectomy with special reference to calcium and folic acid: Part I. Changes in calcium metabolism and the bones. Gut 5, 218 (1964)
18. Bordier, P.H., Matrajt, H., Hioco, D. et al.: Subclinical vitamin D deficiency following gastric surgery. Histological evidence in bone. Lancet I, 437 (1968)
19. Whittle, H., Blair, A., Neale, G., et al.: Intravenous vitamin D in the detection of vitamin D deficiency Lancet I, 747 (1969)
20. Eddy, R.L.: Metabolic bone disease after gastrectomy. Am. J. Med. 50, 442 (1971)
21. Nordin, B.E.C., Fraser, R.: A calcium infusion test. I. Urinary excretion data for recognition of osteomalacia Lancet I, 823 (1956)
22. Wastell, C.. Long-term clinical and metabolic effects of vagotomy with either gastrojejunostomy or pyloroplasty. Ann. R. Coll. Surg. Engl. 45, 193 (1969)
23. Wheldon, E.J., Venables, C.W., Johnston, I.D.A.: Late metabolic sequelae of vagotomy and gastroenterostomy. Lancet I, 437 (1970)
24. Schofield, P.E., Watson-Williams, E.J., Sorrell, V.F.: Vagotomy and pyloric drainage for chronic duodenal ulcer. Arch. Surg. 95, 615 (1967)
25. Garrick, R., Ireland, A.W., Posen, S.: Bone abnormalities after gastric surgery. A prospective histological study. Ann. Int. Med. 75, 221 (1971)
26. Schoen, M.S., Lindenbaum, J., Roginsky, M.S., Holt, R.R.: Significance of serum level of 25-hydroxycholecalciferol in gastrointestinal disease. Am. J. Dig. Dis. 23, 137 (1978)
27. Gertner, J.M., Lilburn, M., Domenech, M.: 25-hydroxycholecalciferol absorption in steatorrhea and postgastrectomy osteomalacia. Brit. Med. J. 1, 1310 (1977)
28. Lilienfeld-Toal, H.V., Mackes, K.G., Kodrat, G.: Plasma 25-hydroxyvitamin D and urinary cyclic AMP in German patients with subtotal gastrectomy (Billroth II). Am. J. Dig. Dis. 22, 633 (1977)

29. Sitrin, M., Rosenberg, I.H.: Vitamin D deficiency and bone disease in gastrointestinal disorders. Arch. int. Med. *138*, 886 (1978)

30. Adams, J.F.: The clinical and metabolic consequences of total gastrectomy: II. Notes on metabolic function, deficiency states, changes in intestinal histology and radiology. Scand. J. Gastroent. *3*, 152 (1968)

31. Alhava, E.M., Aukee, S., Karjalainen, P., et al.: The influence of calcium and calcium + vitamin D$_2$ treatment on bone mineral after partial gastrectomy. Scand. J. Gastroent. *10*, 689 (1975)

21 Special Aspects of Total Gastrectomy

The indications for total gastrectomy and methods for alimentary reconstruction after this operation have changed since Schlatter performed the first successful one in 1897. In the early years thereafter, total gastrectomy was undertaken almost exclusively for gastric malignancy. Pack and McNeer [1] reviewed all cases reported up to 1942 and found an operative mortality in the previous decade of 34% and a 5-year survival rate of 0.5%. It was later proposed by Longmire that total gastrectomy should be performed for all potentially curable gastric cancers [2], regardless of the location or the extent of the primary lesion.

Other influential surgeons agreed [3, 4] and for almost a decade total gastrectomy was used in many surgical units as the standard procedure for gastric cancer. Enthusiasm for this aggressive approach declined in the late 1950s as four facts became apparent [5–7]:
1) Lesions could often be cured by subtotal gastrectomy as well as by total gastrectomy.
2) Operative mortality for total gastrectomy remained about twice as high as for subtotal gastrectomy.
3) Nutritional disabilities were frequent even if the cancer was cured.
4) Total gastrectomy performed for palliation seldom improved or lengthened the life of patients with advanced disease.

Consequently most surgeons performed total gastrectomy only for cure or removal of all visible tumour. End-to-side anastomosis of the oesophagus to a loop of jejunum was the first and predominant method of reconstruction in the early years [1, 7]. Many patients were troubled by malnutrition and postcibal symptoms, however, and other techniques were tried to avoid these troublesome side-effects. Among the surgical approaches introduced were the following:
1) Side-to-side anastomosis of the afferent and efferent limbs of the jejunal loop to minimise oesophagitis by diverting alkaline duodenal juice from the anastomosis
2) oesophagoduodenostomy
3) interposition of transverse or right colon
4) jejunal interposition or Roux-en-Y oesophagojejunostomy.

Pouches were constructed from plicated jejunal loops to provide a substitute food reservoir [8, 9] which would allow patients to eat larger meals. Two decades ago the Zollinger-Ellison syndrome emerged as a new disease best treated by

Table 42. Nutrition after total gastrectomy. (After Schrock et al., 1978)

Method of reconstruction	Patients	Nutrition	
		Adequate	Inadequate
Oesophagojejunostomy	1	0	1
Oesophagojejunostomy with jejunojejunostomy	1	0	1
Oesophagoduodenostomy	5	1 (20%)	4
Colonic interposition	2	1 (50%)	1
Jejunal interposition	7	7 (100%)	0
Roux-en-Y oesophagojejunostomy	18	16 (89%)	2
Total	34	25 (69%)	9

total gastrectomy [10, 11]. In many centres total gastrectomy was more frequently performed to treat Zollinger-Ellison syndrome than to cure gastric cancer. As prolonged survival is the rule in Zollinger-Ellison syndrome, nutritional problems have been a more prolonged and serious problem than in patients undergoing total gastrectomy for gastric cancer. Total gastrectomy nowadays may even be avoided in Zollinger-Ellison syndrome, thanks to the potent antisecretory action of histamine H_2 receptor blocking agents such as cimetidine. The overall operative mortality after total gastrectomy performed between 1940 and 1975 has been reported to be 12.5% [12]; if the last 5 years are considered, in which relatively fewer patients were operated for gastric carcinoma than for Zollinger-Ellison syndrome, operative mortality was 5.3% [12]. Nutrition usually is uniformly poor in patients who die of gastric cancer. Of 34 patients with a total gastrectomy who survived for more than 4 years after operation and were free of cancer, six gained weight after total gastrectomy, five remained at their previous weight and 23 lost weight [12]. If nutrition is judged on the basis of ideal weight corrected for height, age and sex, 69% (20 out of 34) were categorized as nutritionally adequate (Table 42). If benign disease or Zollinger-Ellison syndrome is the indication for total gastrectomy and a jejunal interposition or a Roux-en-Y oesophago-jejunostomy reconstruction procedure is performed, it may be expected that 89%–100% of patients will maintain adequate nutrition [12].

Thus it may be concluded that the status of postoperative nutrition is determined less likely by adverse effects of the operation itself than by the persistence of the tumor. Nutrition after total gastrectomy is determined mainly by two factors: the amount of food consumed and the efficiency of inestinal absorption.

Malabsorption after total gastrectomy has been reported to occur in the range from 10%–20%, which is rarely enough of clinical significance [13–15]. Insufficient caloric intake, not malabsorption, accounts more frequently for the nutritional insufficiency after total gastrectomy [14–16]. The inadequate intake may result from postcibal symptoms due to early satiety (loss of reservoir), the dumping syndrome and oesophagitis.

References

1. Pack, G.T., McNeer, G.: Total gastrectomy for cancer. A collective review of the literature and an original report of twenty cases. Int. Abstract. Surg. *77*, 265 (1943)
2. Longmire, W.P., Jr.: Total gastrectomy for carcinoma of the stomach. Surg. Gynecol. Obstet. *84*, 21 (1947)
3. Lahey, F.H., Marshall, S.F.: Should total gastrectomy be employed in early carcinoma of the stomach? Ann. Surg. *132*, 540 (1950)
4. McNeer, G., VandenBerg, H., Jr., Donn, F.Y., et al.: A critical evaluation of subtotal gastrectomy for the cure of cancer of the stomach. Ann. Surg. *131*, 2 (1951)
5. Rush, B.R., Jr., Brown, M.W., Ravitch, M.M.: Total gastrectomy: an evaluation of its use in the treatment of gastric cancer. Cancer *13*, 643 (1960)
6. Marshall, S.F.: Total versus radical partial resection for cancer of the stomach. Surg Gyneol. Obstet. *104*, 497 (1957)
7. Fly, O.A., Jr., Priestley, J.T., Comfort, M.W., et al.: Total gastrectomy: mortality and survival. Ann. Surg. *147*, 760 (1958)
8. Hunt, C.J : Construction of food pouch from segment of jejunum as substitute for stomach in total gastrectomy. Arch. Surg. *64*, 601 (1952)
9. Lawrence, W., Jr.: Reservoir construction after total gastrectomy: an instructive case. Ann. Surg. *155*, 191 (1962)
10. Zollinger, R.M., Ellison, E.H.: Primary peptic ulcerations of the jejunum associated with islet cell tumors of the pancreas. Ann. Surg. *142*, 709 (1955)
11. Way, L.W., Goldman, L., Dunphy, J.E.: Zollinger-Ellison syndrome. Am. J. Surg. *116*, 293 (1968)
12 Schrock, T.R., Way, L.W.: Total gastrectomy. Am. J. Surg. *135*, 348–355 (1978)
13. Scott, H.W., Jr., Law, D.H. IV, Gobbel, W.G., Jr., et al.: Clinical and metabolic studies after total gastrectomy with a Hunt-Lawrence jejunal food pouch. Am. J. Surg. *115*, 148 (1968)
14. Bradley, E.L. III, Isaacs, J., Hersh, Z., et al.: Nutritional consequences of total gastrectomy. Ann. Surg. *182*, 415 (1975)
15. Adams, J.F.: The clinical and metabolic consequences of total gastrectomy. I. Morbidity, weight, and nutrition Scand. J. Gastroenterol. *2*, 137 (1967)
16. Scott, H.W., Jr., Gobbel, W.G., Jr., Law, D.H. IV: Clinical experience with a jejunal pouch (Hunt-Lawrence) as a substitute stomach after total gastrectomy. Surg. Gynecol. Obstet. *121*, 1231 (1965)

Part IV
Postvagotomy Syndromes

22 Postvagotomy Dysphagia

Postvagotomy dysphagia is a mostly only transient dysphagia beginning between the 7th and 14th days after vagotomy. The degree of the dysphagia can vary considerably and extremely rarely may even reach complete aphagia.

20.1 Incidence, Symptoms and Aetiology

Mild symptoms lasting a few days or weeks after vagotomy may occur in 33% of patients [1], but 10%–15% is a common incidence [2, 3] (Fig. 78). If one considers the reports of several authors [2, 4–7] on 2,891 patients, only 2.6% complained of postvagotomy dysphagia (Table 43). Severe and prolonged dysphagia is uncommon after vagotomy. The incidence varies from one surgeon to another: some do not observe it at all, others recognise it as often as 1% [4]. It may occur not only after truncal vagotomy, but also after selective vagotomy.

One of the characteristic features of postvagotomy dysphagia is that the symptoms usually develop between the 7th and 14th days after operation (Fig. 79) [8, 9]. Sometimes onset may be as early as the 3rd day, and sometimes the initial symptoms may start up to 3 weeks after operation. Dysphagia starts usually with a sensation of slow passage of food down the oesophagus. Then the passage of solids is no longer possible and regurgitation may occur. Liquids are still able to pass, suggesting that stenosis is not complete. Pain is less evident. After a few days, drinking may be difficult. Hot drinks usually do not induce burning sensations, which suggests the absence of oesophagitis. In most cases, dysphagia is only transient and spontaneously disappears in days or weeks (Fig. 80).

The syndrome is clearly the result of the operation for vagal sectioning, but it is debatable whether it is the direct result of vagal section. Some authors [4, 8, 10] attribute dysphagia following vagotomy to an oesophageal spasm or even "cardiospasm", implying a neurogenic origin, induced by damage to the nerval supply, which would result in an abnormal contraction of the oesophagus. Others, however, believe that oesophagitis may be the underlying cause, because oesophagoscopy and biopsy have sometimes shown inflammatory changes of the oesophageal mucosa [2, 12]. Silber [13] pointed out that before operation some

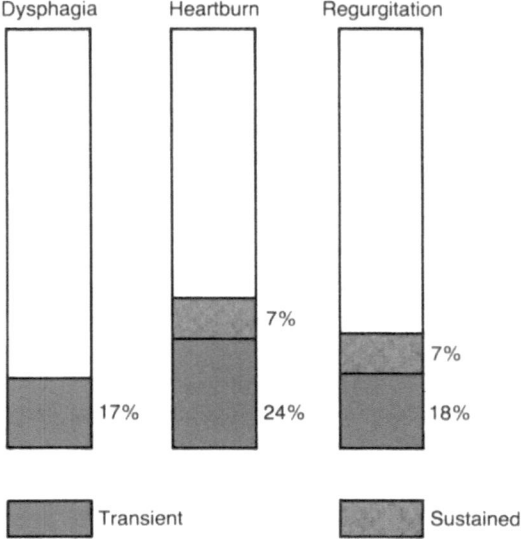

Fig. 78. Incidence of dysphagia, heartburn and regurgitation after vagotomy. (After Williams, J.A., Woodward, D.A.K.; Surg. Clin. North America 47, 1341, 1967)

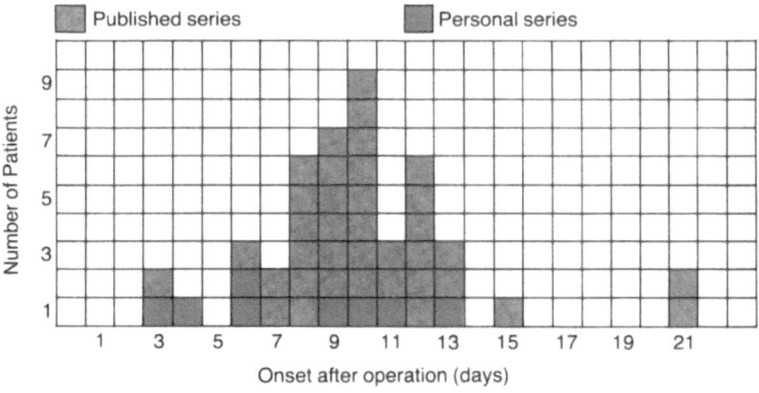

Fig. 79. Onset of postvagotomy dysphagia. (Lancet II, 90, 1970)

Table 43. Frequency of Postvagotomy Dysphagia

Authors	No. of cases	No. of patients with postvagotomy dysphagia	%
Dagradı et al. [4]	1,300	14	1.1
Bruce and Small [2]	116	6	5.2
Grimson et al. [7]	57	21	36.8
Williams and Woodward [6]	150	25	16.7
Anderson et al. [5]	1,268	9	0.7
	2,891	75	2.6

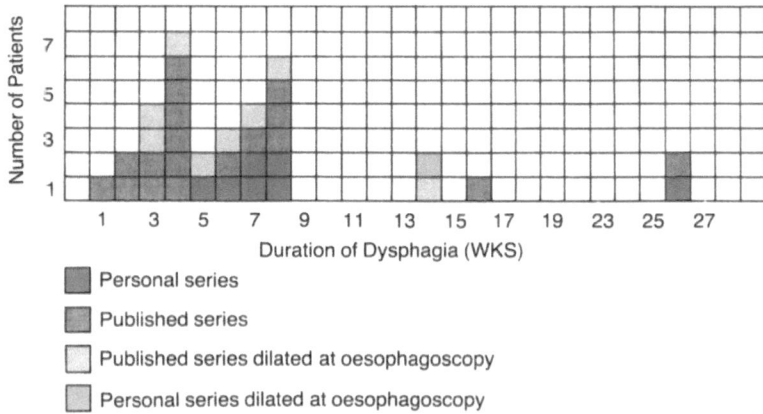

Personal series

Published series

Published series dilated at oesophagoscopy

Personal series dilated at oesophagoscopy

Fig. 80. Duration of postvagotomy dysphagia. (After Edwards, D.A.W., 1970 [8])

of the patients subsequently developing postvagotomy dysphagia already had disturbed motility of the oesophagus, detectable by manometric methods. Finally, oesophageal mucosal damage by a nasogastric tube has been discussed as possibly responsible for postoperative dysphagia. The other, most likely explanation is that postoperative perioesophageal oedema, haemorrhage and fibrosis of the oesophagus are the causative factors [2, 8, 9, 13]. Dysphagia is unlikely to be a direct consequence of cutting the vagus nerve, because it does not follow immediately after operation.

In the patients examined by manometry, Edwards [8, 9] found normal relaxation of the sphincter segment after a swallow. The subsequent contractions were also normal, as was the contracting function of the wall of the oesophagus above the sphincter. Thus Edwards concluded [9, 10] that the innervation mediating both relaxation and contraction was intact and the muscle responded normally to its neural stimuli. Anderson et al. [5], however, made different observations. They observed a lack of relaxation of the oesophageal sphincter and a lack of tone of the oesophagus, on the one hand, and normal relaxation of the sphincter with normal or increased oesophageal muscle tone, on the other hand. They attributed the second type of findings in postvagotomy dysphagia to oesophagitis, perioesophageal oedema or fibrosis. It has been pointed out by Edwards [8, 9] that sectioning of the vagal fibres seems to be the least likely explanation for the relaxation reported by Anderson et al. [5], firstly because the nerve supply to the muscle layers seems to be from the vagal plexus, and secondly because the sectioning is distal and superficial to these intramural fibres; otherwise postvagotomy dysphagia should be much more frequent. It was further pointed out by Edwards [8, 9] that it cannot be explained why and how renervation – which would be implied by the spontaneous recovery from dysphagia – should take place, if the dysphagia was due to denervation; and finally, if dysphagia were due to cutting of the vagus nerve, the symptoms should develop immediately after the operation.

Oesophagitis cannot be completely excluded as a causative factor, since reflux oesophagitis has been reported to occur even after vagotomy. But the symptoms – absence of heartburn and absence of hyperaesthesia after hot drinks or alcohol – are an argument against oesophagitis. Finally, the effect of nasogastric tubes cannot be accepted as a most important factor to explain postvagotomy dysphagia, since dysphagia may also develop in patients with no postoperative intubations. It seems unlikely that sectioning of the vagus is the cause, but dysphagia may be a multifactorial postoperative complication. In some patients, oesophageal oedema, fibrosis and haemorrhage may be the underlying factors; in others, oesophagitis may be considered, if its presence can be proved by oesophagoscopy.

The radiological appearance of the oesophagus in postvagotomy dysphagia resembles achalasia, but its dynamic appearance is clearly different, because normal peristaltic waves are usually seen. These waves can even be seen to flow into and through the narrow segment, demonstrating that the segment has the capacity to contract.

22.2 Experimental Findings

Vagotomy is known to induce a reduction of lower oesophageal sphincter pressure in animal experiments [14–16]. After bilateral cervical vagotomy performed in Rhesus monkeys, Binder et al. [14] observed two distinct pathological results: a syndrome closely resembling achalasia and a radiographic appearance suggestive of oesophageal spasm. Their findings were to some extent supported by Carveth et al. [15], who found that cervical vagotomy performed in dogs resulted in dilatation of the vagotomized segment of the oesophagus and prolonged retention of contrast medium. The resting lower oesophageal sphincter pressure was reduced, and relaxation and contraction of the sphincter with deglutination were only rarely to be observed. Elebute et al. [16] and Lind et al. [17], in addition, found a reduction of sphincter pressure after intra-abdominal supradiaphragmatic vagotomy and gastro-enterostomy in dogs 1–6 months after the operation.

The findings in humans after vagotomy have been different: nearly all groups were unable to observe any remarkable changes of lower oesophageal sphincter pressure. Crispin et al. [18] reported that resting lower oesophageal sphincter pressure was unchanged by vagotomy in man, but the pressure increase following abdominal compression was reduced. Mann and Hardcastle [19] confirmed that distal oesophageal pressure was unchanged in 15 patients who had undergone vagotomy and drainage for duodenal ulcer.

Blackman et al. [20] and Mazur et al. [21] also did not find any effects of transabdominal vagotomy on lower oesophageal sphincter pressure. Thomas [22] described only a slightly reduced high-pressure zone without any functional significance after vagotomy.

22.3 Treatment

Milder forms of dysphagia recover spontaneously. When solid food cannot pass, a liquid or semisolid liquid diet should be taken. Medical therapy including antispasmodic and anticholinergic drugs has been unsuccessful in most instances. This would to some extent support the most likely aetiology of this postoperative disorder. When dysphagia is severe, not permitting liquid diets to pass, oesophagoscopy and repeated bougienage or pneumatic dilatation are usually helpful [4]. Very rarely a thoracotomy with cardiomyotomy or removal of a fibrous sheet has to be performed [2, 12]. Since most patients will recover spontaneously, dilatation will only be necessary in a minority of patients with severe postvagotomy dysphagia.

References

1. Bank, S., Marks, N., Louw, J.H.: Gastric secretory patterns after vagotomy. Lancet *II*, 548 (1966)
2. Bruce, J., Small, W.P.: Dysphagia following vagotomy. J. Royal Coll. Surg. Edinb. *4*, 170 (1969)
3. Williams, J.A., Cox, A.G.: After vagotomy. London: Butterworths 1969
4. Dagradi, A.E., Stempien, S.J., Seifer, H.W., Weinberg, J.A.: Terminal esophageal vestibular spasm after vagotomy. Arch. Surg. *85*, 105 (1962)
5. Anderson, H.A., Schlegel, J.F., Olsen, A.M.: Post-vagotomy dysphagia. Gastroint. Endosc. *12*, 13 (1966)
6. Williams, J.A, Woodward, D.A.L: The effect of supradiaphragmatic vagotomy on the function of the gastrooesophageal sphincter. Surg. Clin. North Amer. *47*, 1321 (1967)
7. Grimson, K.S., Baylin, G.J., Tailor, H.M., et al.: Transthoracic vagotomy: the effects in 57 patients with peptic ulcer and the clinical limitations. J.A.M.A. *134*, 925 (1947)
8. Edwards, D.A.W.: Post vagotomy dysphagia. Lancet *II*, 90 (1970)
9. Edwards, D.A.W : Post-vagotomy dysphagia. In: Handbuch der inneren Medizin Band III/I: Diseases of the esophagus, pp. 367. Berlin, Heidelberg, New York: Springer 1974
10. Harris, J., Miller, C.M : Cardiospasm following vagotomy. Surgery *47*, 568 (1960)

11. Pierandozzi, J S., Ritter, J.H.: Transient achalasia. A complication of vagotomy. Am. J. Surg. *111*, 356 (1966)
12. Guillory, J.R., Clagnett, O.T.: Post vagotomy dysphagia. Surg. Clin. North America *47*, 833 (1967)
13. Silber, W.: Post vagotomy dysphagia. S. Afr. med. J. *43*, 803 (1969)
14. Binder, H.J., Bloom, D.L., Stern, H., et al.: The effect of cervical vagotomy on esophageal function in the monkey. Surgery *64*, 1075 (1968)
15. Carveth, S.W., Schlegel, J.F., Code, C.F., Ellis, F.H., Jr.: Esophageal motility after vagotomy, phrenicotomy, myotomy and myomectomy in dogs. Surg. Gynec. Obstetr. *114*, 31 (1962)
16. Elebute, E., Kelley, M.L., Schwatz, S.I.: Pressure effects of transabdominal supradiaphgramatic vagotomy on the inferior esophageal sphincter of dogs. Surg. Gyn. Obstetr. *123*, 326 (1966)
17. Lind, J.F., Colton, D.J., Blanchard, R., et al.· Effect of thoracic displacement and vagotomy on the canine gastroesophageal junctional zone Gastroenterology *56*, 1078 (1969)
18. Crispin, J.S., McIver, D.K., Lind, J.. Manometric study of the effect of vagotomy on the gastroesophageal sphincter. Can. J. Surg. *10*, 299 (1967)
19. Mann, C.V., Hardcastle, J.D.: The effect of vagotomy on the human gastroesophageal sphincter. Gut *56*, 688 (1968)
20. Blackman, A.H., Rakatansky, H., Nasrullah, M , Thayer, W.R.: Transabdominal vagectomy and lower esophageal function. Arch. Surg. *102*, 6 (1971)
21. Mazur, J.M., Skinner, D.B., Jones, E L., Zuidema, G.D.: Effect of transabdominal vagotomy on the human gastroesophageal high pressure zone. Surgery *73*, 818 (1973)
22. Thomas, P A , Earlam, R.J.: The gastroesophageal junction before and after operation for duodenal ulcer. Brit. J Surgery *60*, 717 (1973)

23 Vagal Denervation Syndrome

23.1 Pathophysiology

The physiology and pathophysiological changes of the motor activity of the stomach are very complex. Besides nervous factors, gastro-intestinal hormones are mainly involved, as is demonstrated in Table 44. Furthermore, receptors in the duodenum represent important regulatory mechanisms; these receptors respond to distention, changes in pH and osmolarity, etc. Three complexes have to be considered separately: (1) motility of the stomach, (2) motor activity of the pylorus, and (3) gastric emptying.

The classical concept included cholinergic vagal stimulation and adrenergic sympathetic inhibition of the smooth muscles of the stomach [2]. Besides these, non-cholinergic, non-adrenergic nerve fibres exist, which are now named peptidergic. At least some of these fibres can be activated by reflexes from oesophagus or stomach.

The anatomical distribution of the stomach in corpus, fundus and antrum cannot be maintained by the motoric physiology of the stomach [3]. Food intake induces a receptive relaxation of the proximal stomach, so that this part acts as a reservoir for solid and liquid food particles [2, 4]. While liquids reach the duodenum mainly by a tonus increase of the middle portion of the stomach, solid food particles are transported to the duodenum above all by contractions of the distal part. The peristaltic activities of the distal stomach originate from a so-called pacemaker, which is located in the upper third of the stomach, close to the greater curvature [5, 6].

Table 44. Control mechanisms acting on gastric motor function. (According to Olbe [1])

Action	Type of agent	Gastric motility	Pyloric sphincter	Gastric emptying
Stimulatory	Nervous	Cholinergic Peptidergic (Vagus, splanchnic)	?	Distention
	Hormonal	Gastrin CCK Motilin	CCK Secretin	?
Inhibition	Nervous	Ganglionic block (adrenergic)	?	—
	Hormonal	Secretin Glucagon GIP CCK	Gastrin	CCK Secretin Gastrin
Relaxation		Vagal	—	—

Each type of vagotomy considerably alters the motor activity of the stomach, influencing both peristalsis and receptive relaxation. After total denervation of the stomach, the regular rhythm of the pacesetter potential is replaced by multiple ectopic pacemakers with ineffective propagation of gastric peristalsis [7, 8]. Whereas in selective gastric and truncal vagotomy all vagal fibres to the stomach are transected, selective proximal vagotomy results only in vagal denervation of the proximal stomach.

While all vagotomy procedures which result in total denervation of the stomach produce a delayed gastric emptying, to some extent of liquids, but mainly of solid food, the findings after selective proximal vagotomy are more complex: gastric emptying of fluids seems to be accelerated during the initial phase, but normal in the later phase [8–10]. Emptying of solid food after selective proximal vagotomy (SPV) is either unchanged [8, 10] or delayed [9]. When SPV is combined with a pyloroplasty, gastric emptying of solid and liquid food is more rapid [10].

Adaptive relaxation of the stomach is abolished after all types of vagotomy, since the reflex areas to the gastric fundus are interrupted. This phenomenon seems to be responsible for the complaints of epigastric fullness observed by most patients; furthermore, it is possible that the initial rapid gastric emptying of fluids is caused by the lack of receptive relaxation of the gastric corpus and fundus.

To what extent the function of the pylorus is altered by vagal denervation is unknown at the moment, since no reliable methods for the measurement of pyloric function are available. After vagal denervation the pylorus is adjusted to a certain diameter, which will not open in co-ordination with antral motor activity; it will thus act as a relative stenosis. This lack of co-ordination causes a further delay of gastric emptying.

However, delayed gastric emptying is also observed during the early post-operative phase in patients with simple gastro-enterostomy, pyloroplasty and partial gastrectomy without vagotomy. The pathophysiological mechanisms are unknown. This phenomenon is particularly observed in patients with organic pyloric stenosis and dilatation of the stomach.

23.2 Treatment

Delayed gastric emptying in the early postoperative phase after vagotomy is common and most patients will not complain of any symptoms. X-ray check-ups demonstrate normalisation in most cases after 3–6 months. A pyloric stenosis immediately after operation is treated best by continous suction of the stomach via a nasogastric tube. In severe prolonged cases a temporary gastrostomy is very beneficial. Medical treatment consists of application of bethanechol chloride (Urecholine) [13] and/or metoclopramide. Parenteral hyperalimentation is indicated in most cases. Continuing this therapy consistently for 3–6 weeks will make a second operation (drainage) unnecessary.

References

1. Olbe, L.: Gastroduodenal physiology and pathophysiology. In: Nyhus, L.M., Wastell, C.: Surgery of the stomach and duodenum. Boston: 3. Ed. Little Brown, 1977
2. Jahnberg, Th.: Gastric adaptive relaxation. Scand. J. Gastroent. Suppl. *12*, 46 (1977)
3. Kelly, K A.. Gastric motility after gastric operation. In: Surgery Annual. New York: Appleton – Century – Crofts, 1974
4. Martinson, J.: Vagal relaxation of the stomach. Experimental re-investigation of the concept of the transmission mechanism. Acta Physiol. Scand. *64*, 453 (1965)
5. Weber, J., Jr., Kohatsu, S.: Pacemaker localisation and electrical conduction patterns in the canine stomach. Gastroenterology *59*, 717 (1970)
6. Kelly, K A , Code, C F · Canine gastric pacemaker Amer. J. Physiol *220*, 112 (1971)
7. Nelsen, T S., Eigenbrodt, E.H , Keoshian et al. Alterations in muscular and electrical activity of the stomach following vagotomy. Arch. Surg. *94*, 821 (1967)
8. Wilbur, B.G., Kelly, K.A.: Effect of proximal gastric, complete gastric and truncal vagotomy on canine gastric electric activity, motility and emptying. Ann. Surg *178*, 295 (1973)
9. Donovan, I.A., Griffen, D.W., Harding, L.K., Alexander-Williams, J.: Paradoxical gastric emptying after gastric surgery in man. Brit. J. Surg. *61*, 916 (1974)
10. Johnston, D.: A new look at vagotomy In: Surgery Annual. New York: Appleton – Century – Crofts, 1974
11. Stadaas, J., Aune, S., Haffner, J., F., W.: Effects of proximal gastric vagotomy on intragastric pressure and adaptation in pigs Scand. J. Gastroent. *9*, 479 (1974)
12. Bushkin, F.L., Woodward, E.R.: Delayed gastric emptying In: Postgastrectomy syndromes. Vol XX. Major problems in Surgery. Philadelphia Saunders 1976
13. Vasconez, L.O., Adams, J T., Woodward, E.R.: Treatment of reductant postvagotomy stoma with bethanechol. Arch. Surg. *100*, 693 (1970)

24 Postvagotomy Diarrhoea

24.1 Definition and Incidence

Most patients have an alteration in bowel habits after gastric surgery, particularly if gastric surgery is accompanied by vagotomy. It is probably because of the close association of diarrhoea with sectioning of the vagus nerves observed by Dragstedt et al. [1] that he term postvagotomy diarrhoea became popular. The exact

Table 45. Incidence of side effects 5–8 years after various elective operations for duodenal ulcer. [Goligher, J.C., et al. (9)]

Symptom	Leeds/York trial			Separate study TV + PY (% of about 161 cases)	Separate study PGV (% of about 117 cases)
	TV + GE (% of about 119 cases)	TV + ANT (% of about 116 cases)	Subtotal gast. (% of about 107 cases)		
Epigastric fullness	40.2	36.3	36.5	37.1	30.8
Early dumping	17.9	8.6	21.5	11.9	0.9
Nausea	12.8	17.2	23.4	17.6	15.4
Bile vomiting	14 5	13.8	13 1	10.1	6 3
Food vomiting	4.3	9.6	5 6	4.4	8.6
Flatulence	17.9	22.8	19.8	20.1	19.2
Heartburn	19.8	15.7	8 4	12.6	13.2
Diarrhoea	→26.3	→23.2	→ 6.5	→21.7	→ 5.1

TV + GE, Truncal vagotomy and gastro-enterostomy, TV + ANT, truncal vagotomy and antrectomy; Gast., gastrectomy;
TV + PY, truncal vagotomy and pyloroplasty; PGV, proximal gastric vagotomy

aetiology is still unknown, but several hypotheses have been put forward to explain the severe, often incapacitating diarrhoea that follows truncal vagotomy especially. Truncal vagotomy has been particularly implicated, but when it is combined with drainage or antrectomy, the incidence of diarrhoea is generally held to be in the region of 25%, of which only 1%–3% of patients find the symptoms troublesome [3–4]. Kronborg [5] found that 64.3% of patients after truncal vagotomy and drainage procedure experienced diarrhoea. Diarrhoea occurring daily was found in 3.7% of patients, weekly in 14.5%, monthly in 22.1% and less frequently in 24%.

Wastell [6] noted that 27% of patients undergoing truncal vagotomy and drainage had episodic diarrhoea, 3% had continuous diarrhoea, 34% had no change, 27% had increased frequency of bowel movements without diarrhoea and 9% noted a decrease of bowel movements.

The less frequent incidence of diarrhoea after gastrectomy without vagotomy compared to gastrectomy with vagotomy (6.5% versus 23.2%) suggests hat vagal denervation is responsible for the diarrhoea [3, 7, 8]. Continuous diarrhoea in the Leeds/York trial did not occur in more than 6% of the patients and was mild to moderate [8]. The incidence of diarrhoea following truncal vagotomy remained constant over the 2 and 5–8 years of observation [7, 8]. The incidence of diarrhoea was considerably less after proximal vagotomy [9] (Table 45). Selective vagotomy in this respect has been shown to be superior to truncal vagotomy, too, when combined with a Finney-type pyloroplasty [10], and there are promising results for the future from highly selective vagotomy without drainage procedure. Johnston [11] reviewed data on 1,130 patients with vagotomy and noted that 24.6% had diarrhoea after truncal vagotomy but only half that number experienced diarrhoea after selective vagotomy.

A very low incidence (2%–3%) of diarrhoea was reported by Burge et al. after selective vagotomy [12]. The authors suggested hat preservation of the hepatic branches of the anterior vagal trunk would prevent diarrhoea. Preservation of the pyloric branches also seems to protect the patient against postoperative diarrhoea, whereas the type of drainage procedure does not influence the incidence of diarrhoea [3, 6–9].

24.2 Aetiology

Several hypotheses have been put forward to explain the cause of postvagotomy diarrhoea (Table 46), Dragstedt and Woodward [13] and others have suggested that the occurrence of postvagotomy diarrhoea might be related to bacterial colonization of the upper small intestine. It was assumed that bacteria could flourish in a stomach rendered hypotonic and hypochlorhydric by vagotomy and then flood the small intestine, causing enteritis and diarrhoea.

Tinker et al. [14], however, were unable to find any relation between diarrhoea and bacterial counts in the stomach and small intestine of vagotomised patients.

Browning and his colleagues [15] studied small-bowel flora in 25 patients for an average of 18 months after truncal vagotomy with drainage procedure. They found significant colonization of the small bowel in 50% of patients with gastrojejunostomy and 9% of those with pyloroplasty. They were, however, unable to establish any relationship between bacterial colonization of the small bowel and diarrhoea. In a later study, Browning et al. [16] reported on 32 patients with postvagotomy diarrhoea following truncal vagotomy. There was no difference in the incidence of bacterial colonization in the upper small intestine of postvagotomy patients with diarrhoea and without diarrhoea (Table 47). Patients with a gastro-enterostomy had a higher incidence of bacterial colonization than those with a pyloroplasty. Colonization was associated with significantly lower levels of gastric acid secretion.

Although 13 of the 32 patients with diarrhoea had an abnormal faecal fat excretion, no correlation could be found between this and the severity of the diarrhoea or bacterial colonization.

Thus bacterial overgrowth with subsequently increased deconjugation of conjugated bile acids seems unlikely to be responsible for vagotomy diarrhoea. The onset of the diarrhoea, mostly within minutes after food intake, would also argue against this hypothesis.

A second theory is that impaired function of the denervated pancreas, biliary system and small intestine leads to diarrhoea. If this is correct the underlying mechanism of the diarrhoea might be due to malabsorption or altered motility. The episodic type of diarrhoea is, however, inconsistent with the steady-state function of a denervated system.

McKelvey [17] studied 18 patients with postvagotomy diarrhoea and compared them with 27 asymptomatic patients who had had a vagotomy, using a liquid test meal. He concluded that following vagotomy there is an alteration in the duodenal regulation of gastric emptying by the physicochemical characteristics of the meal. Emptying could be altered by posture. The stomach

Table 46. Pathophysiology of postvagotomy diarrhoea: suggested mechanisms

---

I. Disturbed motility
   → Rapid gastric emptying
   → Decreased intestinal transit time
   → Hypomotility, stasis

II. Reduced gastric acid secretion
   → Bacterial overgrowth
   → Bacterial action on bile acids
      triglycerides or fatty acids
      amino acids
      carbohydrates

III. Alteration of bile acid metabolism
   → Increase of free (more toxic) bile acids
   → Decrease of conjugated bile acids required for micelle formation
   → Increased loss of bile acids by decrease in small-intestinal transit time and high bile acid load
      (contraction of dilated gall bladder)

IV. Enterohormonal dysregulation

Table 47. Maximal acid output in mEq/peak half-hour analysed according to colonisation. Patients with diarrhoea after vagotomy had a peak half-hour secretion similar to those without diarrhoea. When analysed in relation to colonisation, those patients who were colonised had a significantly lower level of acid secretion than those who were not. (After Browning et al., 1974 [16])

Group	Total No.	All patients	Noncolonised patients	Colonised patients
Diarrhoea	32	6.1 ± 1.8	8.1 ± 2.1	2.7 ± 2.7
No diarrhoea	24	5.3 ± 1.0	6.2 ± 1.5	40 ± 1.5
Total	56	5.2 ± 0.9	6.7 ± 1.2	3.5 ± 1.3

Values are for means ± 1 standard error

subjected to total denervation would behave as an incontinent viscus. By incontinence it was meant that the stomach no longer emptied in an orderly fashion under the co-ordinated control of muscles of the antrum, pylorus and duodenum (Fig. 81). For certain positions they observed a very rapid gastro-intestinal transit time and diarrhoea. As a result, the concept of proximal gastric vagotomy is attractive because it involves preservation of an intact nerve supply to the muscle which controls gastric emptying.

More recent gastric-emptying studies with a ^{99m}Tc-tagged solid test meal (chicken liver) revealed that there may be patients who empty their stomach faster or slower than controls after a vagotomy [18].

A third hypothesis originates from observations of the beneficial therapeutic effect of cholestyramine on postvagotomy diarrhoea. Postvagotomy diarrhoea is in most cases watery in nature, like cholereic enteropathy which results from bile acid malabsorption due to ileal dysfunction. Bile acids, especially deconjugated secondary bile acids, induce a secretion of water and electrolytes into the colon

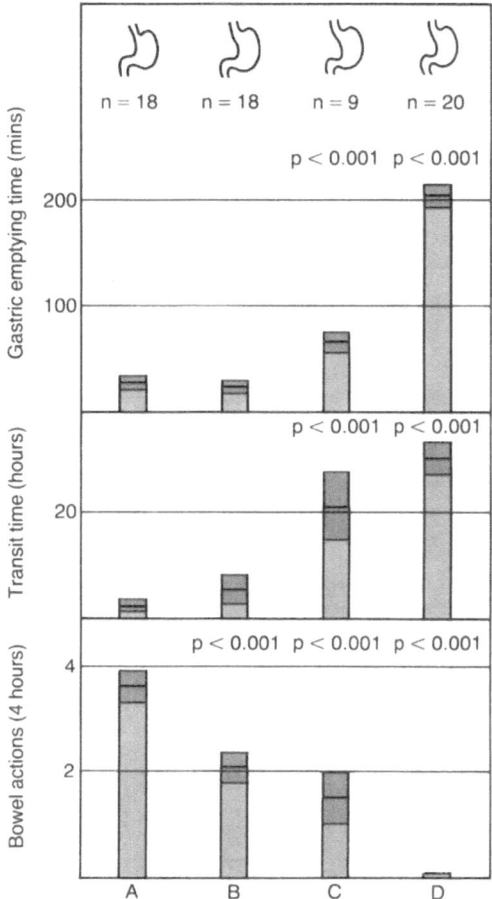

Fig. 81. Response of gastric emptying time, transit time and bowel actions to a balanced fluid meal. The diarrhoea group served as basis for comparison: *A* postvagotomy diarrhoea; *B* less constipated patients; *C* no change in bowel habits; *D* preoperative. Patients with postvagotomy diarrhoea had a markedly decreased gastric emptying time and transit time (After McKelvey, 1970 [17])

[19–21]. It was therefore assumed that bile acid malabsorption might be one of the main mechanisms responsible for watery diarrhoea in the postvagotomy syndrome. Allan, Gerskowitch and Russell [22, 23] indeed observed a markedly increased total bile acid excretion in the faeces of patients with postvagotomy diarrhoea (Table 48). This increase of faecal bile acid excretion was more than three fold, compared to normal controls (2,538 versus 799 mg/day). Analysis of the individual bile acids revealed a significant increase of chenodeoxycholic acid (CDCA) excretion (460 versus 82 mg/day; Table 49). CDCA, which is used as an effective cholelitholytic agent, causes diarrhoea as the most serious side-effect of conservative treatment for cholesterol gall-stone dissolution. Since patients with truncal vagotomy without diarrhoea did not have significantly increased faecal losses of bile acids, it seems plausible at the moment that the

Table 48. Total bile acid excretion (After Allan et al., 1974 [22])

A. Postvagotomy diarrhoea	B. Postvagotomy without diarrhoea	C. Normal controls
1,044	1,049	1,235
1,529	1,140	663
3,914	1,679	1,059
3,576	319	860
1,241	482	901
1,241	1,173	565
5,223	1,406	311
Mean ± s.e.m.		
2,538 ± 632	1,030 ± 482	799 ± 117

A versus B: $P > 0.05$. B versus C: $P > 0.05$. C versus A: $P < 0.025$

Table 49. Excretion of individual bile acids (mg/24 h) measured in normal controls and in patients with vagotomy, with and without diarrhoea. (After Allan et al., 1974 [22])

Bile acid	A.	B.	C.
Cholic acid	321 ± 143	7.68 ± 7 68	36 ± 17
Chenodeoxycholic acid [a]	460 ± 66	170 ± 38	82 ± 23
Deoxycholic acid	1,222 ± 381	499 ± 75	436 ± 74
Lithocholic acid	791 ± 251	366 ± 71	202 ± 47

[a] Statistical analysis of chenodeoxycholic acid excretion: A versus B. $P < 0.005$, B versus C $P > 0 05$, A versus C. $P < 0.001$. All other differences are not significant

cathartic action of bile acids might be mainly responsible for the incapacitating watery diarrhoea complicating truncal vagotomy [22–28].

The beneficial therapeutic effect of cholestyramine reported by several groups would support this third hypothesis.

Diabetic diarrhoea often complicating long-standing diabetes is considered to be induced by a vagal neuropathy of the small intestine. This denervation of the small intestine, resulting in severe, unpredictable diarrhoea, also favourably responded to the treatment of cholestyramine [26]. The question remains: What are the reasons for the increased bile acid excretion in postvagotomy diarrhoea? It has been suggested that vagotomy has little effect on small-intestinal motility [27, 28a], but results on small-intestinal motility responding to rapid gastric emptying of a meal are lacking. A local effect of vagotomy on the ileocaecal valve, resulting in a loss of the damming effect in the terminal ileum, with a consequent rush of intestinal contents directly into the colon, has been discussed [22]. Dilatation of the gall bladder with apparent increase of volume after vagotomy has been reported by several groups [29, 30]. Condon et al. [25] proposed that a dilated gall bladder may play a causal role in postvagotomy diarrhoea by storing excessive volumes of bile acids, which swamp the reabsorptive capacity of the small intestine on contraction during a meal.

Table 50. Therapy of postvagotomy diarrhoea

Medical	Diet·	1. Limitation of liquid meals 2. Small, frequent feedings 3. Reduction of free carbohydrates or disaccharides (e.g. milk) 4. Diet rich in fibre content by addition of carbohydrate gelling agents like guar or pectin
	Drugs.	Antispasmodics Antidiarrhoeals Opiates (loperamide, diphenoxylate) Cholestyramine 4×4 g/day $Al(OH)_3$-containing antacids
Surgical	Jejunal interposition	

24.3 Therapy (Tab. 50)

It was therefore suggested that cholecystectomy might eliminate the symptoms. A positive response to cholecystectomy was not, however, observed [27]. A positive therapeutic response of postvagotomy diarrhoea to cholestyramine and recently to $Al(OH)_3$-containing antacids [31], which are known to bind bile acids very potently [32, 33], suggests at the moment that bile acid malabsorption may be the main important mechanism responsible for the watery diarrhoea following truncal vagotomy. A consistent therapeutic approach with cholestyramine (4×4 g, with meals) or a course with $Al(OH)_3$-containing antacids seems therefore to be indicated in postvagotomy diarrhoea.

Ayulo reported an 80%–100% improvement within 1–4 weeks of treatment with cholestyramine in all responsive cases [24]. The dose recommended was 3×4 g cholestyramine, with meals. The symptom responding most consistently to treatment with cholestyramine was urgency. Since cholestyramine interacts with other drugs, attention has to be paid to other medications the patient is taking.

A variety of other agents has been tried, such as antibiotics, atropine, diphenoxylate and anticholinergics, but their effectiveness is less well established. McKelvey [17] suggested that patients should lie down after meals. The majority of his patients improved when they ingested a meal with a low fluid content.

References

1. Dragstedt, L.R., Harper, P.V., Jr., Tovee, E.B., Woodward, E.R.: Section of the vagus nerve of the stomach in the treatment of peptic ulcer. Complications and end results after four years. Ann. Surg. *126*, 687 (1947)
2. Cox, A.G., Bond, M.R.: Bowel habit after vagotomy and gastrojejunostomy. Brit. Med. J. *1*, 460 (1964)
3. Goligher, J.C., Pulvertaft, C.N., De Dombal, F.T., et al.: Five to eight year results of Leeds/York controlled trial of elective surgery for duodenal ulcer. Brit. Med. J. *2*, 781 (1968)
4. Duthie, H.L, Kwong, N.K.: Vagotomy or gastrectomy for duodenal ulcer. Brit. Med. J. *4*, 79 (1973)

5. Kronborg, O.: Clinical results 6 to 8 years after truncal vagotomy and drainage for duodenal ulcer in 500 patients. Acta chirurg. Scand. *141*, 657 (1975)

6. Wastell, C.: Long-term clinical and metabolic effects of vagotomy with either gastrojenunostomy or pyloroplasty. Ann. Roy. Coll. Surg. Engl. *44*, 193 (1969)

7. Goligher, J.C., Pulvertaft, C.N., De Dombal, F.T., et al.: Clinical comparison of vagotomy and pyloroplasty with other forms of elective surgery for duodenal ulcer. Brit. Med. J. *2*, 787 (1968)

8. Goligher, J.C., Pulvertaft, C.N., Irvin, T.T., et al.: Five- to eight-year results of truncal vagotomy and pyloroplasty for duodenal ulcer. Brit. Med. J. *1*, 7 (1972)

9. Goligher, J.C., Hill, G.L., Kenny, T.E., Nutter, E.: Proximal gastric vagotomy without drainage for duodenal ulcer: results after 5–8 years. Brit. J. Surg. *65*, 145 (1978)

10. Kennedy, T., Connell, A.M., Love, A.H.G., et al.: Selective or truncal vagotomy? Five year results of a double-blind randomized, controlled trial. Brit. J. Surg. *60*, 944 (1973)

11. Johnston, D., Humphrey, C.S., Walker, B.E., et al.: Vagotomy without diarrhea Brit. Med. J. *3*, 788 (1972)

12. Burge, H., Hutchinson, J.S.F., Longland, C.J.: Selective nerve section in the prevention of post-vagotomy diarrhoea. Lancet *I*, 577 (1964)

13. Dragstedt, L.R., Woodward, E.R.: Appraisal of vagotomy for peptic ulcer after seven years J. Am Med. Ass. *145*, 795 (1951)

14. Tinker, J., Hoffbrand, A.V., Mitchison, R.S., et al.: Gastrointestinal flora and diarrhoea after vagotomy. South African Med. J. *45*, 1258 (1971)

15. Browning, G.G., Buchan, K.A., Mackay, C.: Small bowel flora and bowel habit studied at intervals following vagotomy and drainage. Gut *13*, 908 (1972)

16. Browning, G.G., Buchan, K.A., Mackay, C.: Clinical and laboratory study of postvagotomy diarrhoea. Gut *15*, 644 (1974)

17. McKelvey, S.T.D.: Gastric incontinence and post-vagotomy diarrhea. Brit. J. Surg. *57*, 781 (1970)

18. MacGregor, I.L., Martin, P., Meyer, J.H.: Gastric emptying of solid food in normal man and after subtotal gastrectomy and truncal vagotomy with pyloroplasty. Gastroenterology *72*, 206 (1977)

19. Hofmann, A.F.: Bile acid malabsorption caused by ileal resection. Arch. int. Med. *130*, 597 (1972)

20. Hofmann, A.F., Poley, J.R.: Role of bile acid malabsorption in the pathogenesis of diarrhea and steatorrhea in patients with ileal resection. Gastroenterology *62*, 918 (1972)

21. Mekkjian, H.S., Phillips, S.F., Hofmann, A.F.: Colonic secretion of water and electrolytes induced by bile acids: perfusion studies in man. J. Clin. Invest *50*, 1564 (1971)

22. Allan, J.G., Gerskowitch, V.P., Russell, R.I.: The role of bile acids in the pathogenesis of post-vagotomy diarrhea. Brit. J. Surg. *61*, 516 (1974)

23. Allan, J.G., Gerskowitch, V.P., Russell, R.I.: A study of the role of bile acids in the pathogenesis of postvagotomy diarrhoea. Gut *14*, 423 (1973)

24. Ayulo, J.A.: Cholestyramine in postvagotomy syndrome. Amer. J. Gastroent. *57*, 207 (1972)

25. Condon, J.R., Robinson, V., Suleman, M.I., et al.: The cause and treatment of postvagotomy diarrhoea. Brit. J. Surg. *62*, 309 (1975)

26. Condon, J.R., Suleman, M.I., Fan, Y.S., McKeown, M.D.: Cholestyramine and diabetic and postvagotomy diatthoea. Brit. Med. J. *4*, 423 (1973)

27. Duncombe, V.M., Bolin, T.D., Davis, A.E.: Double-blind trial of cholestyramine in postvagotomy diarrhoea. Gut *18*, 531 (1977)

28. Gerskowitch, V.P., Allan, J.G., Russell, R.I.: Increased faecal excretion of bile acids in post-vagotomy diarrhoea. Brit. J. Surg. *60*, 912 (1973)

28 a. Ross, B., Watson, B.W., Kay, A.W.: Studies on the effect of vagotomy on small intestinal motility using the radiotelementry capsule. Gut *4*, 77 (1963)

29. Johnson, F.E., Boyden, E.A.: The effect of double vagotomy on the motor activity of the human gallbladder. Surgery *32*, 591 (1952)

30. Rudick, J., Hutchinson, J.S.F.: Effects of vagal nerve section on the biliary system. Lancet *I*, 579 (1964)

31. Sali, A., Murray, W.R., Mackay, C.: Aluminium hydroxide in bile salt diarrhoea. Lancet *II*, 1051 (1977)

32. Caspary, W.F., Graf, S.: Bindung von Gallensauren an Antazida. Dtsch. Med. Wschr. *103*, 825 (1978)

33 Clain, J.E., Malagelada, R.R., Chadvick, V.S., Hofmann, A.F.: Binding properties in vitro of antacids for conjugated bile acids. Gastroenterology *73*, 556 (1977)

25 Cholelithiasis after Vagotomy

25.1 Incidence

Many observations in the past have suggested that interruption of the vagus should result in a higher incidence of cholelithiasis, possibly due to a decreased biliary flow [1–8], but whether a sequence of a higher incidence of gallstones after gastric surgery really exists remains to be proven [9–10]. A number of reports incriminated vagotomy as a causal factor in cholelithiasis. Clave and Gaspar [3] reported an increased frequency of cholelithiasis in 116 patients who had undergone truncal vagotomy. Unfortunately many of these studies are open to criticism. Thus in the study of Clave and Gaspar [3] no control group was analysed, and the significance of 22.8% for those developing gallstones after vagotomy may not be much greater than the frequency in the control population.

Nobles [4], Nielsen [5], and Miller [6] have recorded the increased clinical appearance of gallstones in postvagotomy patients. Miller [6] reported on six patients in whom cholelithiasis developed 17–30 months after he had performed truncal vagotomy. Nielsen [5] reported four well-documented cases strongly indicting vagus section as the cause of cholelithiasis. Nobles [4] presented a 15-year follow-up study on 110 patients who had undergone vagotomy and gastro-enterostomy. In 20 (18.2%), clinical gallbladder disease developed in the follow-up periods.

Clave and Gaspar [3] reported in 1969 another 21 cases. In their series of 116 patients who had a truncal vagotomy and pyloroplasty, 92 were submitted to routine postoperative roentgenography. Radiographic evidence of gallbladder disease was found in 22.8%, in contrast to the 8.22% probability determined by studies in the general population. More importantly, of 52 patients who had a normal cholecystogram preoperatively and a normal palpable gall-bladder at the time of vagotomy and pyloroplasty, 23.5% had postoperative X-ray evidence of gallbladder disease. There has been reported to be no increased incidence of stone formation following selective vagotomy in which the vagal innervation of the biliary tree is preserved [7]. It is not clear in what manner operations on the stomach may affect the biliary tree and various suggestions have been put forward. Among the most prominent has been the idea that vagal denervation is likely to induce hypotonicity of the gallbladder and thus encourage biliary stasis [11, 12]. Johnson and Boyden [13] were among the first to implicate vagotomy as a cause of biliary dysfunction in man. Their studies on the motor activity of the gallbladder following vagotomy serve as a basis for the bile stasis theory of stone formation following this procedure.

25.2 Pathogenesis

Truncal vagotomy has also been shown, by others, to produce dilatation of the gallbladder in man [3, 13–17], whereas according to three reports selective vagotomy does not [16–18]. In addition, truncal vagotomy leads to a diminished

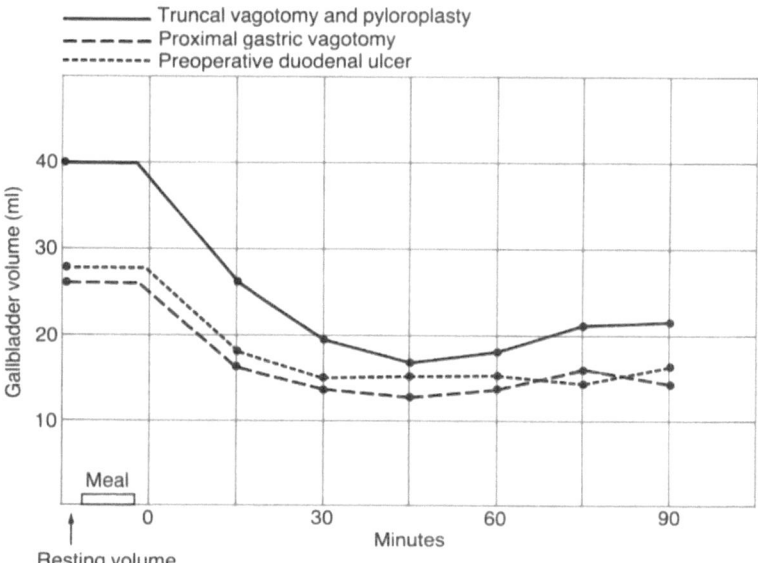

Fig. 82. Gall-bladder contraction after a meal in preoperative duodenal ulcer patients and patients after truncal vagotomy and pyloroplasty or proximal gastric vagotomy. Truncal vagotomy and pyloroplasty is followed by a significant dilatation of the gall-bladder (volume increased), but there is no impairment of gall-bladder contraction following a meal in truncal vagotomy and pyloroplasty (After Parkin et al., 1973 [21])

bile flow [9, 15, 19] and to the production of a potentially lithogenic bile [9, 15, 20] in dogs and may predispose to the formation of gallstones in man [3–6]. Parkin et al. [21] measured the gallbladder volume contractility in patients after truncal, selective and highly selective (parietal cell) vagotomy in man. The resting volume of the gallbladder was markedly increased in patients with truncal vagotomy and pyloroplasty compared to duodenal ulcer patients before the operation, but unaltered in highly selective and selective vagotomy (Fig. 82). Thus it may be concluded that the gallbladder is abnormally large after truncal vagotomy. It was to be expected that highly selective vagotomy should not increase the volume of the gallbladder, since in this kind of operation vagotomy is confined to the parietal cell mass. In selective vagotomy the hepatic and coeliac branches are preserved. The gallbladder has been shown to dilate progressively in the course of the first year after truncal vagotomy [13], which may explain why Glanville and Duthie [22], who measured the volume of the gallbladder less than 1 year after truncal vagotomy, did not find significant dilatation. That the vagally dernerved gallbladder contracts vigorously in response to fat in the intestine has been known for many years [22, 23, 13, 24]. It has been shown that stimulation of the vagi leads to an increase in bile flow, both in man [25] and in dogs [15, 26]. Stimulation of bile flow thus cannot occur after truncal vagotomy. In dogs, truncal vagotomy leads to diminution of bile flow [9, 19, 20]. Thus increased lithogenicity and stasis in a large gall bladder could be causative factors, predisposing patients after truncal vagotomy to form gallstones.

Indeed, stasis of bile in a hypotonic denervated gallbladder as a cause of postoperative gallstone disease is an attractive theory, but may not represent a complete assessment of the physiological effects of vagotomy on the biliary mechanism. Changes in the enterohepatic circulation of an imperfectly contracting gallbladder have been shown to alter the composition of liver bile in such a way that precipitation of cholesterol gallstones is favoured [25]. Formation of gallstones may occur if bile is supersaturated with cholesterol. Since the lithogenicity of bile is determined by the relative concentration of bile acids, phospholipids (lecithin) and cholesterol, alterations to one or more of the constituents may result in supersaturated bile, a prerequisite for cholesterol gallstone formation [28]. Fletcher and Clark [9] observed, following administration of a fatty meal to vagotomized dogs, a reduction of bile flow and a reduced cholate/cholesterol ratio, but normal phospholipid concentrations. Thus with the decrease in cholate it may be assumed that the bile became lithogenic. It cannot be decided whether this effect was mediated by impairment of gallbladder contraction, resulting in a retardation of the enterohepatic circulation, or by direct alteration of the composition of bile formed by the hepatic cells.

More recently animal studies have been performed by White et al. [29] and Wilbur et al. [30]. White et al. reported an increase of bile acid pool size in the dog after vagotomy. The concentration of cholic acid in bile dropped after vagotomy. However, since the dog's bile is so markedly undersaturated with cholesterol, the lithogenic range was never reached. Wilbur et al. [30] compared the effect of proximal gastric vagotomy, truncal vagotomy and truncal vagotomy with pyloroplasty on the concentration of the main constituents of gallbladder in bile in dogs. Both truncal vagotomy groups showed marked increases in aspirate volumes at subsequent laparotomies. As in the study of White et al. [29], the lithogenic range was not reached. Nevertheless, two dogs in each truncal vagotomy group were found to have gallstones. Griffith and Holmes [7] and Amdrup and Griffith [31] also did not observe changes in bile salt, phospholipid and cholesterol concentrations after various forms of hepatic, coeliac and gastric denervation in dogs. Bile salt pool size has been found to be unchanged in Rhesus monkeys [32].

Various groups have carried out studies on dog's bile following vagotomy. They all studied only the concentration of the different elements in bile and performed the experiments in different ways. Fletcher and Clark [9] used an external by-pass for the bile and found a decreased concentration of cholates after vagotomy, which might be the cause of cholesterol precipitation. Inberg et al. [33] noted no changes in the total bile acid content in the gallbladder following vagotomy, but a decrease in the deoxycholate secretion after pyloroplasty alone or vagotomy and pyloroplasty. There was no change in the phospholipid and cholesterol concentrations. Tomkins et al. [34] have shown that cutting the posterior vagus and pyloroplasty did not significantly alter the concentrations of cholesterol and phospholipids. On the other hand, truncal vagotomy produced a significant decrease in phospholipids immediately after

Table 51. Lipid composition of gallbladder bile from healthy controls and patients after truncal vagotomy and pyloroplasty. The reduction in relative cholesterol content of bile was accompanied by higher molar per cent of both bile acid and phospholipid in the vagotomy group relative to controls. The mean lithogenic index calculated on the solubility limits of Admirand and Small was 0.62 in the vagotomy patients and 0.81 in the control group ($p < 0.51$). (After Stempel and Duane, 1978)

	Cholesterol		Phospholipid		Bile acid	
	Control	Vagotomy	Control	Vagotomy	Control	Vagotomy
Molar per cent	5.34	5.13	15.5	19.5	79.2	75.4
	5.31	6.16	18.7	18.8	76.0	75.0
	5.23	4.01	16.4	18.4	78.3	77.6
	7.25	4.49	20.8	15.0	71.0	80.5
	8.66	5.37	22.6	17.8	68.7	76.8
	6.60	5.38	21.4	18.6	72.0	76.0
	6.65	7.65	20.2	18.3	73.2	74 1
	11.40	9 48	24.8	18.6	63.9	72.0
Mean	7.06	5.96	20.0	18.1	72 9	75.9
	$P < 0.05$		$P < 0.10$		$P < 0.10$	

vagotomy, followed by a slight decrease. There was no change in either instance in the concentration of cholates. Sheen [35] showed an increase in both phospholipids and cholesterol, and no change in cholates.

More recently, Smith et al. [36] compared gallbladder bile in patients with gallstones and in patients with duodenal ulcer before and after vagotomy. They did not observe an increase of the lithogenic index of patients after vagotomy.

Clear evidence against a predisposition to cholesterol gallstone formation after vagotomy has been presented recently. Stempel and Duane [37] found in eight male subjects who had undergone vagotomy and pyloroplasty a significantly larger bile acid pool size than in a group of matched controls. Associated with these expanded pools was a significantly lower molar per cent cholesterol of gallbladder bile in the vagotomy group (Table 51). These findings were the opposite of those expected in a group predisposed to cholesterol cholelithiasis, suggesting that vagotomy, at least in males, does not predispose to cholesterol gallstones. One disadvantage of the study is that biliary lipids and bile acid pool size were not examined pre- and postoperatively in the same subjects, nevertheless a lithogenic bile was not observed after vagotomy. The possibility that an increased formation of non-cholesterol cholelithiasis may develop after vagotomy, owing to dilatation of the gall bladder, has not yet been totally excluded.

In conclusion, vagotomy may alter bile flow and the size of the contracting gall bladder; biochemical evidence, however, of the formation of a more lithogenic bile after truncal vagotomy has not been presented. Thus it also seems unlikely that following vagotomy an increased formation of cholesterol gall-stones may appear. The clinical data in the literature are rather anecdotal, in that most studies do not incorporate a control group. We therefore cannot accept at the moment the notion that truncal vagotomy leads to an increased incidence of gallstone formation.

References

1. Krause, U.: Long-term results of medical and surgical treatment of peptic ulcer. Acta chirurg. Scand. Suppl. *310*, 1 (1963)
2. Lundman, P., Orinius, E., Thorsén, G.· Incidence of gallstone disease following partial gastric resection. Acta chirurg. Scand. *127*, 130 (1964)
3. Clave, R.A., Gaspar, M.R.: Incidence of gallbladder disease after vagotomy. Am. J. Surg. *118*, 169 (1969)
4. Nobles, E.R.: Vagotomy and gastroenterostomy: 15-year follow-up in 175 patients. Am. Surg *32*, 177 (1966)
5. Nielsen, J.R.: Development of cholelithiasis following vagotomy. Surgery *56*, 909 (1964)
6. Miller, M.C.: Cholelithiasis developing after vagotomy: a preliminary report. Canad. Med. Assoc. J. *98*, 350 (1968)
7. Griffith, J.M.T., Holmes, G.: Cholecystitis following gastric surgery. Lancet *II*, 780 (1964)
8. Horwith, A., Kirson, S M . Cholecystitis and cholelithiasis as a sequel to gastric surgery. Am. J. Surg. *109*, 760 (1965)
9. Fletcher, D.M., Clark, C.G.. Changes in canine bile-flow and composition after vagotomy. Brit. J. Surg. *56*, 103 (1969)
10. Bouchier, I A.D.· The vagus, the bile and gallstones. Gut *11*, 799 (1970)
11. Berndt, O.. Gallensteinbildung nach Magenresektion. Dtsch. Gesundheitsw. *15*, 402 (1960)
12. Delgado-Pereira, B., Zerbino, V.: Pancreatitis postoperatoria en la cirurgia biliar. A propósito de observaciones. Rev. Cirurg. Urug. *35*, 154 (1965)
13. Johnson, F.E., Boyden, E.A.: The effect of double vagotomy on the motor activity of the human gallbladder. Surgery *32*, 591 (1952)
14. Fagerberg, S., Grevsten, S., Johannson, H., Krause, U.: Vagotomy and gallbladder function. Gut *11*, 789 (1970)
15. Fritz, M.E., Brooks, F.P.: Control of bile flow in the cholecystectomized dog Am. J. Physiol. *204*, 825 (1963)
16. Rudick, J , Hutchinson, J.S.F. Effects of vagal nerve section on the biliary system. Lancet *I*, 579 (1964)
17. Rudick, J., Hutchinson, H S.F.: Evaluation of vagotomy and biliary function by combined oral cholecystography and intravenous cholangiography. Ann. Surg. *162*, 234 (1965)
18. Inberg, M V., Vuorio, M.: Human gallbladder function after selective gastric and total abdominal vagotomy. Acta chirurg Scand. *135*, 625 (1969)
19. Cowie, A., Clark, C.G.. The lithogenic effect of vagotomy. Brit. J. Surg. *59*, 365 (1972)
20. Schein, C J , Rosen, R.C., Warren, A., Gliedman, M.L. A vagal factor in cholecystitis. Surgery *66*, 345 (1969)
21. Parkin, G.J., Smith, R B , Johnson, D.: Gallbladder size and contractility after truncal, selective and highly selective vagotomy in man. Ann. Surg *178*, 581 (1973)
22. Glanville, J N , Duthie, H.L : Contraction of the gallbladder before and after total abdominal vagotomy. Clin. Radiol. *15*, 350 (1964)
23. Boyden, E A., Van Buskirk, C.· Rate of emptying of biliary tract following section of vagi or of all intrinsic nerves. Proc Soc. Exptl. Biol. Med. *53*, 174 (1943)
24. Whitacker, L.R. The mechanism of the gallbladder. Am J. Physiol. *78*, 411 (1926)
25. Baldwin, J., Heer, F.W., Albo, R., et al.. Effect of vagus nerve stimulation on hepatic secretion of bile in human subjects. Am. J. Surg. *111*, 66 (1966)
26. Tanturi, C.A., Ivey, A.C. On the existence of secretory nerves in the vagi for reflex excitation and inhibition of bile secretion. Am. J. Physiol. *121*, 270 (1938)
27. Heaton, K.W.: Bile salts in health and disease. London: Churchill Livingstone, Edinburgh 1972

28. Admirand, W.H., Small, D.M.: The physicochemical basis of cholesterol gallstone formation in man. J. Clin. Invest. 47, 1043
29. White, T.T., Tournat, R.A., Scharplate, D., et al.: The effect of vagotomy on biliary secretion and bile salt pools in dogs. Ann. Surg 179, 406 (1974)
30. Wilbur, B.G., Gomez, F.C., Tomkins, R.K.: Canine gallbladder bile Effects of proximal vagotomy, truncal vagotomy and truncal vagotomy with pyloroplasty. Arch. Surg. 110, 792 (1975)
31. Amdrup, B.M., Griffith, C.A.: The effects of vagotomy upon biliary function in dogs. J. Surg. Res. 10, 209 (1970)
32. Deveney, C W., Gardiner, B.N., Way, L.W.: Effect of truncal vagotomy on bile kinetics in the rhesus monkey. Surg Forum 25, 402 (1974)
33. Inberg, M.V., Ahonen, J Scheinin, T.M.: Bile composition in the gallbladder after selective gastric and truncal vagotomy. Ann Chir. Gynaecol Fenn. 58, 329 (1969)
34. Tomkins, R.K., Kraft, A.R., Zollinger, R.M.: Alterations in biliary phospholipid: cholesterol ratios following vagotomy. Surgical Forum 21, 396 (1970)
35. Sheen, P C.. Developing cholelithiasis after vagotomy. Jap. J. Surg. 1, 19 (1971)
36. Smith, D.C., Crook, J.N., McAllister, R., MacKay, C.: The comparison of gallbladder bile in patients with gallstones and in patients with duodenal ulcer before and after vagotomy. Brit. J Surg 59, 306 (1972)
37. Stempel, J.M., Duane, W.C.. Biliary lipids and bile acid poolsize after vagotomy in man. Gastroenterology 75, 608–611 (1978)

26 Recurrent Ulcer After Vagotomy

After different types of vagotomy a certain number of patients will develop recurrent ulceration. These patients will make high demands on differential diagnosis and therapy, since very complex pathophysiological facts may be involved. As in gastric resection, an inadequate initial surgical technique is responsible for the majority of cases. On the other hand some rare factors may be involved, which have to be differentiated.

26.1 Incidence

Reports about the incidence of recurrent ulcer after vagotomy show it to be very variable. Furthermore, the incidence may vary according to the type of vagotomy. In Table 49 some representative results of vagotomy in duodenal ulcer patients are compiled. These numbers seem to indicate that, in particular, patients with truncal vagotomy may have a higher recurrence rate than patients with selective gastric or selective proximal vagotomy. Addition of antrectomy (combined operation) reduces the recurrence rate. In patients with gastric ulcer, the recurrence rate after selective proximal vagotomy seems to be much higher than in duodenal ulcer patients [11].

As demonstrated before, in patients with gastric resection there is a great variance in the time interval between operation and recurrence in the different operations: the mean interval after vagotomy and gastro-enterostomy was 3.6 years, after vagotomy plus resection 2.8 years and after vagotomy and pyloroplasty 5 years.

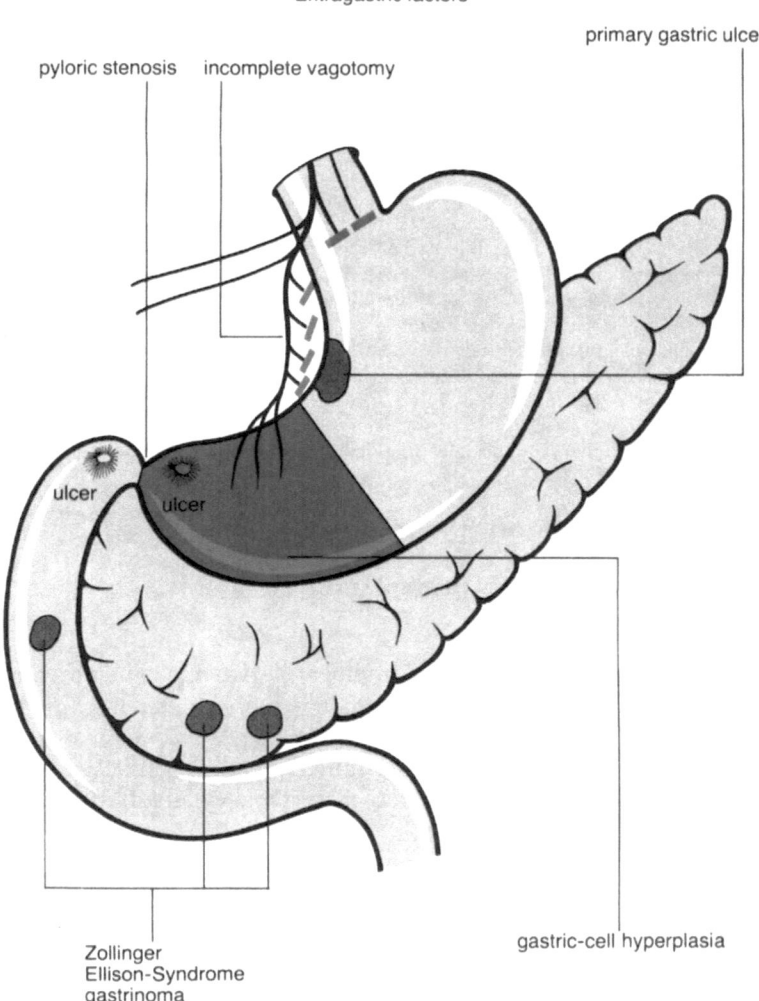

Extragastric factors

primary gastric ulcer

pyloric stenosis   incomplete vagotomy

ulcer

ulcer

Zollinger
Ellison-Syndrome
gastrinoma

gastric-cell hyperplasia

Fig. 83. Pathogenetic factors in recurrent ulcer after vagotomy

26.2 Pathogenetic Factors

Where vagotomy has been combined with resection, all the pathogenetic factors discussed in Chap. 16.2 have to be considered. The most important factor responsible for recurrent ulcers after vagotomy is incomplete vagotomy. Because of the large number of anatomical varieties of abdominal vagal fibres, incomplete dissection is possible if an inadequate technique is used. The rate of incomplete vagotomies is difficult to estimate, since no absolutely reliable method is available for measuring the completeness of a vagotomy (problems of the insulin test are discussed in Chap. 5.2).

Besides a technically incomplete vagotomy, several other factors may be responsible for the development of recurrent ulcers after vagotomy; these have

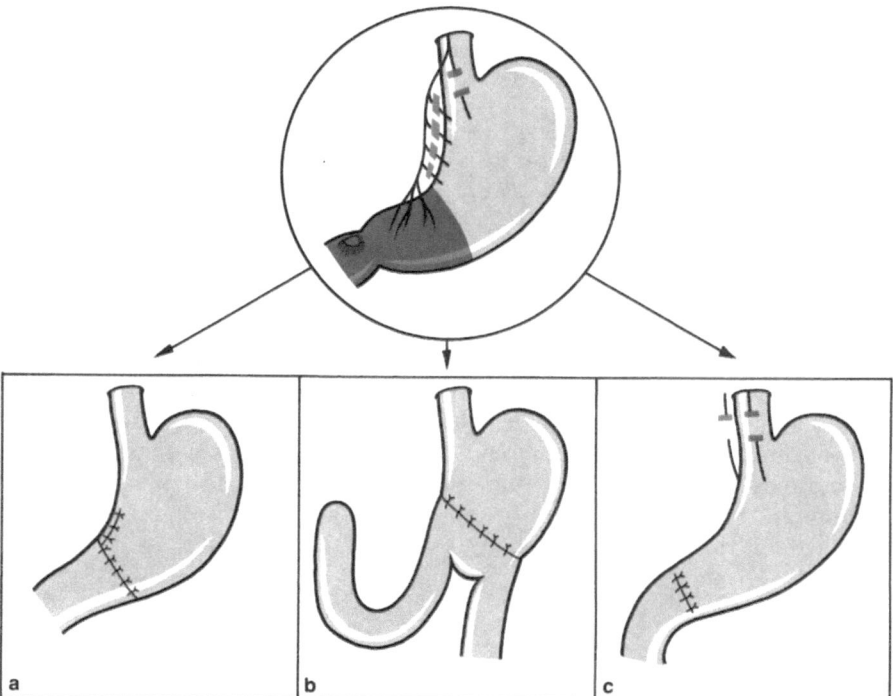

Fig. 84. Therapeutic approach to recurrent ulcer after vagotomy

already been listed and discussed (Fig. 83; Tab. 37; Chap. 16). G-cell hyperplasia of the gastric antrum may be of special importance, since in vagotomy the antrum is left intact. Furthermore, organic pyloric stenosis may be difficult to substantiate, since clinically relevant methods for measurement of delay in gastric emptying are not availaible at the moment [12, 13].

26.3 Diagnostic Procedure

For recurrences after vagotomy the same criteria are effective as after gastric resection. Of great importance is the estimation of completeness of vagotomy; in most cases the insulin test is used (see Chap. 5.2). Since the interpretation of the insulin test involves a lot of problems, its discriminatory effect is relatively small. The efficiency of the insulin test is exceeded by the pentagastrin gastric acid analysis, provided pre- and postoperative measurements are available. In general it can be assumed that after a reduction of BAO and MAO of 60% and more, recurrent ulcers will be observed in a very low percentage.

Serum gastrin determination in patients with recurrences after vagotomy is dubious, since all types of vagotomy induce hypergastrinaemia [14]. Furthermore, vagotomy induces an increase in the G-cell number of the gastric antrum [15], which may imitate the syndrome of G-cell hyperplasia. Differentiation between the different types of increased antral G-cells is impossible, since G-cell hyperplasia without previous vagotomy does not behave like a Zollinger-Ellison syndrome, i.e. differentiation by provocation tests is impossible.

Table 52. Results of surgery for recurrent ulcer after vagotomy and resection [15]

Operative procedure	No. of patients	Operative mortality	Second recurrences
Revagotomy	8	0	0
Resection	21	0	6
Revagotomy plus resection	16	1	1

26.4 Treatment (Fig. 84)

Data concerning results of reoperation for recurrences after vagotomy are rare; a compilation of reported results is presented in Table 52.

In recurrences after truncal vagotomy and drainage revagotomy has a low mortality, but a high recurrence rate. The operative procedure of choice seems to be the combinaton of vagotomy and resection. In patients with recurrences after vagotomy plus resection as the original surgical procedure, a repeated vagotomy plus resection gives best results; in certain cases revagotomy alone, which may be performed intrathoracally, shows promising results.

References

1. Goligher, J.C., Pulvertaft, C.N., Irvin, T.T., Johnston, D., Walker, B., Hall, R.A., Willson-Pepper, J., Matheson, T.S.: Five-to-eight year results of truncal vagotomy and pyloroplasty for duodenal ulcer. Brit. med. J. 1, 7 (1972)
2. Postlethwait, R.W.: Five year follow-up results of operations for duodenal ulcer. Surg. Gynec. Obstet. 137, 387 (1973)
3. Jordan, P.H.: A follow-up report of a prospective evaluation of vagotomy-pyloroplasty and vagotomy antrectomy for treatment of duodenal ulcer. Ann. Surg. 180, 259 (1974)
4. Kronborg, O., Malmström, J., Christiansen, P.M : A comperison between the results of truncal and selective vagotomy in patient with duodenal ulcer. Scand. J. Gastroent. 5, 519 (1970)
5. Kennedy, T., Connell, A.M., Lova, A.H.G., Mac Rae, K.D., Spencer, E.F.: Selective or truncal vagotomy? Brit. J. Surg. 60, 944 (1973)
6. Sawyers, J.L., Scott, H.W.: Selective gastric vagotomy with antrectomy or pyloroplasty. Ann. Surg. 174, 541 (1971)
7. Jordan, P.H.: A prospective study of parietal cell vagotomy and selective vagotomy-antrectomy for treatment of duodenal ulcer. Ann. Surg. 183, 619 (1976)
8. Bauer, H., Brückner, W., Welsch, K.H., Holle, F.: Die nicht-resezierende Chirurgie des Gastro-Duodenal-Ulkus. III. Klinische Resultate. Münch. med. Wschr. 118, 785 (1976)
9. Kronborg, O., Madsen, P.: A controlled randomised trial of highly selective vagotomy vesus selective vagotomy and pyloroplasty with treatment of duodenal ulcer. Gut 16, 268 (1975)
10. Amdrup, E., Jensen, H.E., Johnston, D., Walker, B.E., Goligher, J.C.: Clinical results of parietal cell vagotomy (highly selective vagotomy) two of four years after operation. Ann. Surg. 180, 269 (1974)
11. Madsen, P., Kronborg, O , Hart Hasen, O., Pedersen, T : Billroth I gastric resection versus truncal vagotomy and pyloroplasty in the treatment of gastric ulcer. Acta chir. scad. 142, 151 (1976)
12. Cleator, JGM, Holubitsky, J.B., Harrison, R.C.: Anastomotic ulceration. Ann. Surg. 1979, 339 (1974)
13. Becker, H.D., Reeder, D.D., Thompson, J.C.: Vagal control of gastrin release. In: Thompson, J.C.: Gastrointestinal hormones. Univ. Texas Press, Austin (1975)
14. Becker, H.D., Arnold, R., Börger, H.W., Creutzfeldt, C., Schafmayer, A., Creutzfeldt, W.: Influence of truncal vagotomy on serum and antral gastrin and G cells. Gastroenterology 72, 811 (1977)
15. Stabile, B.E., Passaro, E.: Recurrent peptic ulcer. Gastroenterology 70, 124 (1976)

Subject Index

Gastric Cancer

Editors: C. Herfarth, P. Schlag

1979. 161 figures, 144 tables. XV, 374 pages
ISBN 3-540-09467-9

Contents: Epidemiology and Pathogenesis. – Experimental Gastric Cancer. – Precancerous Lesions of Gastric Cancer. – Risk Factors for Gastric Cancer. – Diagnostic Procedures for Classification of Gastric Cancer. – Prognostic Factors of Gastric Cancer. – Surgical Therapy. – The Patient After Total Gastrectomy. – Experiences with Various Reconstructive Methods After Total Gastrectomy. – Adjuvant Therapeutic Measures. – Subject Index.

K. Kawai, H. Tanaka

Differential Diagnosis of Gastric Diseases

1974. 102 color photos, 422 black and white photos, 31 figures.
VI, 262 pages
ISBN 3-540-06579-2
Distribution rights for Japan: Igaku Shoin Ltd., Tokyo

Contents: General Section: On the concepts of protruding and excavated lesions. The fundamentals of an x-ray diagnosis. General remarks on the technique of x-ray diagnosis; X-ray findings on examination; Technical details of x-ray examination; How to diagnose protuberant lesions. The fundamentals of endoscopic diagnosis. Basic problems of endoscopic examination; Clinical application of endoscopy; Technical details of endoscopy; Special remarks on endoscopic examination. – Case presentations: Producting type. Typical cases of gastric polypous lesions; Indistinguishable cases; Rare cases. Excavated type. Typical cases of gastric excavated lesions; Indistinguishable cases; Rare cases.

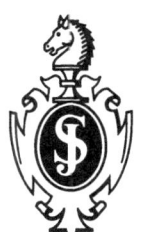

Springer-Verlag
Berlin
Heidelberg
New York

Vagotomy

Latest Advances with Special Reference to Gastric and Duodenal Ulcers Disease

Editors: F. Holle, S. Andersson

1974. 124 figures, including 16 colored, 51 tables. XII, 244 pages
ISBN 3-540-06801-5

Information: The latest research confirms the importance of the vagus nerve in the anatomy, functional pathology, and pathophysiology of stomach secretion and motility. The clinical part of this book deals with vagotomy, particularly for the relief of gastric and duodenal ulcer. Experimental and clinical data are quoted to show the advantages of selective proximal vagotomy with pyloroplasty as appropriate to preserve function.

Comprehensive Manuals of Surgical Specialties

Editor: R. H. Egdahl

A. T. K. Cockett, K. Koshiba

Manual of Urologic Surgery

Illustrated by I. Takamoto
1979. 532 color illustrations. XVIII, 284 pages
ISBN 3-540-90423-9

A. J. Edis, L. A. Ayala, R. H. Egdahl

Manual of Endocrine Surgery

1975. 266 figures, mostly in color, 242 color plates.
XIII, 274 pages
ISBN 3-540-07064-8

B. J. Harlan, A. Starr, F. M. Harwin

Manual of Cardiac Surgery

Volume 1
1980. Approx. 180 figures. Approx. 290 pages
ISBN 3-540-90393-3

R. E. Hermann

Manual of Surgery of the Gallbladder, Bile Ducts and Exocrine Pancreas

With contributions by A. M. Cooperman,
C. B. Esselstyn jr., E. Steiger, R. T. Holzbach
1979. 197 color figures (123 figures in black and
white), 16 tables. XIV, 306 pages
ISBN 3-540-90351-8

W. P. Longmire

Manual of Liver Surgery

1980. Approx. 150 figures. Approx. 250 pages
ISBN 3-540-90212-0

W. S. McDougal, C. L. Slade, B. A. Pruitt jr.

Manual of Burns

Medical Illustrators: M. Williams, C. H. Boyter,
D. P. Russell
1978. 214 color figures, 4 tables. X, 165 pages
ISBN 3-540-90319-4

B. J. Masterson

Manual of Gynecologic Surgery

With contributions by K. E. Krantz,
W. J. Cameron, J. W. Daly, J. A. Fayez,
E. W. Franklin
Illustrator: D. McKeown
1979. 204 figures, 192 in color, 12 tables.
XV, 256 pages
ISBN 3-540-90372-0

C. E. Welch, L. W. Ottinger, J. P. Welch

Manual of Lower Gastrointestinal Surgery

1980. 215 figures, approx. 138 figures in color.
XIV, 274 pages
ISBN 3-540-90205-8

E. J. Wylie, R. J. Stoney, W. K. Ehrenfeld

Manual of Vascular Surgery, Part 1

1980. Approx. 540 figures, mostly in color.
Approx. 320 pages
ISBN 3-540-90408-5

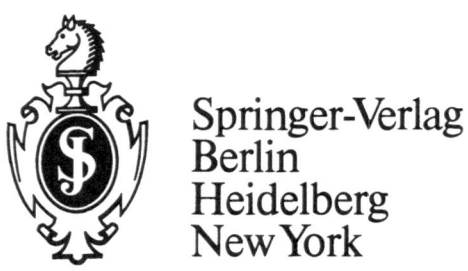

Springer-Verlag
Berlin
Heidelberg
New York